Injury & Trauma Sourcebook

Learning Disabilities Sourcebook, 3rd Edition

Leukemia Sourcebook

Liver Disorders Sourcebook

Medical Tests Sourcebook, 4th Edition

Men's Health Concerns Sourcebook, 3rd Edition

Mental Health Disorders Sourcebook, 4th Edition

Mental Retardation Sourcebook

Movement Disorders Sourcebook, 2nd Edition

Multiple Sclerosis Sourcebook

Muscular Dystrophy Sourcebook

Obesity Sourcebook

Osteoporosis Sourcebook

Pain Sourcebook, 3rd Edition

Pediatric Cancer Sourcebook

Physical & Mental Issues in Aging Sourcebook

Podiatry Sourcebook, 2nd Edition

Pregnancy & Birth Sourcebook, 3rd Edition

Prostate & Urological Disorders Sourcebook

Prostate Cancer Sourcebook

Rehabilitation Sourcebook

Respiratory Disorders Sourcebook, 2nd Edition

Sexually Transmitted Diseases Sourcebook, 4th Edition

Sleep Disorders Sourcebook, 3rd Edition

Smoking Concerns Sourcebook

Sports Injuries Sourcebook, 4th Edition

Stress-Related Disorders Sourcebook, 2nd Edition

Stroke Sourcebook, 2nd Edition

Surgery Sourcebook, 2nd Edition

Thyroid Disorders Sourcebook

Transplantation Sourcebook

Traveler's Health Sourcebook

Urinary Tract & Kidney Diseases & Disorders Sourcebook, 2nd Edition

Vegetarian Sourcebook

Women's Health Concerns Sourcebook, 3rd Edition

Workplace Health & Safety Sourcebook

Worldwide Health Sourcebook

Teen Health Series

Abuse & Violence Information for Teens

Accident & Safety Information for Teens

Alcohol Information for Teens, 2nd Edition

Allergy Information for Teens

Asthma Information for Teens, 2nd Edition

Body Information for Teens

Cancer Information for Teens, 2nd Edition

Complementary & Alternative Medicine Information for Teens

Diabetes Information for Teens, 2nd Edition

Diet Information for Teens, 3rd Edition

Drug Information for Teens, 3rd Edition

Eating Disorders Information for Teens, 2nd Edition

Fitness Information for Teens, 2nd Edition

Learning Disabilities Information for Teens

Mental Health Information for Teens, 3rd Edition

Pregnancy Information for Teens, 2nd Edition

Sexual Health Information for Teens, 3rd Edition

Skin Health Information for Teens, 2nd Edition

Sleep Information for Teens

Sports Injuries Information for Teens, 2nd Edition

Stress Information for Teens

Suicide Information for Teens, 2nd Edition

Tobacco Information for Teens, 2nd Edition

Sports
Injuries
SOURCEBOOK

Fourth Edition

Health Reference Series

Fourth Edition

Sports Injuries
SOURCEBOOK

Basic Consumer Health Information about Sprains, Fractures, Tendon Injuries, Overuse Injuries, and Injuries to the Head, Spine, Shoulders, Arms, Hands, Trunk, Legs, Knees, and Feet, and Facts about Sports-Specific Injuries, Injury Prevention, Protective Equipment, Children and Sports, and the Diagnosis, Treatment, and Rehabilitation of Sports Injuries

Along with a Glossary of Related Terms and a Directory of Resources for More Information

Edited by
Laura Larsen

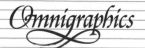

155 W. Congress, Suite 200, Detroit, MI 48226

Bibliographic Note

Because this page cannot legibly accommodate all the copyright notices, the Bibliographic Note portion of the Preface constitutes an extension of the copyright notice.

Edited by Laura Larsen

Health Reference Series

Karen Bellenir, *Managing Editor*
David A. Cooke, MD, FACP, *Medical Consultant*
Elizabeth Collins, *Research and Permissions Coordinator*
Cherry Edwards, *Permissions Assistant*
EdIndex, Services for Publishers, *Indexers*

* * *

Omnigraphics, Inc.

Matthew P. Barbour, *Senior Vice President*
Kevin M. Hayes, *Operations Manager*

* * *

Peter E. Ruffner, *Publisher*

Copyright © 2012 Omnigraphics, Inc.

ISBN 978-0-7808-1226-0

Library of Congress Cataloging-in-Publication Data

Sports injuries sourcebook : basic consumer health information about sprains, fractures, tendon injuries, overuse injuries, and injuries to the head, spine, shoulders, arms, hands, trunk, legs, knees, and feet, and facts about sports- specific injuries, injury prevention, protective equipment, children and sports, and the diagnosis, treatment, and rehabilitation of sports injuries ... / edited by Laura Larsen. -- 4th ed.
    p. cm.
  Summary: "Provides basic consumer health information about sports injuries in various parts of the body, protective equipment and preventive measures, treatment options, and a special section on sports injuries in children and teens. Includes index, glossary of related terms, and other resources"-- Provided by publisher.
  Includes bibliographical references and index.
  ISBN 978-0-7808-1226-0 (hardcover : alk. paper) 1. Sports injuries. 2. Sports medicine. 3. Wounds and injuries. I. Larsen, Laura.
  RD97.S736 2012
  617.1'027--dc23
                                                            2011043876

∞

Table of Contents

Visit www.healthreferenceseries.com to view *A Contents Guide to the Health Reference Series*, a listing of more than 16,000 topics and the volumes in which they are covered.

Part III: Head and Facial Injuries

Part IV: Back, Neck, and Spine Injuries

Part V: Shoulder and Upper Arm Injuries

Part VII: Injuries to the Trunk, Groin, Upper Legs, and Knees

Part VIII: Injuries to the Lower Legs, Ankles, and Feet

Part IX: Diagnosis, Treatment, and Rehabilitation of Sports Injuries

Part X: Sports Injuries in Children and Young Athletes

Part XI: Additional Help and Information

Preface

About This Book

Although the health benefits of participation in sports and exercise far outweigh the risks, sports injuries can occur in athletes of all ages and levels of experience and in many different activities. According to the Centers for Disease Control and Prevention, each year 38 million youth participate in organized sports and 170 million adults participate in leisure-time physical activity. Overuse and sudden, traumatic injuries often lead to short- and long-term consequences for athletes. With proper training, warm-up, and equipment, many of these injuries can be prevented. Many others can be treated and rehabilitated.

Sports Injuries Sourcebook, Fourth Edition, describes the basic types of sports injuries, including overuse injuries, tendonitis, heat illness, and skin disorders as well as traumatic injuries such as fractures, sprains, strains, spinal injuries, sudden cardiac arrest, concussion, and injuries to parts of the body, including the head, spine, torso, arms, hands, legs, and feet. The book discusses protective equipment and injury prevention strategies for specific activities and provides facts about nutrition and hydration, supplements, diagnosis and treatment, and specific risks and prevention strategies for children and young athletes. The book concludes with a glossary of related terms and a directory of resources for additional help and information. OVER 1 Million Injuries.

How to Use This Book

This book is divided into parts and chapters. Parts focus on broad areas of interest. Chapters are devoted to single topics within a part.

Part I: Health and Sports provides an introduction to basic sports injuries such as sprains, tendon injuries, overuse injuries, and sudden cardiac arrest, and it details the connection between sports injuries and arthritis, breathing disorders, and skin disease. Sports nutrition and performance-enhancing substances are also discussed.

Part II: Preventing Sports Injuries offers guidance for injury prevention and first aid, along with facts about protective equipment and safety tips for a wide variety of team and individual sports and recreation activities. It also discusses safety when engaging in sports in various weather conditions.

Part III: Head and Facial Injuries details traumatic brain injuries, concussions, and injuries to the face, including the eyes.

Part IV: Back, Neck, and Spine Injuries offers facts about back pain in athletes as well as spinal and cervical injuries, degenerative conditions, and nerve damage.

Part V: Shoulder and Upper Arm Injuries discusses common sports injuries affecting the shoulder, including problems with motion loss, instability, and muscle and tendon injuries. It also offers details about collarbone fractures and biceps tendon injury.

Part VI: Injuries to the Elbows, Wrists, and Hands explores injuries such as sprains and fractures that can affect arms, hands, fingers, and elbows, as well as other sports-related conditions that have an impact on the hands and elbows of athletes.

Part VII: Injuries to the Trunk, Groin, Upper Legs, and Knees provides facts about trunk and groin injuries, injuries to the hip, and leg injuries such as fractures and tendon strains or ruptures. It details injuries sustained by athletes to the knee cartilage, ligaments, and patella and patellar tendon, as well as other painful knee conditions and injuries.

Part VIII: Injuries to the Lower Legs, Ankles, and Feet discusses Achilles tendon and other injuries, including sprains and fractures, that affect the lower legs, ankles, feet, or toes of athletes.

Part IX: Diagnosis, Treatment, and Rehabilitation of Sports Injuries offers details on tests used to diagnose sports injuries, medications used for the management of sports injuries, and treatments involving surgical procedures and physical therapies.

Part X: Sports Injuries in Children and Young Athletes provides specific details about the effect of sports injuries on young athletes, including details about sports physicals, prevention, overtraining, and other forms of abuse that can occur in youth sports programs. It details several growth conditions or injuries that specifically affect children and offers guidance on returning to play after an injury.

Part XI: Additional Help and Information contains a glossary of terms related to sports injuries and a list of resources providing information about sports injury topics.

Bibliographic Note

This volume contains documents and excerpts from publications issued by the following U.S. government agencies: Centers for Disease Control and Prevention (CDC); Consumer Product Safety Commission (CPSC); Federal Citizens Information Center; National Cancer Institute (NCI); National Highway Traffic Safety Administration (NHTSA); National Institute of Arthritis and Musculoskeletal and Skin Diseases (NIAMS); National Institute of Diabetes and Digestive and Kidney Diseases (NIDDK); National Institute of Neurological Disorders and Stroke (NINDS); National Institute on Drug Abuse (NIDA); National Institutes of Health (NIH); National Oceanic and Atmospheric Administration, National Weather Service (NOAA, NWS); and the President's Council on Physical Fitness and Sports.

In addition, this volume contains copyrighted documents from the following organizations and individuals: About.com; A.D.A.M., Inc.; American Academy of Orthopaedic Surgeons; American Chiropractic Association; American College of Sports Medicine; American Orthopaedic Foot and Ankle Society; American Orthopaedic Society for Sports Medicine; American Red Cross; American Society for Surgery of the Hand; Association for Applied Sport Psychology; Asthma and Allergy Foundation of America; AthleticAdvisor.com; Barnes-Jewish Hospital and Washington University Physicians; Beth Israel Deaconess Medical Center; California Dental Association; Center for Orthopaedics and Sports Medicine; Children's Healthcare of Atlanta; Children's Memorial Hospital; DePuy Companies; Georgia High School Association;

Hughston Foundation; iHealthSpot, Inc.; Indiana Podiatry Group; Iowa State University Extension; Kingsley Physiotherapy; Mayfield Clinic; MomsTeam.com; National Athletic Trainers' Association; National Center for Sports Safety; National Spinal Cord Association; National Strength and Conditioning Association; Nemours Foundation; New England Musculoskeletal Institute at the University of Connecticut Health Center; NY SportsMed & Physical Therapy; Orthosports; Prevent Blindness America; Rachel S. Rohde, MD; Raymond Chiropractic and Sports Injury Center; Richard Stockton College Athletic Training; Rothman Institute; Royal Australian and New Zealand College of Radiologists; Safe Kids Worldwide; Skin Cancer Foundation; SportsMD; St. Elizabeth Community Hospital; St. John's Hospital; Tri-Valley Orthopedic Specialists; and University of Southern California–Center for Spinal Surgery.

Full citation information is provided on the first page of each chapter or section. Every effort has been made to secure all necessary rights to reprint the copyrighted material. If any omissions have been made, please contact Omnigraphics to make corrections for future editions.

Acknowledgements

Thanks go to the many organizations, agencies, and individuals who have contributed materials for this *Sourcebook,* to medical consultant Dr. David Cooke, and to prepress services provider WhimsyInk. Special thanks go to managing editor Karen Bellenir and research and permissions coordinator Liz Collins for their help and support.

About the Health Reference Series

The *Health Reference Series* is designed to provide basic medical information for patients, families, caregivers, and the general public. Each volume takes a particular topic and provides comprehensive coverage. This is especially important for people who may be dealing with a newly diagnosed disease or a chronic disorder in themselves or in a family member. People looking for preventive guidance, information about disease warning signs, medical statistics, and risk factors for health problems will also find answers to their questions in the *Health Reference Series*. The *Series*, however, is not intended to serve as a tool for diagnosing illness, in prescribing treatments, or as a substitute for the physician/patient relationship. All people concerned about medical symptoms or the possibility of disease are encouraged to seek professional care from an appropriate health care provider.

A Note about Spelling and Style

Health Reference Series editors use *Stedman's Medical Dictionary* as an authority for questions related to the spelling of medical terms and the *Chicago Manual of Style* for questions related to grammatical structures, punctuation, and other editorial concerns. Consistent adherence is not always possible, however, because the individual volumes within the *Series* include many documents from a wide variety of different producers and copyright holders, and the editor's primary goal is to present material from each source as accurately as is possible following the terms specified by each document's producer. This sometimes means that information in different chapters or sections may follow other guidelines and alternate spelling authorities. For example, occasionally a copyright holder may require that eponymous terms be shown in possessive forms (Crohn's disease *vs.* Crohn disease) or that British spelling norms be retained (leukaemia *vs.* leukemia).

Locating Information within the Health Reference Series

The *Health Reference Series* contains a wealth of information about a wide variety of medical topics. Ensuring easy access to all the fact sheets, research reports, in-depth discussions, and other material contained within the individual books of the *Series* remains one of our highest priorities. As the *Series* continues to grow in size and scope, however, locating the precise information needed by a reader may become more challenging.

A *Contents Guide to the Health Reference Series* was developed to direct readers to the specific volumes that address their concerns. It presents an extensive list of diseases, treatments, and other topics of general interest compiled from the Tables of Contents and major index headings. To access *A Contents Guide to the Health Reference Series*, visit www.healthreferenceseries.com.

Medical Consultant

Medical consultation services are provided to the *Health Reference Series* editors by David A. Cooke, MD, FACP. Dr. Cooke is a graduate of Brandeis University, and he received his M.D. degree from the University of Michigan. He completed residency training at the University of Wisconsin Hospital and Clinics. He is board-certified in Internal Medicine. Dr. Cooke currently works as part of the University of Michigan Health System and practices in Ann Arbor, MI. In his free time, he enjoys writing, science fiction, and spending time with his family.

Our Advisory Board

We would like to thank the following board members for providing guidance to the development of this *Series*:

- Dr. Lynda Baker, Associate Professor of Library and Information Science, Wayne State University, Detroit, MI

- Nancy Bulgarelli, William Beaumont Hospital Library, Royal Oak, MI

- Karen Imarisio, Bloomfield Township Public Library, Bloomfield Township, MI

- Karen Morgan, Mardigian Library, University of Michigan-Dearborn, Dearborn, MI

- Rosemary Orlando, St. Clair Shores Public Library, St. Clair Shores, MI

Health Reference Series *Update Policy*

The inaugural book in the *Health Reference Series* was the first edition of *Cancer Sourcebook* published in 1989. Since then, the *Series* has been enthusiastically received by librarians and in the medical community. In order to maintain the standard of providing high-quality health information for the layperson the editorial staff at Omnigraphics felt it was necessary to implement a policy of updating volumes when warranted.

Medical researchers have been making tremendous strides, and it is the purpose of the *Health Reference Series* to stay current with the most recent advances. Each decision to update a volume is made on an individual basis. Some of the considerations include how much new information is available and the feedback we receive from people who use the books. If there is a topic you would like to see added to the update list, or an area of medical concern you feel has not been adequately addressed, please write to:

Editor
Health Reference Series
Omnigraphics, Inc.
155 W. Congress, Suite 200
Detroit, MI 48226
E-mail: editorial@omnigraphics.com

Part One

Health and Sports

Chapter 1

An Introduction to Sports Injuries and Exercise

"Sports injuries" are injuries that happen when playing sports or exercising. Some are from accidents. Others can result from poor training practices or improper gear. Some people get injured when they are not in proper condition. Not warming up or stretching enough before you play or exercise can also lead to injuries. The most common sports injuries are the following:

- Sprains and strains
- Knee injuries
- Swollen muscles
- Achilles tendon injuries
- Pain along the shin bone
- Fractures
- Dislocations

There are two kinds of sports injuries: acute and chronic. Acute injuries occur suddenly when playing or exercising. Sprained ankles, strained backs, and fractured hands are acute injuries. Signs of an acute injury include these symptoms:

- Sudden, severe pain

This chapter excerpted from "Fast Facts: Sports Injuries," National Institute of Arthritis and Musculoskeletal and Skin Diseases (www.niams.nih.gov), June 2009.

- Swelling
- Not being able to place weight on a leg, knee, ankle, or foot
- An arm, elbow, wrist, hand, or finger that is very tender
- Not being able to move a joint as normal
- Extreme leg or arm weakness
- A bone or joint that is visibly out of place

Chronic injuries happen after you play a sport or exercise for a long time. Signs of a chronic injury include these symptoms:

- Pain when you play
- Pain when you exercise
- A dull ache when you rest
- Swelling

What should I do if I get injured?

Never try to "work through" the pain of a sports injury. Stop playing or exercising when you feel pain. Playing or exercising more only causes more harm. Some injuries should be seen by a doctor right away. Others you can treat yourself.

Call a doctor if any of the following occur:

- The injury causes severe pain, swelling, or numbness
- You can't put any weight on the area
- An old injury hurts or aches
- An old injury swells
- The joint doesn't feel normal or feels unstable

If you don't have any of these signs, it may be safe to treat the injury at home. If the pain or other symptoms get worse, you should call your doctor. Use the RICE (Rest, Ice, Compression, and Elevation) method to relieve pain, reduce swelling, and speed healing. Follow these four steps right after the injury occurs and do so for at least 48 hours:

- **Rest:** Reduce your regular activities. If you've injured your foot, ankle, or knee, take weight off of it. A crutch can help. If your right foot or ankle is injured, use the crutch on the left side. If your left foot or ankle is injured, use the crutch on the right side.

4

- **Ice:** Put an ice pack to the injured area for 20 minutes, four to eight times a day. You can use a cold pack or ice bag. You can also use a plastic bag filled with crushed ice and wrapped in a towel. Take the ice off after 20 minutes to avoid cold injury.

- **Compression:** Put even pressure (compression) on the injured area to help reduce swelling. You can use an elastic wrap, special boot, air cast, or splint. Ask your doctor which one is best for your injury.

- **Elevation:** Put the injured area on a pillow, at a level above your heart, to help reduce swelling.

How are sports injuries treated?

Treatment often begins with the RICE method. Here are some other things your doctor may do to treat your sports injury.

- **Nonsteroidal anti-inflammatory drugs (NSAIDs):** Your doctor will suggest that you take a nonsteroidal anti-inflammatory drug such as aspirin, ibuprofen, ketoprofen, or naproxen sodium. These drugs reduce swelling and pain. You can buy them at a drug store. Another common drug is acetaminophen. It may relieve pain, but it will not reduce swelling.

- **Immobilization:** Immobilization is a common treatment for sports injuries. It keeps the injured area from moving and prevents more damage. Slings, splints, casts, and leg immobilizers are used to immobilize sports injuries.

- **Surgery:** In some cases, surgery is needed to fix sports injuries. Surgery can fix torn tendons and ligaments or put broken bones back in place. Most sports injuries don't need surgery.

- **Rehabilitation (exercise):** Rehabilitation is a key part of treatment. It involves exercises that step by step get the injured area back to normal. Moving the injured area helps it to heal. The sooner this is done, the better. Exercises start by gently moving the injured body part through a range of motions. The next step is to stretch. After a while, weights may be used to strengthen the injured area.

  As an injury heals, scar tissue forms. After a while, the scar tissue shrinks. This shrinking brings the injured tissues back together. When this happens, the injured area becomes tight or stiff. This is when you are at greatest risk of injuring the area again. You should stretch the muscles every day. You should always stretch as a warm-up before you play or exercise.

Don't play your sport until you are sure you can stretch the injured area without pain, swelling, or stiffness. When you start playing again, start slowly. Build up to full speed.

- **Rest:** Although it is good to start moving the injured area as soon as possible, you must also take time to rest after an injury. All injuries need time to heal; proper rest helps the process. Your doctor can guide you on the proper balance between rest and rehabilitation.

- **Other therapies:** Other common therapies that help with the healing process include mild electrical currents (electrostimulation), cold packs (cryotherapy), heat packs (thermotherapy), sound waves (ultrasound), and massage.

What can people do to prevent sports injuries?

- Don't bend your knees more than half way when doing knee bends.
- Don't twist your knees when you stretch. Keep your feet as flat as you can.
- When jumping, land with your knees bent.
- Do warm-up exercises before you play any sport.
- Always stretch before you play or exercise.
- Don't overdo it.
- Cool down after hard sports or workouts.
- Wear shoes that fit properly, are stable, and absorb shock.
- Use the softest exercise surface you can find; don't run on asphalt or concrete.
- Run on flat surfaces.

Adults should follow these tips:

- Don't be a "weekend warrior." Don't try to do a week's worth of activity in a day or two.
- Learn to do your sport right. Use proper form to reduce your risk of "overuse" injuries.
- Use safety gear.
- Know your body's limits.
- Build up your exercise level gradually.

- Strive for a total body workout of cardiovascular, strength-training, and flexibility exercises.

Parents and coaches should follow these tips:

- Group children by their skill level and body size, not by their age, especially for contact sports.
- Match the child to the sport. Don't push the child too hard to play a sport that she or he may not like or be able to do.
- Try to find sports programs that have certified athletic trainers.
- See that all children get a physical exam before playing.
- Don't play a child who is injured.
- Get the child to a doctor, if needed.
- Provide a safe environment for sports.

Children should follow this advice:

- Be in proper condition to play the sport.
- Get a physical exam before you start playing sports.
- Follow the rules of the game.
- Wear gear that protects, fits well, and is right for the sport.
- Know how to use athletic gear.
- Don't play when you are very tired or in pain.
- Always warm up before you play.
- Always cool down after you play.

What research is being done on treating sports injuries?

Today, treating a sports injury is much better than in the past. Most people who get sports injuries play sports and exercise again. Doctors have many new ways to treat sports injuries, including the following:

- Arthroscopy (fiber optic scopes put through small cuts in the skin to see inside joints)
- Tissue engineering (using a person's own tissues or cells to help heal injuries)

- Targeted pain relief (pain-reducing drug patches put directly on the injured area)

- Advanced imaging techniques (like X-rays) that will lead to better diagnosis and treatment

Chapter 2

Sprains and Strains

The Difference between a Sprain and a Strain

A sprain is a stretch and/or tear of a ligament (a band of fibrous tissue that connects two or more bones at a joint). One or more ligaments can be injured at the same time. The severity of the injury will depend on the extent of injury (whether a tear is partial or complete) and the number of ligaments involved.

A strain is an injury to either a muscle or a tendon (fibrous cords of tissue that connect muscle to bone). Depending on the severity of the injury, a strain may be a simple overstretch of the muscle or tendon, or it can result from a partial or complete tear.

Sprains

A sprain can result from a fall, a sudden twist, or a blow to the body that forces a joint out of its normal position and stretches or tears the ligament supporting that joint. Typically, sprains occur when people fall and land on an outstretched arm, slide into a baseball base, land on the side of their foot, or twist a knee with the foot planted firmly on the ground.

This chapter excerpted from "Sprains and Strains," National Institute of Arthritis and Musculoskeletal and Skin Diseases (www.niams.nih.gov), April 2009.

9

Where Sprains Usually Occur

Although sprains can occur in both the upper and lower parts of the body, the most common site is the ankle. More than 25,000 individuals sprain an ankle each day in the United States.

The ankle joint is supported by several lateral (outside) ligaments and medial (inside) ligaments. Most ankle sprains happen when the foot turns inward as a person runs, turns, falls, or lands on the ankle after a jump. This type of sprain is called an inversion injury. The knee is another common site for a sprain. A blow to the knee or a fall is often the cause; sudden twisting can also result in a sprain.

Sprains frequently occur at the wrist, typically when people fall and land on an outstretched hand. A sprain to the thumb is common in skiing and other sports.

Signs and Symptoms of a Sprain

The usual signs and symptoms include pain, swelling, bruising, instability, and loss of the ability to move and use the joint (called functional ability). However, these signs and symptoms can vary in intensity, depending on the severity of the sprain. Sometimes people feel a pop or tear when the injury happens.

Doctors closely observe an injured site and ask questions to obtain information to diagnose the severity of a sprain. In general, a grade I or mild sprain is caused by overstretching or slight tearing of the ligaments with no joint instability. A person with a mild sprain usually experiences minimal pain, swelling, and little or no loss of functional ability. Bruising is absent or slight, and the person is usually able to put weight on the affected joint.

A grade II or moderate sprain is caused by further, but still incomplete, tearing of the ligament and is characterized by bruising, moderate pain, and swelling. A person with a moderate sprain usually has more difficulty putting weight on the affected joint and experiences some loss of function. An X-ray may be needed to help the health care provider determine if a fracture is causing the pain and swelling. Magnetic resonance imaging is occasionally used to help differentiate between a significant partial injury and a complete tear in a ligament, or it can be recommended to rule out other injuries.

People who sustain a grade III or severe sprain completely tear or rupture a ligament. Pain, swelling, and bruising are usually severe, and the patient is unable to put weight on the joint. An X-ray is usually taken to rule out a broken bone. When diagnosing any sprain, the health care provider will ask the patient to explain how the injury happened. He or she will examine the affected area and check its stability and its ability to move and bear weight.

Seeing a Health Care Provider for a Sprain

You should see a health care provider for a sprain in these circumstances:

- You have severe pain and cannot put any weight on the injured joint.
- The injured area looks crooked or has lumps and bumps (other than swelling) that you do not see on the uninjured joint.
- You cannot move the injured joint.
- You cannot walk more than four steps without significant pain.
- Your limb buckles or gives way when you try to use the joint.
- You have numbness in any part of the injured area.
- You see redness or red streaks spreading out from the injury.
- You injure an area that has been injured several times before.
- You have pain, swelling, or redness over a bony part of your foot.
- You are in doubt about the seriousness of the injury or how to care for it.

Strains

A strain is caused by twisting or pulling a muscle or tendon. Strains can be acute or chronic. An acute strain is associated with a recent trauma or injury; it also can occur after improperly lifting heavy objects or overstressing the muscles. Chronic strains are usually the result of overuse: prolonged, repetitive movement of the muscles and tendons.

Where Strains Usually Occur

Two common sites for a strain are the back and the hamstring muscle (located in the back of the thigh). Contact sports such as soccer, football, hockey, boxing, and wrestling put people at risk for strains. Gymnastics, tennis, rowing, golf, and other sports that require extensive gripping can increase the risk of hand and forearm strains. Elbow strains sometimes occur in people who participate in racquet sports, throwing, and contact sports.

Signs and Symptoms of a Strain

Typically, people with a strain experience pain, limited motion, muscle spasms, and possibly muscle weakness. They also can have localized swelling, cramping, or inflammation and, with a minor or moderate strain, usually some loss of muscle function. Patients typically have pain in the injured area and general weakness of the muscle when they attempt to move it. Severe strains that partially or completely tear the muscle or tendon are often very painful and disabling.

Treating Sprains and Strains

Reduce Swelling and Pain

Treatments for sprains and strains are similar and can be thought of as having two stages. The goal during the first stage is to reduce swelling and pain. At this stage, health care providers usually advise patients to follow a formula of rest, ice, compression, and elevation (RICE) for the first 24 to 48 hours after the injury. The health care provider also may recommend an over-the-counter or prescription nonsteroidal anti-inflammatory drug (NSAID), such as aspirin or ibuprofen, to help decrease pain and inflammation.

For people with a moderate or severe sprain, particularly of the ankle, a hard cast may be applied. This often occurs after the initial swelling has subsided. Severe sprains and strains may require surgery to repair the torn ligaments, muscle, or tendons. Surgery is usually performed by an orthopedic surgeon.

It is important that moderate and severe sprains and strains be evaluated by a health care provider to allow prompt, appropriate treatment to begin. A person who has any concerns about the seriousness of a sprain or strain should always contact a health care provider for advice.

RICE Therapy

- **Rest:** Reduce regular exercise or activities of daily living as needed. Your health care provider may advise you to put no weight on an injured area for 48 hours. If you cannot put weight on an ankle or knee, crutches may help. If you use a cane or one crutch for an ankle injury, use it on the uninjured side to help you lean away and relieve weight on the injured ankle.

- **Ice:** Apply an ice pack to the injured area for 20 minutes at a time, four to eight times a day. A cold pack, ice bag, or plastic bag filled with crushed ice and wrapped in a towel can be used. To avoid cold injury and frostbite, do not apply the ice for more than 20 minutes.

- **Compression:** Compression of an injured ankle, knee, or wrist may help reduce swelling. Examples of compression bandages are elastic wraps, special boots, air casts, and splints. Ask your health care provider for advice on which one to use and how tight to apply the bandage safely.

- **Elevation:** If possible, keep the injured ankle, knee, elbow, or wrist elevated on a pillow, above the level of the heart, to help decrease swelling.

Begin Rehabilitation

The second stage of treating a sprain or strain is rehabilitation, with the overall goal of improving the condition of the injured area and restoring its function. The health care provider will prescribe an exercise program designed to prevent stiffness, improve range of motion, and restore the joint's normal flexibility and strength. Some patients may need physical therapy during this stage. When the acute pain and swelling have diminished, the health care provider will instruct the patient to do a series of exercises several times a day. These are very important because they help reduce swelling, prevent stiffness, and restore normal, pain-free range of motion. The health care provider can recommend many different types of exercises, depending on the injury. The duration of the program depends on the extent of the injury, but the regimen commonly lasts for several weeks.

Another goal of rehabilitation is to increase strength and regain flexibility. Depending on the patient's rate of recovery, this process begins about the second week after the injury. The health care provider will instruct the patient to do a series of exercises designed to meet these goals. During this phase of rehabilitation, patients progress to more demanding exercises as pain decreases and function improves.

The final goal is the return to full daily activities, including sports when appropriate. Patients must work closely with their health care provider or physical therapist to determine their readiness to return to full activity. Sometimes people are tempted to resume full activity or play sports despite pain or muscle soreness. Returning to full activity before regaining normal range of motion, flexibility, and strength increases the chance of reinjury and may lead to a chronic problem.

The amount of rehabilitation and the time needed for full recovery after a sprain or strain depend on the severity of the injury and individual rates of healing. For example, a mild ankle sprain may require 3–6 weeks of rehabilitation; a moderate sprain could require 2–3 months. With a severe sprain, it can take 8–12 months to return to full activities.

Preventing Sprains and Strains

People can do many things to help lower their risk of sprains and strains:

- Avoid exercising or playing sports when tired or in pain.
- Maintain a healthy, well-balanced diet to keep muscles strong.
- Maintain a healthy weight.
- Practice safety measures to help prevent falls. For example, keep stairways, walkways, yards, and driveways free of clutter; anchor scatter rugs; and salt or sand icy sidewalks and driveways in the winter.
- Wear shoes that fit properly.
- Replace athletic shoes as soon as the tread wears out or the heel wears down on one side.
- Do stretching exercises daily.
- Be in proper physical condition to play a sport.
- Warm up and stretch before participating in any sport or exercise.
- Wear protective equipment when playing.
- Run on even surfaces.

Chapter 3

Tendon Injuries

Chapter Contents

Section 3.1

Tendonitis

Overview

Early intervention is the key to treating tendonitis. Tendonitis can be successfully treated but it is important to note that the treatment protocol for tendonitis is unique and different than treating other acute injuries. The wrong treatment can exacerbate the condition, increasing the time for recovery.

Tendonitis can affect many body segments. Although the body segments may differ, the structural damage and healing process are the same. Understanding the basic structure and function of a tendon will give the athlete a better understanding of why the treatment protocol for tendonitis is different than other types of acute injuries.

What is the structure and function of a tendon?

The purpose of a tendon is to connect muscle to bone. While the specific structure of a tendon may vary from tendon to tendon, the components are the same. A tendon is primarily made up of collagen fibers, water, and ground substance. It is the components in the ground substance that give the tendon its viscoelastic properties (ability to stretch and return to its original shape).

In a resting state, a tendon has a wavy appearance. When the muscle attached to the tendon contracts, the tendon straightens out and becomes tighter.

Some tendons are wrapped in synovial sheaths (Achilles and biceps tendons). In tendons where a sheath is present, the blood supply for the tendon comes primarily from the synovial sheath. The synovial sheath also contains a very small amount of fluid to help reduce friction between the tendon and sheath while the tendon elongates.

As with muscle tissue, a tendon has a structural breaking point. Initially, when stress is applied to the tendon, the tendon will elongate.

16

If the force continues beyond what the tensile strength of the tendon can handle, the tendon will eventually rupture.

Symptoms

What are the classifications of tendonitis?

There are six classifications of tendonitis ranging from mild to severe. Each classification is based on the amount of pain the athlete experiences before, during, and after exercise and is correlated to the athlete's functional ability.

Mild tendonitis (levels 1 and 2) is usually associated with pain with extreme exertion that stops when activity stops. The athlete can usually continue to compete with mild tendonitis without any functional impact to his/her ability to perform.

Moderate tendonitis (levels 3 and 4) is usually associated with pain with extreme exertion that lasts several hours after the activity. Moderate tendonitis may begin to affect the athlete's ability to perform at high levels. As the inflammation increases towards level 4, the athlete's ability to perform at a normal level may begin to be impacted.

Severe tendonitis (levels 5 and 6) is usually associated with pain during the activity that may continue to last throughout the day and night. The athlete may also have pain in the affected region during everyday activities and not just during athletic performance.

Causes

What causes tendonitis?

Tendonitis is considered an overuse injury caused by repetitive loading of a tendon exceeding the ability of the tendon to handle the load. Repetitive loading of a tendon can break down otherwise normal tissue resulting in pain, swelling, and decreased functional ability of the associated joint.

Common causes of tendonitis include the following:

- Excessive increases in training load, distances, and speed
- Mechanical errors from improper technique
- Structural abnormalities
- Inappropriate equipment or play or work conditions
- Training surfaces (surfaces that do not give)
- Muscle imbalances

- Inadequate time for tendon recovery

What happens to the structure of the tendon when it is overloaded?

The initial response of the tendon is inflammation. In fact, when you break down the word tendonitis, "itis" means inflammation. Add "itis" to tendon and you have inflammation of a tendon.

Initially, the tendon becomes painful to the touch and begins to weaken. If the tendon is continuously overloaded, the tissue begins to break down.

A number of structural changes can occur during this process including thickening of the synovial sheath surrounding the tendon, areas of abnormal tissue known as fibrosis laid down within the tendon, thickening of connective tissue, and adhesions (scar tissue laid down in and around the tendon). The longer the condition goes untreated, the more structural changes occur.

Treatment

What is the first step in treating tendonitis?

The first step in treating tendonitis is to identify the cause. This step cannot be overemphasized because even if you treat the tendonitis, the condition will return if the cause has not been identified and dealt with.

Identifying the possible causes of tendonitis begins with a detailed history of the athlete specifically looking at specific load increases. These may include significant increases in the amount of activity (number of repetitions), distance (mileage) increases, and/or speed increases.

For example, in a softball pitcher suffering from bicipital tendonitis in her throwing shoulder, one would specifically look at the number of pitches thrown, the types of pitches thrown, the distances of pitches thrown, and the intensity of pitches thrown. If there was an identifiable jump in the number, type, distance, or intensity of pitches thrown that triggered the tendonitis, then the therapist can work with the coach to reduce the workout to one in which the athlete can compete safely and without damage to her tendon.

If there is not an obvious increase in the athlete's history that triggered the tendonitis, an analysis of the athlete's mechanics may be in order. If the sports medicine professional is not proficient in the athlete's sport, the professional may need to consult with the athlete's coach.

In order to ensure that the tendonitis does not return, the causative factors must be identified and changed prior to the athlete returning to sport.

How is tendonitis treated?

The initial phase in treating tendonitis is to get the inflammation under control. If the tendon is acutely inflamed (tender to the touch, swollen, and painful with movement), the treatment needs to focus on reducing the inflammation.

Acute inflammation can be treated using the P.R.I.C.E. principle of Protection, Rest, Ice, Compression, and Elevation with the focus on rest and ice. Rest is absolutely crucial in treating tendonitis and is the most difficult component to get an athlete to adhere to. However, athletes who continue to push through pain risk moving their injury from the acute inflammation phase to a chronic tendonitis which is much harder to treat.

Once again, the longer an athlete plays with tendonitis, the more structural changes and damage there will be to the tendon. As the tendon worsens, the time frame for healing the tendon significantly increases.

If complete rest from the activity is not possible, the athlete needs to accommodate his/her activities to reduce the amount of stress on the tendon. For example, the softball pitcher with bicipital tendonitis can perform wrist work for ball rotation rather than full arm rotation pitches. The pitcher can also reduce the number and intensity of pitches thrown focusing more on mechanics than speed.

When trying to reduce inflammation in a tendon, the initial treatment focus is not on exercises, but on calming down the inflamed tendon. This is the key difference between treating a sprain or a strain versus treating tendonitis. While traditional rehabilitation protocols for most acute injuries focus on increasing range of motion and strengthening the surrounding muscles, tendons, and ligaments, initial treatment for tendonitis focuses on reducing inflammation.

Early exercise for an individual with tendonitis can make the condition worse. The patient will have an increase in pain and swelling the day after treatment rather than a reduction in symptoms. This is one way to tell if the treatment is too aggressive.

During early tendonitis treatment, the sports medicine professional may also prescribe anti-inflammatory medication to help reduce the inflammation. Rest, ice, and anti-inflammatory medications are the primary treatment protocol during early rehabilitation for tendonitis.

When can I proceed to range of motion and strengthening exercises?

As pain and swelling dissipate, the athlete can then move carefully into a progression of exercises to improve the range of motion of the affected tendon and strengthen the tendon. However, because of the delicate nature of the tendon, these exercises need to be carefully monitored to ensure that the athlete does not digress in his/her symptoms.

Flexibility exercises should focus on gradually elongating the tendon without causing an increase in pain. If fibrosis or adhesions are noted in the tendon by the sports medicine professional, he/she may apply one or more soft tissue techniques to help release the adhesions that may be interfering with the tendon's ability to elongate.

Strengthening exercises should focus on light intensity and higher repetitions so as not to place too much stress on the tendon. Research has also supported the use of eccentric strength exercises (lengthening contraction) early in the rehabilitation process because eccentric exercises place less stress on the tendons than other types of strengthening exercises.

When eccentric exercises are applied to the joint, the exercises should be initiated within a shortened range of motion. Again, this is to ensure that the tendon is not placed in a position of stress during the earlier rehabilitation phases.

For example, when treating bicipital tendonitis, eccentric exercises should begin with the shoulder in a position of flexion. The arm is loaded in a position of flexion. The athlete resists moving the arm into extension, but the resistance is ended before the athlete's shoulder is in full extension.

As the athlete's strength improves, the athlete can move from endurance and eccentric types of strength exercises to concentric (shortening contraction) exercises focusing on gradually higher loads or intensities and less repetitions.

When can I begin functional sports training?

When strength exercises can be performed pain free and equal in intensity to the uninjured side, then the athlete can begin agility and functional sports specific training exercises. These exercises should be carefully selected to match the demands of the athlete's sport.

For athletes recovering from lower extremity tendonitis, agility drills are introduced to ensure that the athlete's body can respond quickly to demands for changes in direction. These drills should include a variety of directional changes and distances that mimic the demands of the athlete's sport.

For example, an athlete competing in the sport of basketball recovering from patellar tendonitis should include agility drills that include the components of quickly shifting directions from side-to-side, front-to-back and back-to-front, and diagonal changes of directions all within small distances that would mimic the size of a basketball court.

Once agility drills can be performed pain free and at a maximum intensity, functional sports specific drills can be performed. The keys to these drills is that they need to include all of the primary skills that the athlete needs to perform within their sport and that they gradually progress from low intensity to high intensity over time.

The basketball player recovering from patellar tendonitis should include non-contact sports specific drills like the following: defensive slides, line drills, shooting drills starting from shots close to the basket increasing to shots behind three point line, lay-ups, defensive drills, and offensive drills.

Once the athlete can complete all of these skills without pain, the athlete can then progress to contact drills. Once controlled contact drills can be performed without pain, the athlete can be released to full competition with no restrictions.

When can I return to sport?

The athlete can return to participation in sport when he/she has been released to participate by his/her sports medicine professional and is pain free during full activity.

Chronic tendonitis is very difficult to treat. The goal for the athlete is to catch the tendonitis and treat it early before it becomes a chronic problem.

The keys to successfully treating tendonitis and returning an athlete to sport are early diagnosis, identification of the cause, addressing the cause, and following a careful progression of rehabilitation focusing initially on rest and reducing inflammation.

If you suspect that you have a tendonitis, it is critical to seek the urgent consultation of a local sports injuries doctor for appropriate care.

Reference

Houglum, P.A. (2005). Therapeutic Exercise for Musculoskeletal Injuries (2nd Ed.). Human Kinetics: Champaign, IL.

Section 3.2

Tendinopathy

It's Not Just Tendonitis

Overuse or degeneration of tendons occurs not only with sport and physical activity, but may occur in everyday life. This is sometimes known as tendinopathy or tendinosis. Tendinopathy is notorious for being difficult to treat as the tendon has often been failing under a physical load for years. It tends to be an ongoing problem, and even if it subsides, there is a high risk of recurrence.

What Is a Tendon?

A tendon is part of a muscle. The fleshy part of the muscle is known as its "belly." The ends of a muscle are called tendons and these attach usually to bones. A tendon is a cord of fibrous tissue in which the fundamental building block is a protein called collagen. There are many different types of collagen and it is likely that certain types of collagen are strong while others are weak and fail more rapidly under a load. This may explain why some individuals are prone to certain injuries or may be slower in their healing of certain injuries. There is a genetic tendency to tendon disorders and injury patterns may occur, in which tendinopathy may exist in more than one body area (e.g., the elbow and the Achilles tendon).

Why Does a Tendon Wear Down? Tendinosis, Not Tendonitis.

A tendon works hard to transfer force. If a tendon is overloaded it may become inflamed and this is known as tendonitis. This is a short-term inflammation which responds to simple measures such as ice, activity reduction, anti-inflammatory medications, and physical treatment. Sometimes cortisone injections are given.

Over time, if a tendon is repeatedly overloaded or if there have been previous injuries, tendinopathy may develop. In this circumstance, the typical features within the tendon are that it begins to split or tear internally, it becomes thickened, it weakens, and a range of chemicals are released causing inflammation. Scar tissue develops within the tendon and there is irritation of the nerve endings, causing pain.

Common Areas for Tendinopathy

Tendinopathy may occur in a number of areas around the body:

- **Shoulder:** Rotator cuff; supraspinatus tendon; biceps tendon (long head)

- **Elbow:** Common extensor tendon (tennis elbow), common flexor tendon (golfer's elbow); biceps tendon

- **Hip/groin region:** Gluteus medius; adductor and hamstring origin tendons

- **Knee:** Patellar tendon (jumper's knee); quadriceps tendon

- **Foot and ankle:** Achilles and tibialis posterior tendon

Management of Tendinopathy

A step-by-step management plan is critical to avoid aggravation and also frustration during what is always a long-term process. The correct diagnosis is essential. Sometimes imaging of the tendon is indicated with a high quality ultrasound or an MRI [magnetic resonance imaging] scan. Activity should be modified to avoid aggravation and an appropriate rehabilitation program to strengthen the area is required.

Strengthening exercises are commonly referred to as eccentric exercises. Eccentric exercises use a tendon and muscle over their full length in a functional capacity. An experienced sports physiotherapist is helpful in this regard.

The use of ice may alleviate the pain, and a range of medication and other treatment options are available and have been researched. Simple analgesics (e.g., paracetamol) may reduce pain. Anti-inflammatory medications and cortisone injections do not improve the healing of a tendon and indeed may impair healing. The use of repeated cortisone injections in the management of tendinopathy should be discouraged, even though it may reduce pain for a short period.

Some treatments options include:

- **Glyceryl trinitrate:** This may involve using "nitrate patches" or creams. This alters the chemistry at the site of tendinosis.

23

Many patients experience headache with this treatment and the dose needs to be carefully adjusted by the doctor.

- **Aprotinin injections:** This medication has been used in surgery from time to time. It alters and inhibits the activity of certain chemicals which contribute to the chronic tendinopathy. Its side effects include allergy (usually an itch), rash, and some degree of localized pain.

- **Autologous blood injection (ABI):** This interesting option uses the patient's own blood which is injected into the tendon site under local anesthetic. The research and theories for its use suggest that the patient's own growth factors and healing chemicals may be injected to promote healing of the tendon. This does make sense as chronic tendon injuries generally don't have good blood circulation. A course of three injections coupled with exercises is the usual protocol. Tennis elbow and jumper's knee are the more common areas for this treatment.

- **Dry needling, shock wave therapy, calcium gluconate injections, and prolotherapy (dextrose/sugar injections)** have also been studied.

- **Surgery:** Repair or "reinforcement" of tendons and removal (excision) of scar tissue and calcium deposits is sometimes required in severe cases.

Prognosis and Long-Term Outlook

Chronic tendon injury is always a difficult problem. There is no "quick fix." Understanding the nature of the condition is critical as a number of different treatments may need to be applied with an appropriate rehabilitation regime. As a general rule, tendinopathy requires at least two or three months of treatment before normal activities are possible. Maintenance exercises and strategies to prevent a recurrence of the tendon injury are essential.

Chapter 4

Overuse and Repetitive Stress Injuries

Introduction

Overuse injuries occur, as the name states, as a result of overuse. These injuries can occur in virtually any part of the body. Unlike other injuries, there is not a specific incident that causes harm. Overuse injuries occur over a prolonged period and are the result of an accumulation of very minor injuries.

Onset

Overuse injuries typically occur in individuals who perform repetitive activities such as typing, factory work, running, golf, or racquet sports. Symptoms usually start out as minor soreness after activity. As the injury progresses, the individual experiences pain with activity, and eventually the ability to perform the task is impaired. Overuse injuries can also occur with a sudden increase in a person's activity level. The athlete that drastically increases his or her training regimen and the weekend warrior who goes from sitting on the couch to playing softball or golf three times a week are both at risk.

Types of Overuse Injuries

The following is a list of some common overuse injuries.

Tennis elbow (lateral epicondylitis): Pain at the outside of the elbow that is produced by grasping objects with the hand and by extending the wrist. This injury is caused by trauma to the muscles that bend the wrist back.

Golfer's elbow (medial epicondylitis): Similar to tennis elbow, but this injury occurs on the inside of the elbow. Pain is produced by grasping objects with the hand and by flexing the wrist.

Shin splints (medial tibial stress syndrome): Pain along the inside of the shin that occurs frequently in running athletes. This syndrome is the result of excessive stress being placed on the calf musculature. Precipitating factors include inappropriate footwear and having flat feet.

Jumper's knee (patellar tendonitis): Pain in the front of the knee that is produced by jumping. This condition is caused by excessive stress being placed on the tendon that straightens the knee.

Stress fractures: Very small fractures that can occur in weight-bearing bones. Typically, stress fractures occur in the feet of an athlete that increases his or her activity level. Stress fractures will not show up on an X-ray immediately, but will show on a bone scan within 24 hours.

Prevention

Prevention is the best treatment of overuse injuries. Maintaining flexibility by stretching before and after activity is critical in reducing the stress placed upon muscles and tendons. Stretches should be held for 30 seconds and repeated three times for each muscle group. While stretching, it is important to do long, sustained stretches without bouncing.

Adequate strength is also necessary to improve the body's ability to resist and absorb force. Strength training should focus on using light weighs and performing high repetitions. The appropriate weight is one that can be lifted between 8 and 12 repetitions for at least three sets.

An additional preventative measure is to increase training gradually. This is necessary for the body to be able to adapt to increased workload. A general rule is to increase training distance or weight by no more than 10% every week.

High-quality equipment to absorb force and shock can also greatly reduce the risk of overuse injuries. Athletes who participate in racquet sports should purchase shock-reducing devices. Runners should purchase new shoes every 500 miles. This can be between three and six months, depending upon distance and frequency of running.

Conclusion

Overuse injuries are common among athletes and can result in a significant loss of playing time when not managed properly. The best treatment, as with any injury, is prevention. Nevertheless, if symptoms of pain after activity do develop, these symptoms should be treated immediately. Being aware of overuse injuries and taking a few simple precautions against them will significantly reduce your risk of suffering an overuse injury.

Chapter 5

Sudden Cardiac Arrest (SCA) in Athletes

Preventing Sudden Death in Young Athletes

The sudden death of a young athlete is a tragic event that has devastating effects on families and communities. Sudden death in young athletes is usually due to unsuspected heart disease or other heart problems that are not detected by routine screening measures.

Prevalence of Sudden Death in Athletes

There are approximately 75 deaths per year in both male and female athletes between the ages of 13 and 25. Most sudden deaths occur during or immediately after exercise.

Mechanism of Sudden Death in Athletes

Certain heart conditions react adversely to exercise. Exercise causes the heart to fibrillate, usually ventricular fibrillation, and then stop. The athlete collapses suddenly and if not resuscitated dies within minutes.

Cardiac Causes of Sudden Death

- Hypertrophic cardiomyopathy: 36%

- Coronary anomalies: 17%
- Myocarditis: 6%
- Arrhythmogenic right ventricular dysplasia: 4%
- Long QT syndrome: 4%

Coronary Anomalies

Coronary anomalies occur when the arteries originate and/or course in an abnormal way. If the left coronary artery originated from the site of the right coronary artery, for example, it would have to course across the heart to reach its intended heart muscle. This abnormal course could result in compression of the artery between the aorta and the pulmonary artery during exertion resulting in chest pain, shortness of breath, or sudden death.

The diagnosis can only be made if an athlete with chest pain or shortness of breath undergoes a detailed echocardiogram looking at the coronary arteries, a CAT [computerized (axial) tomography] scan of the heart, or a MRI [magnetic resonance imaging] of the heart.

Other Causes of Sudden Death

Myocarditis: Myocarditis is a virus that affects the heart. Symptoms include fever, chest pain, and shortness of breath. Treatment involves bed rest until it resolves. Athletes with a fever or viral illness should not exercise.

Arrhythmogenic right ventricular dysplasia (ARVD): ARVD accounts for 4% of cardiac deaths in the U.S. ARVD is a genetic condition causing the heart to be replaced by fat and fibrous tissue. Symptoms include palpitations or passing out. Diagnosis is made by family history of ARVD and echocardiogram (ECG). ARVD is difficult to detect in routine athletic screening.

Commotio cordis: Commotio cordis accounts for 3% of deaths in athletes. The mean age of the athlete is 14 years. When a hockey puck, a baseball, or blow strikes the chest, the heart can be hit at a vulnerable point of its electrical cycle causing the heart to fibrillate and stop. Softer baseballs and chest barriers may protect the athlete.

Pre-Participation History and Exam

The goal of screening is to detect an abnormal medical condition that could harm or kill the athlete when they exert themselves. The

American Heart Association has recommendations on screening athletes that should be followed by all medical providers. The recommendations include a focused medical history and physical examination. This should be repeated every two years for high school athletes and every three years for college athletes.

Questions to Ask Athletes

- Chest discomfort
- Dizziness or passing out
- Shortness of breath
- Heart murmur
- Elevated blood pressure
- Family history of a serious heart condition

Examination

- Blood pressure
- Listen for a heart murmur lying down, standing, and squatting
- Check pulses in all extremities
- Look for signs of Marfan's syndrome including long limbs and mobile joints

Pitfalls in Screening Athletes

There are millions of athletes that need screening and there are an inadequate number of trained medical personnel. Screening is often performed by medical personnel who have not been trained to screen athletes and the American Heart Association guidelines are not adhered to. Many of the deadly heart conditions are difficult to detect.

Preventative Measures

- Ensure that athletes with chest pain, shortness of breath, palpitations, or passing out undergo a thorough medical evaluation.
- Train athletes with a graded program gradually building up their fitness level.
- Keep athletes well hydrated.
- Respond immediately to an athlete who has collapsed and be aware that the athlete may have suffered a cardiac arrest.

- Train your staff to perform cardiac life support and have trained staff available at every practice and sporting event.

- Purchase a defibrillator and ensure it is readily accessible.

Chapter 6

Arthritis and Sports Injuries

Americans of all ages are increasingly participating in sporting activities. This is a healthy trend, as sports are well known to be helpful for cardiopulmonary fitness and weight-control. However, with the benefits does come some risk, namely sports injuries. Most sports injuries are mild and temporary, with no long-term effects. Minor sprains and bruises or overuse injuries treated properly may be nuisances but do not necessarily cause any permanent problems. Some injuries, however, may lead to arthritis later in life.

Millions of Americans are affected by arthritis, a potentially painful and debilitating condition. Arthritis is the result of disease or damage to articular cartilage, the white glistening surface of our bones found in the joints. Articular cartilage is found in all major joints of the body, including the hips, knees, and shoulders, as well as the smaller joints of the upper and lower extremities and even the spine and pelvis. When this normally smooth gliding surface is no longer intact, pain, swelling, and stiffness may result. This is what is referred to as arthritis.

Arthritis is usually seen in older people, but is also seen in younger people who either have a less common form of the disease or have suffered an injury. The most common form is osteoarthritis, also referred to as degenerative arthritis. It usually occurs naturally, without any specific prior injury, in older people. However, this form of arthritis is also the type seen after injury. In this case, it may be referred to as post-traumatic osteoarthritis, or wear-and-tear arthritis. Whatever the name, the result is the same—a painful, swollen, stiff, and sometimes enlarged or deformed joint. It can be mild in some people, offering only an occasional reminder of an old sports injury, or it can be severe, causing daily suffering and degrees of disability.

It is important to understand the types of injury that can go on to cause arthritis in later life. The types of injuries that lead to arthritis include direct injury to the cartilage (as in fractured joints) or injuries that alter joint mechanics, increasing the stress on the articular surface. The first type is less common in sports, more often seen in motor vehicle accidents or falls from a great height. In these instances, severe bruising of the cartilage surface may lead to permanent injury and eventual arthritis. It may also occur from a fracture of the bone through the cartilage in the joint. In these cases the joint may heal with irregularity causing the cartilage to wear unevenly and eventually erode, resulting in arthritis. A key factor is that, while cartilage is a living tissue and does respond to injury, its reparative capacity is limited, and any significant damage usually results in a permanent alteration.

The more common way a sports injury leads to arthritis is when a ligament or supporting structure is damaged, causing abnormal mechanics in the joint. This greatly increases the stress on the articular surface, which, over time, wears out and causes arthritis. One of the most known examples of this type of this injury is in the knee. With the increased attention of media to the injuries sustained by star athletes, most people have heard of an ACL injury. ACL stands for anterior cruciate ligament, one of the major stabilizers of the knee. The ACL is in the center of the joint and keeps the tibia (lower leg bone) from moving forward on the femur (thigh bone). Commonly an athlete injures the ACL trying to pivot. The result of a torn ACL is generally an unstable knee, one that buckles occasionally, especially with strenuous activities or further participation in sports. This instability abuses the knee, and over time, the articular surfaces are damaged by the abnormal stresses. Once again, the result is eventual arthritis, although the timetable ranges from a short time to many years.

Another knee injury that results in arthritis is torn cartilage. The menisci are a different form of cartilage found in the knee. They are roughly semicircular wedges, two in each knee, that function to cushion the joint, absorbing a great deal of stress, and also more evenly distribute stress across the joint. A torn meniscus alone can be painful and cause swelling and stiffness, leading a patient to seek early surgical treatment. Historically, the entire torn meniscus was removed. We now know that, while this treatment relieves the acute pain and swelling, it eventually predisposes the patient to premature arthritis due to the absence of the protective effects of the menisci. Currently, attempts are made to repair a torn meniscus to remove only the torn part, leaving as much healthy meniscus as possible. Despite these efforts, an injured meniscus may still lead to earlier arthritis.

The next issue is treatment of arthritis due to sports injuries. As is true in most cases, the best treatment is prevention of the injuries. There are a few different methods to prevent sports injuries. The first is proper conditioning. When someone is poorly conditioned or fatigued, the muscles do not protect the joints, and an injury is more likely. It is important for athletes at any level to be properly conditioned for their sport, not only with regards to stamina but also strength and flexibility. Proper nutrition and hydration also come into play. The next aspect of prevention is proper form and technique in the specific sport, assured in part by following the rules of the game. Finally, certain sports offer protective equipment, and this may be of benefit in injury prevention.

Once an injury has been sustained, there are still measures that may prevent arthritis. Avoiding strenuous or demanding activities may decrease the chances of arthritis. In many cases, as in the torn ACL, the problem can be surgically corrected, restoring proper mechanics and thereby hopefully preventing arthritis.

If arthritis does result, there are also many ways to treat the symptoms. The first is activity modification. Occasionally, orthotics or braces may help. Medications such as acetaminophen (Tylenol) or anti-inflammatory medicines such as ibuprofen may offer relief. Physical therapy, including exercises, is sometimes helpful. New over-the-counter nutritional supplements have also shown promise. Occasional joint injections may give some relief. When all other measures have failed, surgery ranging from arthroscopy to joint replacement can be performed. Unfortunately, there is no cure for arthritis, and that is why prevention is the best treatment.

Editor's Note

Glucosamine, chondroitin, and MSM (methylsulfonylmethane) are nutritional supplements frequently recommended for arthritis. While some individual patients report excellent results, most large studies of the supplements, alone and in combination, have shown no effects on arthritis or pain. Their role in treatment, if any, remains unclear.

Chapter 7

Athletes and Skin Disorders

Chapter Contents

Section 7.1

Preventing Skin Diseases in Athletes

"National Athletic Trainers' Association (NATA) Releases Position Statement Guidelines on the Prevention of Skin Diseases in Athletics," June
23, 2010. © 2010 National Athletic Trainers' Association (www.nata.org).
Reprinted with permission.

NATA annual meeting and clinical symposium offers comprehensive recommendations for avoiding, identifying, and treating fungal,
viral, and bacterial skin infections in athletes at all levels.

Drexel University Wrestler Discusses Battle with MRSA [Methicillin-Resistant Staphylococcus Aureus]

As part of an ongoing effort to reduce the incidence of skin diseases among athletes at all levels, today at its 61st annual meeting
and clinical symposium at the Pennsylvania Convention Center in
Philadelphia, the National Athletic Trainers' Association (NATA)
released a position statement on Preventing Skin Diseases in Athletics. The statement, which will be published in the July 2010 issue
of the *Journal of Athletic Training*, NATA's scientific publication,
includes comprehensive recommendations for avoiding, identifying, and treating fungal, viral, and bacterial skin infections, some
of which are life threatening. An electronic version of the complete
statement is available at http://www.nata.org/statements/position
-statements.

A recent review of infectious disease outbreaks reported that skin
diseases accounted for more than half (56%) of all infectious diseases
in competitive sports from 1922 through 2005. Close quarters that
promote skin-to-skin and bodily secretion contact make athletes
particularly vulnerable to contracting skin diseases—some of which
(e.g., MRSA) can be life threatening. Understanding basic preventive
measures, identifying clinical features, and swift management of skin
diseases is essential in preventing the spread of common and serious
skin infections.

Guidelines for Skin Disease Prevention

Steven M. Zinder, PhD, ATC, assistant professor of exercise and sport science at the University of North Carolina at Chapel Hill and chair of the position statement writing group, provided an overview of the statement. His presentation included seven key guidelines for preventing the spread of skin diseases, as follows:

1. Institutions must provide adequate financial and human resources to implement a comprehensive infectious disease control policy.

2. Maintenance of clean facilities is paramount in limiting the spread of infectious diseases.

3. Adequate hand hygiene including frequent hand washing and showering after every sport activity may be one of the biggest factors in reducing the spread of infectious diseases.

4. Athletes and coaches must be educated about, and encouraged to follow, good overall hygiene practices.

5. Athletes must be discouraged from sharing towels, athletic gear, water bottles, disposable razors, and hair clippers.

6. All clothing and equipment should be laundered and/or disinfected on a daily basis.

7. Athletes should be encouraged to complete daily skin surveillance and report any suspicious lesions for treatment.

"The burden of skin diseases extends far beyond the financial toll for medical services and lost productivity," Zinder said. "We should concentrate our efforts on preventing these diseases rather than expending our resources attempting to treat them."

Education: The First-Line Defense against Skin Diseases

Jack Foley, ATC, assistant athletic director and director of sports medicine, Lehigh University and part of the position statement writing group, believes that education is the fundamental first step in halting the spread of skin diseases. "It is necessary to have well informed personnel and athletes in order to promote our best line of defense against skin infection outbreaks," Foley said. "Putting a strategic plan in place, and using a team approach with the latest clinical knowledge available to us, is the absolute best insurance against skin infections in athletics."

David B. Vasily, MD, FAAD, team physician/dermatologist at Lehigh University, president of Lehigh Valley Dermatology Associates and writing group member, agreed with Foley that a preemptive, forward-looking plan is also essential in preventing skin diseases among athletes and teams. "Until now the medical field has been by necessity focused on the reactive development of treatment regimens and drugs, rather than on prevention," Vasily said. "It's now clear that we need to re-focus our efforts in a more proactive and preventive way to achieve the greatest benefits."

Mitigating MRSA

Skin diseases fall into the following three categories, based on the type of infectious agent: fungal (e.g., tinea pedis or athlete's foot); viral (e.g., herpes simplex or cold sores); and bacterial (e.g., *Staphylococcus a* or impetigo). One of the most insidious, dangerous, and even life-threatening bacterial skin diseases athletes are dealing with today is the explosion of the common antibiotic-resistant pathogen known as methicillin-resistant *Staphylococcus aureus* (MRSA). According to data from the U.S. Centers for Disease Control and Prevention (CDC), in 1974 MRSA accounted for just 2% of all infections; however, by 2004 MRSA accounted for 63% of all infections.

James J. Leyden, MD, FAAD, emeritus professor of dermatology at the University of Pennsylvania and position statement reviewer, believes it's crucial that athletes, coaches, parents, and health care providers be made aware of MRSA, among other infectious diseases, as a major disease risk among athletes, since it can result in serious long-term illness or even death. "Everybody on the team and on the sidelines must follow infection control protocols, understand how MRSA spreads, and act in ways that will reduce the risk of contagion," Leyden said. "Careful decisions regarding the safe and effective use of antibiotics will help slow or halt the development of additional drug resistant strains of this very serious pathogen."

"There is nothing more important to coaches than the health and safety of their athletes," according to Mike Moyer, executive director of the National Wrestling Coaches Association. "Skin infections can not only sideline the athlete from play, but also cause removal from school classes and social activities. MRSA and other skin conditions can be passed along from athlete to athlete very quickly, sometimes with fatal consequences, so prevention and detection efforts aren't just nice to have. They're imperative."

A Successful Battle with Infection Reinforces Recommendations

Kyle Frey, 21, a junior and wrestler at Drexel University in Philadelphia, shared with the audience his own battle with MRSA while competing in January of this year. What started as a small "pimple" grew to the size of his left bicep in just two days. He was diagnosed with MRSA, spent five days in quarantine at Hahnemann University Hospital, and was given antibiotics which he was initially resistant to. He was then given a different set of antibiotics and had his arm surgically cleaned to control infection. He remained on these drugs and his arm was stitched and bandaged so he could return to play.

"The whole experience taught me the importance of prevention and early treatment when it comes to skin infections," said Frey. "My athletic trainer, coach, and doctors knew immediately what do to. My mom and teammates provided additional support and we are all much more aware of our personal hygiene in the locker room and with team equipment and mats."

Section 7.2

Athletes and Skin Cancer Risk

"Outdoor Activities: Don't Feel the Burn,"
© 2011 Skin Cancer Foundation (www.skincancer.org).

Athletes worry about speed, endurance, and staying in form—but they should also be concerned about sun damage. Training outdoors without taking protective measures could result in premature skin aging and skin cancers. Learn how to protect yourself while staying in shape.

Everyone knows it's important to get regular exercise. A game of tennis, a bike ride, or a brisk walk all go a long way towards keeping healthy. But these activities can result in the ravages of sun exposure—premature skin aging and increased risk of skin cancer.

Triathletes are a good example. Competing in three endurance sports in a row—swimming, bicycling, and running—they face long hours of training.

Scott B. Phillips, MD, in the Department of Dermatology at St. Elizabeth's Hospital in Chicago, IL, studied the skin injuries faced by endurance athletes. Of 100 triathletes surveyed, about half responded, all but one describing skin problems.

"Sun overexposure and sunburn are a major concern for endurance athletes," says Dr. Phillips.

"During races, triathletes can run into problems even when they use sunscreen, because it tends to wash off during swimming." Then, they may go on racing unprotected when back on land. Another problem in races for endurance athletes is that, for the sake of speed, they wear less clothing than they do in workouts, exposing more skin. "But overall, the greatest amount of exposure occurs during training, since athletes may work out several hours daily," says Dr. Phillips.

Fortunately, experienced competitors learn a host of methods to help avoid these threats. Dr. Phillips provides some key strategies for anyone who exercises in the sun:

Train early and/or late in the day, even if it means breaking workouts into two sessions. From 10:00 a.m. to 4:00 p.m., try to stay out of the sun. Do the bulk of your exercise before and after work, and sometimes during lunch hour, says Dr. Phillips. "But if you're out for hours on weekends, perhaps on a five- or six-hour bike ride, always use sun protection."

- Although you can't choose the time of day when races are run, encourage race promoters to take sun exposure into consideration in scheduling.

- During training, cover as much skin as possible, wearing sweatpants or at least long shorts, and a long-sleeved shirt or sweatshirt. Wear socks to soak up sweat and absorb impact as well as block the sun; wear them as high up on your leg as possible. And shield your eyes with UV-blocking sunglasses.

- While wide-brimmed hats are too unwieldy for endurance sports, wear a baseball-type cap whenever you can. It protects the forehead and front of the face. And always wear a helmet when biking, for both sun protection and crash protection.

- For extended exposure outdoors, use a broad-spectrum SPF 30 or higher water-resistant sunscreen on all exposed skin, up to 6:30 p.m. or later on a summer's day, even when it is cloudy. (The sun's harmful ultraviolet rays go through clouds.) "I recommend alcohol-based sunscreens for the face, because they're more resistant to sweating," says Dr. Phillips. "I also like to apply stick sunscreens around the eyes, since they are almost impervious to sweating. And I'm a big fan of lip balm."

- Even if sunscreen is labeled "water-resistant" or "waterproof," some washes off during swimming and heavy sweating. Replenish it when you come out of the water, and at least every two hours after. In races, triathletes should keep sunscreen handy in the transition areas. Or, if you're bicycling next, keep sunscreen taped to the bike and reapply it to the arms, face, and neck while pedaling.

"Taking these few moments makes a big difference in sun protection, and little difference in your competitiveness," says Dr. Phillips.

Chapter 8

Athletes and Exercise-Induced Asthma and Allergies

Chapter Contents

Section 8.1

Exercise-Induced Asthma

"Exercise-Induced Asthma," reprinted with permission from the
Asthma and Allergy Foundation of America (www.aafa.org), © 2005.
Revised by David A. Cooke, MD, FACP, August 2011.

Everyone needs to exercise, even people with asthma! A strong
healthy body is one of your best defenses against disease. But some
people with asthma have "exercise-induced asthma" (EIA). But with
proper medical prevention and management you should be able to
walk, climb stairs, run, and participate in activities, sports, and
exercise without experiencing symptoms. You don't have to let EIA
keep you from leading an active life or from achieving your athletic
dreams.

What Is Exercise-Induced Asthma?

Exercise is a common cause of asthma symptoms. This is usually
called exercise-induced asthma (EIA) or exercise-induced bronchospasm (EIB). It is estimated that 80% to 90% of all individuals who
have allergic asthma will experience symptoms of EIA with vigorous
exercise or activity. For teenagers and young adults this is often the
most common cause of asthma symptoms. Fortunately with better
medications, monitoring, and management you can participate in
physical activity and sports and achieve your highest performance
level.

What Are the Symptoms of EIA?

Symptoms of exercised-induced asthma include coughing, wheezing, chest tightness, and shortness of breath. Coughing is the most
common symptom of EIA and may be the only symptom you have.
The symptoms of EIA may begin during exercise and will usually
be worse 5 to 10 minutes after stopping exercise. Symptoms most
often resolve in another 20 to 30 minutes and can range from
mild to severe. Occasionally some individuals will experience "late

phase" symptoms 4 to 12 hours after stopping exercise. Late-phase symptoms are frequently less severe and can take up to 24 hours to go away.

What Causes EIA?

When you exercise you breathe faster due to the increased oxygen demands of your body. Usually during exercise you inhale through your mouth, causing the air to be dryer and cooler than when you breathe through your nasal passages. This decrease in warmth and humidity are both causes of bronchospasm. Exercise that exposes you to cold air such as skiing or ice hockey is therefore more likely to cause symptoms than exercise involving warm and humid air such as swimming. Pollution levels, high pollen counts, and exposure to other irritants such as smoke and strong fumes can also make EIA symptoms worse. A recent cold or asthma episode can cause you to have more difficulty exercising.

How Is EIA Diagnosed?

It is important to know the difference between being out of condition and having exercise-induced asthma. A well-conditioned person will usually only experience the symptoms of EIA with vigorous activity or exercise. To make a diagnosis, your doctor will take a thorough history and may perform a series of tests. During these tests, which may include running or a treadmill test, your doctor will measure your lung functions using a spirometer before, during, and after exercise. Monitoring your peak flows before, during, and after exercise can also help you and your doctor detect narrowing of your airways. Then, using guidelines established by your doctor, you can help prevent asthma symptoms and participate in and enjoy physical activity. Your doctor will also tell you what to do should a full-blown episode occur.

Treatment and Management of EIA

With proper treatment and management people with EIA can participate safely and achieve their full potential. Proper management requires that you take steps to prevent symptoms and carefully monitor your respiratory status before, during, and after exercise. Taking medication prior to exercising is important in preventing EIA. Proper warm up for 6 to 10 minutes before periods of exercise or vigorous activity will usually help. Individuals who can tolerate continuous exercise with minimal symptoms may find that proper warm-up may prevent the need for repeated medications.

What Types of Medications Treat/Prevent EIA?

There are four types of medications to prevent or treat the symptoms of EIA. Your health care provider can help you determine the best treatment program for you based on your asthma condition and the type of activity or exercise.

The first medication is a short-acting beta2-agonist, also called a bronchodilator. This medication can prevent symptoms and should be taken 10 to 15 minutes before exercise. It will help prevent symptoms for up to four hours. This same medication can also be used to treat and reverse the symptoms of EIA should they occur.

The second medication is a long-acting bronchodilator. It needs to be taken 30 to 60 minutes prior to activity and only once within a 12-hour period. Salmeterol can help prevent EIA symptoms for 10 to 12 hours. This medication should only be used to prevent symptoms and should never be used to relieve symptoms once they occur because it does not offer any quick relief.

The third type of medication is cromolyn or nedocromil. They also need to be taken 15 to 20 minutes prior to exercise. There is also some evidence that taking these medications will also help to prevent the late-phase reaction of EIA that is experienced by some individuals. These medications also should only be used as a preventative measure because they do not relieve symptoms once they begin. Some individuals use one of these medications in combination with a short-acting bronchodilator.

The fourth type of medication is montelukast, which is a leukotriene inhibitor. This reduces the tendency of airways to constrict and can work well for some people with exercise-induced asthma. Unlike the other medications discussed here, montelukast is taken on a daily basis, rather than before exercise.

If you have frequent symptoms with usual activity or exercise, talk to your doctor. An increase in your long-term control medications may help. Long-term anti-inflammatory medications such as inhaled steroids can reduce the frequency and severity of EIA.

Teachers and coaches should be informed if a child has exercise-induced asthma. They should be told that the child should be able to participate in activities, but that they may require medication prior to activity. Athletes should also disclose their medications and adhere to standards set by the U.S. Olympic Committee. Approved and prohibited medications can be obtained from the committee hotline (800-233-0393).

What Types of Sports Are Best for People with EIA?

Activities that involve only short bursts of exercise or intermittent periods of activity are usually better tolerated. Such sports include walking, volleyball, basketball, and gymnastics or baseball. Swimming that involves breathing warm and moist air is often well tolerated. Aerobic sports such as distance running, soccer, or basketball are more likely to cause symptoms. In addition cold air sports such as ice hockey or ice-skating may not be tolerated as well.

It is important to consult with your health care provider prior to beginning any exercise program and to pace yourself. With effective management people with EIA can perform and excel in a variety of sports. Many Olympic athletes and professional athletes with exercise-induced asthma have excelled in their sports, many winning Olympic gold medals.

Remember, with proper medical management you should be able to walk, climb stairs, run, and participate in activities, sports, and exercise without experiencing symptoms. Do not let EIA keep you from leading an active life or from achieving your athletic dreams.

Section 8.2

Exercise-Induced Urticaria (Hives) and Anaphylaxis

What is exercise-induced anaphylaxis?

Exercise-induced anaphylaxis (EIA) is a form of chronic hives that is caused by exercise. However, people can also experience symptoms of a more severe allergic reaction, called anaphylaxis. Other than hives, people with EIA may have breathing difficulties (shortness of breath, wheezing), circulatory problems (lightheadedness, low blood pressure), and gastrointestinal symptoms (nausea, vomiting, and diarrhea).

As its name implies, EIA occurs as a result of exercise. Exercise can be of any form, including jogging, tennis, swimming, walking, or even strenuous chores such as shoveling snow. Symptoms may start as tiredness, warmth, itching, and redness, usually within a few minutes of starting exercise. If exercise continues, hives begin to occur, and may include swelling of the face, lips, eyes, and throat (angioedema), and ultimately anaphylaxis.

Cholinergic urticaria is similar to EIA in that exercise, or anything that increases body temperature, triggers hives. However, in EIA, only exercise triggers symptoms, while other increases in body temperature, such as hot showers, will not.

What causes exercise-induced anaphylaxis?

Like other types of chronic urticaria, EIA's cause is unknown. However, many people have another trigger that, along with exercise, causes the symptoms. These triggers include various medications, a variety of foods, alcohol, cold weather, and menstruation. Typically, either exercise or the specific trigger alone will not cause symptoms. But, if the person is exposed to the trigger and exercise, then symptoms of EIA may occur.

Medications that have reported to cause EIA include aspirin, ibuprofen, and other non-steroidal anti-inflammatory drugs (NSAIDs). It is possible that any medication may trigger EIA when taken before exercising.

A variety of foods, when eaten 24 hours prior to exercising, may cause EIA. However, a person may be able to eat these foods without symptoms if they do not exercise. A long list of foods have been associated with EIA, including cereal grains, seafood, nuts, fruits, vegetables, dairy, and alcohol. Some people have EIA associated with eating, but there is no specific food that triggers the symptoms.

How is exercise-induced anaphylaxis diagnosed?

Typically, the diagnosis of EIA is based on a person's history of symptoms that occur only with exercise. If symptoms occur outside of exercise, such as with any increase in body temperature, it is more likely that cholinergic urticaria is the reason for the symptoms.

It is not usually necessary to attempt to trigger symptoms of EIA with having a person exercise under medical supervision. This may be required in special circumstances if the diagnosis is in question. Only a physician skilled in the diagnosis and treatment of anaphylaxis should perform such a test under close medical supervision, with equipment immediately available to treat a potentially life-threatening reaction.

Once a diagnosis of EIA is made, it is important to assess for other triggers as previously mentioned. This may include allergy testing to a variety of foods. A negative skin test to a particular food nearly rules out the possibility of that food as the cause of the EIA. A positive food skin test, especially to a food that was eaten within 24 hours before the person experienced symptoms, may represent the food that caused the reaction.

How is exercise-induced anaphylaxis treated?

Immediate symptoms of EIA should be treated in much the same way as anaphylaxis from any cause (such as from a food or insect sting allergy). This may require the use of injectable epinephrine, such as with an Epi-Pen or Twin-Ject device.

Prevention of EIA symptoms is the most important goal of treatment. People with EIA should avoid exercising alone, avoid exercising in cold weather, only exercise on an empty stomach, and should avoid eating any causative food (as determined by skin testing) for at least 24 hours before exercise. In addition, avoidance of NSAIDs and alcoholic beverages for 24 hours prior to exercise is also advised.

It may be important for women to avoid exercising during their menstrual period.

It would be reasonable for a person with EIA to carry an Epi-Pen and wear a Medic-Alert bracelet describing their medical condition and potential need for injectable epinephrine. An exercising buddy, one who is familiar with how to recognize and treat the person's EIA, would be ideal.

Want to learn more? Find out the basics of food allergies [at allergies .about.com/od/foodallergies/a/foodbasic.htm].

Sources

Dice, JP. Physical Urticaria. *Immunol Allergy Clin N Am*. 2004;24:225–246.

Perkins DN, Keith PK. Food- and Exercise-Induced Anaphylaxis: Importance of History in the Diagnosis. *Ann Allergy Asthma Immnuol*. 2002;89:15–23.

Chapter 9

Sports Nutrition, Weight Maintenance, and Hydration

Chapter Contents

Section 9.1

Basic Facts about Sports Nutrition

"Questions Most Frequently Asked about Sports Nutrition," President's Council on Physical Fitness and Sports (www.fitness.gov), April 23, 2008.

What diet is best for athletes?

It's important that an athlete's diet provides the right amount of energy, the 50-plus nutrients the body needs, and adequate water. No single food or supplement can do this. A variety of foods are needed every day. But, just as there is more than one way to achieve a goal, there is more than one way to follow a nutritious diet.

Do the nutritional needs of athletes differ from non-athletes?

Competitive athletes, sedentary individuals, and people who exercise for health and fitness all need the same nutrients. However, because of the intensity of their sport or training program, some athletes have higher calorie and fluid requirements. Eating a variety of foods to meet increased calorie needs helps to ensure that the athlete's diet contains appropriate amounts of carbohydrate, protein, vitamins, and minerals.

Are there certain dietary guidelines athletes should follow?

Health and nutrition professionals recommend that 55%–60% of the calories in our diet come from carbohydrate, no more than 30% from fat, and the remaining 10%–15% from protein. While the exact percentages may vary slightly for some athletes based on their sport or training program, these guidelines will promote health and serve as the basis for a diet that will maximize performance.

How many calories do I need a day?

This depends on your age, body size, sport, and training program. For example, a 250-pound weight lifter needs more calories than a 98-pound gymnast. Exercise or training may increase calorie needs by

54

as much as 1,000 to 1,500 calories a day. The best way to determine if you're getting too few or too many calories is to monitor your weight. Keeping within your ideal competitive weight range means that you are getting the right amount of calories.

Which is better for replacing fluids—water or sports drinks?

Depending on how muscular you are, 55%–70% of your body weight is water. Being "hydrated" means maintaining your body's fluid level. When you sweat, you lose water that must be replaced if you want to perform your best. You need to drink fluids before, during, and after all workouts and events.

Whether you drink water or a sports drink is a matter of choice. However, if your workout or event lasts for more than 90 minutes, you may benefit from the carbohydrates provided by sports drinks. A sports drink that contains 15–18 grams of carbohydrate in every eight ounces of fluid should be used. Drinks with a higher carbohydrate content will delay the absorption of water and may cause dehydration, cramps, nausea, or diarrhea. There are a variety of sports drinks on the market. Be sure to experiment with sports drinks during practice instead of trying them for the first time the day of an event.

What are electrolytes?

Electrolytes are nutrients that affect fluid balance in the body and are necessary for our nerves and muscles to function. Sodium and potassium are the two electrolytes most often added to sports drinks. Generally, electrolyte replacement is not needed during short bursts of exercise since sweat is approximately 99% water and less than 1% electrolytes. Water, in combination with a well-balanced diet, will restore normal fluid and electrolyte levels in the body. However, replacing electrolytes may be beneficial during continuous activity of longer than two hours, especially in a hot environment.

What do muscles use for energy during exercise?

Most activities use a combination of fat and carbohydrate as energy sources. How hard and how long you work out, your level of fitness, and your diet will affect the type of fuel your body uses. For short-term, high-intensity activities like sprinting, athletes rely mostly on carbohydrate for energy. During low-intensity exercises like walking, the body uses more fat for energy.

What are carbohydrates?

Carbohydrates are sugars and starches found in foods like breads, cereals, fruits, vegetables, pasta, milk, honey, syrups, and table sugar. Carbohydrates are the preferred source of energy for your body. Regardless of origin, your body breaks down carbohydrates into glucose that your blood carries to cells to be used for energy. Carbohydrates provide four calories per gram, while fat provides nine calories per gram. Your body cannot differentiate between glucose that comes from starches or sugars. Glucose from either source provides energy for working muscles.

Is it true that athletes should eat a lot of carbohydrates?

When you are training or competing, your muscles need energy to perform. One source of energy for working muscles is glycogen, which is made from carbohydrates and stored in your muscles. Every time you work out, you use some of your glycogen. If you don't consume enough carbohydrates, your glycogen stores become depleted, which can result in fatigue. Both sugars and starches are effective in replenishing glycogen stores.

When and what should I eat before I compete?

Performance depends largely on the foods consumed during the days and weeks leading up to an event. If you regularly eat a varied, carbohydrate-rich diet you are in good standing and probably have ample glycogen stores to fuel activity. The purpose of the pre-competition meal is to prevent hunger and to provide the water and additional energy the athlete will need during competition. Most athletes eat two to four hours before their event. However, some athletes perform their best if they eat a small amount 30 minutes before competing, while others eat nothing for six hours beforehand. For many athletes, carbohydrate-rich foods serve as the basis of the meal. However, there is no magic pre-event diet. Simply choose foods and beverages that you enjoy and that don't bother your stomach. Experiment during the weeks before an event to see which foods work best for you.

Will eating sugary foods before an event hurt my performance?

In the past, athletes were warned that eating sugary foods before exercise could hurt performance by causing a drop in blood glucose levels. Recent studies, however, have shown that consuming sugar up to 30 minutes before an event does not diminish performance. In fact, evidence suggests that a sugar-containing pre-competition beverage or snack may improve performance during endurance workouts and events.

What is carbohydrate loading?

Carbohydrate loading is a technique used to increase the amount of glycogen in muscles. For five to seven days before an event, the athlete eats 10–12 grams of carbohydrate per kilogram body weight and gradually reduces the intensity of the workouts. (To find out how much you weigh in kilograms, simply divide your weight in pounds by 2.2.) The day before the event, the athlete rests and eats the same high-carbohydrate diet. Although carbohydrate loading may be beneficial for athletes participating in endurance sports that require 90 minutes or more of nonstop effort, most athletes needn't worry about carbohydrate loading. Simply eating a diet that derives more than half of its calories from carbohydrates will do.

As an athlete, do I need to take extra vitamins and minerals?

Athletes need to eat about 1,800 calories a day to get the vitamins and minerals they need for good health and optimal performance. Since most athletes eat more than this amount, vitamin and mineral supplements are needed only in special situations. Athletes who follow vegetarian diets or who avoid an entire group of foods (for example, never drink milk) may need a supplement to make up for the vitamins and minerals not being supplied by food. A multivitamin-mineral pill that supplies 100% of the Recommended Dietary Allowance (RDA) will provide the nutrients needed. An athlete who frequently cuts back on calories, especially below the 1,800 calorie level, is not only at risk for inadequate vitamin and mineral intake, but also may not be getting enough carbohydrate. Since vitamins and minerals do not provide energy, they cannot replace the energy provided by carbohydrates.

Will extra protein help build muscle mass?

Many athletes, especially those on strength-training programs or who participate in power sports, are told that eating a ton of protein or taking protein supplements will help them gain muscle weight. However, the true secret to building muscle is training hard and consuming enough calories. While some extra protein is needed to build muscle, most American diets provide more than enough protein. Between 1.0 and 1.5 grams of protein per kilogram body weight per day is sufficient if your calorie intake is adequate and you're eating a variety of foods. For a 150-pound athlete, that represents 68–102 grams of protein a day.

Why is iron so important?

Hemoglobin, which contains iron, is the part of red blood cells that carries oxygen from the lungs to all parts of the body, including muscles. Since your muscles need oxygen to produce energy, if you have low iron levels in your blood, you may tire quickly. Symptoms of iron deficiency include fatigue, irritability, dizziness, headaches, and lack of appetite. Many times, however, there are no symptoms at all. A blood test is the best way to find out if your iron level is low. It is recommended that athletes have their hemoglobin levels checked once a year.

The RDA for iron is 15 milligrams a day for women and 10 milligrams a day for men. Red meat is the richest source of iron, but fish and poultry also are good sources. Fortified breakfast cereals, beans, and green leafy vegetables also contain iron. Our bodies absorb the iron found in animal products best.

Should I take an iron supplement?

Taking iron supplements will not improve performance unless an athlete is truly iron deficient. Too much iron can cause constipation, diarrhea, and nausea and may interfere with the absorption of other nutrients such as copper and zinc. Therefore, iron supplements should not be taken without proper medical supervision.

Why is calcium so important?

Calcium is needed for strong bones and proper muscle function. Dairy foods are the best source of calcium. However, studies show that many female athletes who are trying to lose weight cut back on dairy products. Female athletes who don't get enough calcium may be at risk for stress fractures and, when they're older, osteoporosis. Young women between the ages of 11 and 24 need about 1,200 milligrams of calcium a day. After age 25, the recommended intake is 800 milligrams. Low-fat dairy products are a rich source of calcium and also are low in fat and calories.

Section 9.2

Weight Loss in Wrestlers

For more than a half century, rapid weight loss in wrestling has remained a concern among educators, health professionals, exercise scientists, and parents. Since ACSM first published the Position Stand "Weight Loss in Wrestlers" in 1976, numerous research articles have been published on this topic. On a weekly basis, rapid weight loss in high school and collegiate wrestlers has been shown to average four to five pounds and may exceed six to seven pounds among 20% of the wrestlers. One-third of high school and collegiate wrestlers have been reported repeating this practice more than 10 times in a season. These practices have been documented over the past 25 years, and during that time, there appears to be little change in their prevalence.

Wrestlers often justify their choice of weight class with the belief that they have excess fat to lose. However, studies show that in the off-season, high school wrestlers have 8%–11% body fat, well below their high school peers who average 15%. In season, wrestlers typically have 6%–7% body fat. Consequently, loss of fat would contribute minimally to the rapid weekly weight reduction while the primary methods for weight loss (e.g., exercise, food restriction, fasting, and various dehydration methods) affect body water, energy stores, and lean tissue. These weight loss techniques are used by one-quarter to two-thirds of wrestlers.

Most wrestlers practice these weight-loss techniques believing their chances of competitive success will increase. Ironically, weight cutting may impair performance and endanger the wrestler's health. The combination of food restriction and fluid deprivation creates an adverse physiological effect on the body, leaving the wrestler ill prepared to compete. In addition, forms of dehydration, such as sweating and catharsis (laxatives and forced vomiting), contribute to the loss of electrolytes as well as water. Wrestlers hope to replenish body fluids, electrolytes, and glycogen in the brief period between the weigh-in and competition. Reestablishing bodily fluids, however, may take 24–48 hours, replenishing muscle glycogen may take 72 hours, and replacing lean tissue might take even longer. In short, weight cutting appears to influence the wrestler's energy reserves, fluid levels, and electrolyte balances.

Despite repeated warning by the medical community, weight cutting (rapid weight reduction) remains popular among amateur wrestlers. Weight cutting has significant adverse consequences that may affect competitive performance, health, and normal growth and development. To enhance the educational experience and reduce the health risks for the participants, the American College of Sports Medicine (ACSM) recommends the education of coaches and wrestlers toward sound nutrition and weight control behaviors to curtail weight cutting and the enactment of rules that limit weight loss.

Because of the questionable benefits and the potential health risks caused by the procedures used for weight cutting by wrestlers (particularly adolescents), ACSM makes the following recommendations:

1. Educate coaches and wrestlers about the adverse consequences of prolonged fasting and dehydration on physical performance and physical health.

2. Discourage the use of rubber suits, steam rooms, hot boxes, saunas, laxatives, and diuretics for weight cutting.

3. Adopt new state or national governing-body legislation that schedules weigh-ins immediately prior to competition.

4. Schedule daily weigh-ins before and after practice to monitor weight loss and dehydration. Weight loss during practice should be regained through adequate food and fluid intake.

5. Assess the body composition of each wrestler prior to the season using valid methods for this population. Males 16 years old and younger with body fat below 7% or those over 16 with a body fat below 5% need medical clearance before being allowed to compete. Female wrestlers need minimal body fat of 12%–14%.

6. Emphasize the need for daily caloric intake obtained from a balanced diet high in carbohydrates (>55% of calories), low in fat (<30% of calories), and adequate in protein (15%–20% of calories, 1.0–1.5 g/kg body weight) determined on the basis of RDA guidelines and physical activity levels.

The minimal caloric intakes for wrestlers of high school and college age range from 1,700 to 2,500 kcal/day. Rigorous training may increase the requirement by an additional 1,000 calories per day. Wrestlers should be discouraged by coaches, parents, school officials, and physicians from consuming less than their minimal daily needs. Combined with exercise, this minimal caloric intake will allow for gradual weight loss. Once the minimal weight has been attained, caloric intake should be increased to support the normal development needs and training of the young wrestler.

The American College of Sports Medicine encourages:

- permitting more participants per team to compete by adding weight classes between 119 and 151 pounds or by allowing more than one representative at a given weight class just as in swimming and track meets;

- standardizing the eligibility rules for championship tournaments so that severe, rapid weight loss is discouraged at the end of the season (e.g., a wrestler dropping an extra weight class);

- cooperative efforts between coaches, exercise scientists, physicians, dietitians, and wrestlers to use research and education to determine the best medically sound system for selecting a weight class.

Through this Current Comment, ACSM hopes to further the sport of wrestling by providing a positive educational environment for the primary, secondary, or collegiate wrestler. ACSM believes these recommendations will enable the athlete to better focus on skill acquisition, fitness enhancement, psychological preparation, and the social interactions offered by the sport.

Section 9.3

Female Athlete Triad

"Female Athlete Triad: Disordered Eating, Amenorrhea and Osteoporosis," reprinted with permission of the American College of Sports Medicine. Copyright © 2005 American College of Sports Medicine (www.acsm.org). Editor's note added by David A. Cooke, MD, FACP, August 2011.

Active women and girls who are driven to excel in sports risk developing the Female Athlete Triad. Three distinct but interrelated conditions—disordered eating, amenorrhea, and osteoporosis—comprise the Female Athlete Triad. Disordered eating is a range of poor nutritional behaviors. Amenorrhea refers to irregular or absent menstrual periods. Osteoporosis refers to low bone mass and microarchitectural deterioration, which leads to bone fragility and risk of fracture.

Exercise Promotes Good Health

Physical activity should be encouraged since it promotes health, cardiovascular fitness, bone strength, and longevity. Exercise alone is not a risk for development of the Triad. An energy deficit, in which caloric intake doesn't match energy expenditure, is a risk factor, however.

External and Internal Pressure May Foster Development of the Triad

All women face societal pressure that "thin is in." Well-meaning coaches, friends, and parents may encourage weight loss by a female athlete due to a misconception that excessive leanness enhances performance. A young woman or girl who is determined to achieve a lean appearance or athletic success may attempt to excel through dieting and exercise. (Such females are typically goal-oriented, perfectionistic, and compulsive.) This misguided approach may lead to disordered eating, menstrual dysfunction, and lower than normal bone mass formation.

Anyone may be affected, but women and girls participating in activities in which leanness is emphasized are at high risk. Gymnastics, ballet, diving, figure skating, aerobics, and running are examples. Sports with weight classifications such as wrestling, rowing, and martial arts may foster disordered eating in athletes, including males.

Disordered Eating Is a Spectrum of Abnormal Behaviors

In response to pressure to lose weight, women and girls may practice unhealthy weight-control methods, ranging from restricted food intake, self-induced vomiting, consumption of appetite suppressants and diet pills, use of laxatives and compounds to increase urination, to anorexia nervosa and bulimia. Anorexia nervosa refers to weight 15% below normal, obsessive fear of fatness, abnormal body image (i.e., a thin person who think she is fat), and amenorrhea. Bulimia is defined as binge eating at least two times a week for at least three months, loss of control over eating, and purging (i.e., self-induced vomiting or use of diet pills, laxatives, enemas, or excessive exercise to lose weight).

Some warning signs of eating disorders include:

- excessive leanness or rapid weight loss;
- preoccupation with weight, food, mealtime rituals, and body image;
- wide fluctuations in weight;
- daily vigorous exercise in addition to regular training sessions;
- stress fractures (i.e., microfractures of bones that may progress to complete fractures);
- yellowing of the skin;
- soft baby hair on the skin;
- frequent sore throats despite no other signs of respiratory illness (self-induced vomiting);
- chipmunk-like cheek from swollen parotid glands (self-induced vomiting);
- many dental cavities, foul breath (self-induced vomiting);
- fatigue, light-headedness, dizziness;
- depression, low self-esteem.

Disordered Eating Is Often Hidden

Many girls and women hide or deny their eating disorders due to embarrassment, shame, fear of losing control of their dieting, and their mistaken believe that excessive weight loss enhances performance.

Performance in Sport, School, and Work May Decline from Disordered Eating

Disordered eating may cause weakness, dehydration, anemia (i.e., low oxygen-carrying capacity of blood), lack of concentration, impaired coordination, frequent and delayed recovery from illness and injuries, and depression.

Eating Disorders May Be Fatal

Eating disorders are serious, chronic medical and psychological illnesses. Individuals with untreated chronic anorexia or bulimia may die prematurely from heart problems, blood electrolyte (i.e., salt) disorders, suicide, or other health problems. In 1994, Christy Henrich, a member of the U.S. gymnastic team, died at age 21 from consequences of anorexia nervosa. If these disorders are recognized early, however, treatment may be effective.

Amenorrhea Warrants Evaluation

An unbalanced diet, inadequate caloric intake relative to exercise level, and perhaps excessive training may predispose females to menstrual abnormalities. Although women and girls may be relieved to not experience menstrual periods, their absence may be dangerous since lack of menstrual periods may be due to a medical disorder and can be associated with osteoporosis.

Any female who hasn't started menstruating by the age of 16, misses three consecutive periods, or has periods that occur at intervals of greater than 35 days should be evaluated by a physician. Before attributing menstrual abnormalities to exercise, other conditions, such as pregnancy, abnormalities of the reproductive organs, or thyroid disease, must be excluded. Any female without periods who is sexually active may become pregnant, so contraception should be used if pregnancy is not desired.

Osteoporosis May Occur Prematurely

Osteoporosis refers to low bone mass and fragility of the skeleton. Bone mass of women typically peaks in the mid 20s to 30s. A 20-year-old woman without menses during her critical teenage growth period may have bone mass typical of a 70-year-old woman, predisposing her to stress fractures and fractures later in life.

Adequate nutrition, including a balanced diet, adequate calories, relative number of calories spent during exercise, and proper calcium, fosters good bone formation. Calcium requirements for teenage girls and young women with normal menses is 1,200 mg per day. This can be obtained by consuming three to four dairy products per day or calcium supplement tablets. Females with irregular or absent menses require 1,500 mg of calcium and 400 mg of vitamin D per day.

Low estrogen levels and other hormonal changes, which accompany irregular or absent menstrual periods, may predispose females to osteoporosis.

Editor's Note: In 2010, the U.S. Institute of Medicine revised daily intake recommendations for young women to 600 international units per day of vitamin D and 1,300 mg per day of calcium.

The Female Athlete Triad Can Be Prevented

Proper nutritional practices should be taught to women and girls. Athletes and non-athletes should strive for proper caloric intake while eating a well balanced diet.

Emphasis or pressure to achieve unrealistically low body weight should be avoided by coaches, parents, athletic administrators, and health professionals. Out-of-competition "weigh-ins" should be discouraged. Rules governing sports should be examined and eliminated or revised if they encourage excessive leanness. Individuals working with active women and girls should learn the seriousness of each of the disorders comprising the Triad and recognize warning signs.

Early Recognition and Treatment Hastens Recovery

Although individuals with disordered eating or amenorrhea may deny nutritional or health problems and are reluctant to seek care, medical attention is mandatory. An individual may be more likely to seek medical help if the risks of poor nutrition and amenorrhea are explained in a non-judgmental way. An athlete should be reminded that medical care and proper nutrition may enhance performance.

If an eating disorder or amenorrhea is suspected, the involved individual should be strongly encouraged or required to seek medical attention. If the individual refuses, the concerned coach, friend, or parents should consult with a physician directly.

Treatment of the Triad often requires intervention via a team approach. A physician, nutritionist, and psychologist may need to work with the woman or girl, coaches, parents, and close friends. Nutritional monitoring, hormone replacement, and reduced training may be recommended. Early intervention hastens recovery.

Section 9.4

Healthy Hydration for Athletes

"Quench Your Thirst" by Debra Wein, Ms. RD, LDN, © 2003 National Strength and Conditioning Association (NSCA). Reprinted with permission. This article originally appeared in the NSCA's *Performance Training Journal*. To access articles online, visit www.nsca-lift.org/Perform. Reviewed by David A. Cooke, MD, FACP, August 2011.

Long and tough running workouts can be exhausting and also dangerous, if you neglect to "quench your thirst." Replacing the fluids lost from your body when you exercise in the heat is essential to sustain performance, prevent dehydration, and ultimately, to avoid injury. What to drink and when to drink is commanded by how long and how hard you exercise, environmental conditions, and whether or not you have acclimated to the heat. For training and running events less than one hour in duration, good old water is sufficient for optimal rehydration. On the other hand, workouts that last more than an hour increase fluid losses (1–2 quarts/hour) and drain the muscle's energy stores, making sports drinks the optimum replacement.

Sports drinks contain three main ingredients: water, carbohydrate (6%–10%), and sodium, and are precisely formulated for utilization during exercise. The benefits of these drinks include the offset of fluid losses, the replacement of energy (50–80 calories per cup), the boosting of fluid absorption into the blood, and of course the sweeter taste (lemon-lime, etc.).

However, if you dislike the taste of these drinks you may want to try diluting fruit juice, which is about 12%–15% carbohydrate, with an equal amount of water. The drawbacks of sports drinks include the cost and also the excess calories, particularly if you are trying to lose weight rather than win a competition. So taste-test the different brands, but make sure it is while you are exercising, because your taste buds do change, and different drinks will have different effects during exercise. The bottom line is, choose one that you enjoy; the more you like it the more you'll drink it!

Lastly, keep in mind that these beverages are not complete foods; they lack protein, fat, fiber, and some of the essential vitamins and minerals. Therefore, it is still necessary to eat a well-balanced diet—including fruit, vegetables, lean proteins, beans, and whole grains—to provide your body with the nutrients that you need to run and perform your best.

More fluid facts and guidelines for the successful runner:

- Thirst is not always a good indicator of fluid loss. Drink before you are thirsty!

- Avoid caffeine and alcohol, as they increase the rate of fluid loss.

- Drink fluids at a cool temperature.

- Unless you are an ultra-endurance athlete participating in events lasting over eight hours, electrolyte (sodium, potassium, and chloride) losses from exercise are easily overcome by typical intakes from the regular diet. Therefore, salt tablets are not recommended.

Healthy Hydration

For an active person, adequate hydration can mean a difference between moderate dehydration and optimal performance. Follow these sport nutrition guidelines:

Hyper-Hydrate

One to two hours before a run, drink a sports drink or 2½ cups (20 oz.) of water.

An alternative method is to drink 1½ cups (12 oz.) of water 15–20 minutes before exercise. (Do both in very hot conditions, for a total of 4 cups or 32 oz.)

Hydrate

Drink 1 cup (8 oz.) of water or a sports drink every 15–20 minutes during a workout.

Rehydrate

Weigh yourself before and after a workout. For each pound of body weight lost drink 20 ounces of water. If you don't have access to a scale, drink until your urine is clear. Clear urine is a good indication of adequate hydration.

Chapter 10

Performance-Enhancing Substances

Chapter Contents

Section 10.1

Steroids

"NIDA InfoFacts: Steroids (Anabolic-Androgenic),"
National Institute on Drug Abuse (nida.nih.gov), July 2009.

Anabolic-androgenic steroids (AAS) are synthetically produced variants of the naturally occurring male sex hormone testosterone. "Anabolic" refers to muscle building, and "androgenic" refers to increased male sexual characteristics. "Steroids" refers to the class of drugs. These drugs can be legally prescribed to treat conditions resulting from steroid hormone deficiency, such as delayed puberty, as well as diseases that result in loss of lean muscle mass, such as cancer and AIDS.

How are AAS abused?

Some people, both athletes and non-athletes, abuse AAS in an attempt to enhance performance and/or improve physical appearance. AAS are taken orally or injected, typically in cycles rather than continuously. "Cycling" refers to a pattern of use in which steroids are taken for periods of weeks or months, after which use is stopped for a period of time and then restarted. In addition, users often combine several different types of steroids in an attempt to maximize their effectiveness, a practice referred to as "stacking."

How do AAS affect the brain?

The immediate effects of AAS in the brain are mediated by their binding to androgen (male sex hormone) and estrogen (female sex hormone) receptors on the surface of a cell. This AAS-receptor complex can then shuttle into the cell nucleus to influence patterns of gene expression. Because of this, the acute effects of AAS in the brain are substantially different from those of other drugs of abuse. The most important difference is that AAS are not euphorigenic, meaning they do not trigger rapid increases in the neurotransmitter dopamine, which is responsible for the "high" that often drives substance abuse behaviors. However, long-term use of AAS can eventually have an impact on some of the same brain pathways and chemicals—such as dopamine, serotonin, and opioid systems—that are affected by other drugs of abuse. Considering the combined effect of their complex direct and indirect actions, it is not surprising that AAS can affect mood and behavior in significant ways.

AAS and mental health: Preclinical, clinical, and anecdotal reports suggest that steroids may contribute to psychiatric dysfunction. Research shows that abuse of anabolic steroids may lead to aggression and other adverse effects.[1] For example, although many users report feeling good about themselves while on anabolic steroids, extreme mood swings can also occur, including manic-like symptoms that could lead to violence.[2] Researchers have also observed that users may suffer from paranoid jealousy, extreme irritability, delusions, and impaired judgment stemming from feelings of invincibility.

Addictive potential: Animal studies have shown that AAS are reinforcing—that is, animals will self-administer AAS when given the opportunity, just as they do with other addictive drugs.[3,4] This property is more difficult to demonstrate in humans, but the potential for AAS abusers to become addicted is consistent with their continued abuse despite physical problems and negative effects on social relations.[5] Also, steroid abusers typically spend large amounts of time and money obtaining the drug: this is another indication of addiction. Individuals who abuse steroids can experience withdrawal symptoms when they stop taking AAS—these include mood swings, fatigue, restlessness, loss of appetite, insomnia, reduced sex drive, and steroid cravings, all of which may contribute to continued abuse. One of the most dangerous withdrawal symptoms is depression—when persistent, it can sometimes lead to suicide attempts.

Research also indicates that some users might turn to other drugs to alleviate some of the negative effects of AAS. For example, a study of 227 men admitted in 1999 to a private treatment center for dependence on heroin or other opioids found that 9.3% had abused AAS before trying any other illicit drug. Of these, 86% first used opioids to counteract insomnia and irritability resulting from the steroids.[6]

What other adverse effects do AAS have on health?

Steroid abuse can lead to serious, even irreversible health problems. Some of the most dangerous among these include liver damage; jaundice (yellowish pigmentation of skin, tissues, and body fluids); fluid retention; high blood pressure; increases in LDL (low-density lipoprotein, or "bad," cholesterol); and decreases in HDL (high-density lipoprotein, or "good," cholesterol). Other reported effects include renal failure, severe acne, and trembling. In addition, there are some gender- and age-specific adverse effects:

- **For men:** Shrinking of the testicles, reduced sperm count, infertility, baldness, development of breasts, increased risk for prostate cancer

- **For women:** Growth of facial hair, male-pattern baldness, changes in or cessation of the menstrual cycle, enlargement of the clitoris, deepened voice

- **For adolescents:** Stunted growth due to premature skeletal maturation and accelerated puberty changes; risk of not reaching expected height if AAS is taken before the typical adolescent growth spurt

In addition, people who inject AAS run the added risk of contracting or transmitting HIV/AIDS or hepatitis, which causes serious damage to the liver.

What treatment options exist?

There has been very little research on treatment for AAS abuse. Current knowledge derives largely from the experiences of a small number of physicians who have worked with patients undergoing steroid withdrawal. They have learned that, in general, supportive therapy combined with education about possible withdrawal symptoms is sufficient in some cases. Sometimes, medications can be used to restore the balance of the hormonal system after its disruption by steroid abuse. If symptoms are severe or prolonged, symptomatic medications or hospitalization may be needed.

How widespread is AAS abuse?

Monitoring the Future* is an annual survey used to assess drug use among the nation's 8th-, 10th-, and 12th-grade students. While steroid use remained stable among all grades from 2007 to 2008, there has been a significant reduction since 2001 for nearly all prevalence periods (i.e., lifetime, past-year, and past-month use) among all grades surveyed. The exception was past-month use among 12th-graders, which has remained stable. Males consistently report higher rates of use than females: for example, in 2008, 2.5% of 12th-grade males, versus 0.6% of 12th-grade females, reported past-year use.

Table 10.1. Anabolic Steroid Use by Students, 2008 Monitoring the Future Survey

	8th Grade	10th Grade	12th Grade
Lifetime**	1.4%	1.4%	2.2%
Past Year	0.9%	0.9%	1.5%
Past Month	0.5%	0.5%	1.0%

* These data are from the 2008 Monitoring the Future survey, funded by the National Institute on Drug Abuse, National Institutes of Health, Department of Health and Human Services, and conducted by the University of Michigan's Institute for Social Research. The survey has tracked 12th-graders' illicit drug use and related attitudes since 1975; in 1991, 8th- and 10th-graders were added to the study. The latest data are online at www.drugabuse.gov.

** "Lifetime" refers to use at least once during a respondent's lifetime. "Past year" refers to use at least once during the year preceding an individual's response to the survey. "Past month" refers to use at least once during the 30 days preceding an individual's response to the survey.

1. Pope HG Jr, Kouri EM, Hudson JI. Effects of supraphysiologic doses of testosterone on mood and aggression in normal men: A randomized controlled trial. *Arch Gen Psychiatry* 57(2):133–140, 2000.

2. Pope HG Jr, Katz DL. Affective and psychotic symptoms associated with anabolic steroid use. *Am J Psychiatry* 145(4):487–490, 1988.

3. Arnedo MT, Salvador A, Martinez-Sanchis S, Gonzalez-Bono E. Rewarding properties of testosterone in intact male mice: A pilot study. *Pharmacol Biochem Behav* 65:327–332, 2000.

4. DiMeo AN, Wood RI. Self-administration of estrogen and dihydrotestosterone in male hamsters. *Horm Behav* 49(4):519–526, 2006.

5. Brower KJ. Anabolic steroid abuse and dependence. *Curr Psychiatry Rep* 4(5):377–387, 2002.

6. Arvary D, Pope HG Jr. Anabolic-androgenic steroids as a gateway to opioid dependence. *N Engl J Med* 342:1532, 2000.

Section 10.2

Sports Supplements (Ergogenic Aids)

"Supplements," © 2006 Iowa State University Extension (www.extension.iastate.edu). Reprinted with permission. Reviewed by David A. Cooke, MD, FACP, August 2011.

Athletes are known to use substances, commonly dietary supplements, to improve performance. These are referred to as ergogenic aids. Athletes have used ergogenic aids since ancient times. Ancient Greek Olympians ate mushrooms to increase their chances to win the laurel wreath, and Aztec athletes ate human hearts. The ergogenic aid industry is massive, and most sporting magazines contain advertisements for new "revolutionary" ergogenic aids that are sold as dietary supplements. The world of sports is a competitive business. Athletes fear that others are taking something that will give them an advantage. This means that many athletes will try out new substances and supplements on the off chance that it will give them the edge over other competitors. Forgotten in the push to excel are the unknown dangers of unproven substances and the temptations for misuse and abuse. Dietary supplements can be harmful as well as useful.

What Are Supplements?

Prior to 1994, the term "dietary supplement" referred to products made of one or more of the essential nutrients, such as vitamins, minerals, and protein. Congress passed the Dietary Supplement Health and Education Act (DSHEA) in 1994, which expanded the definition so that dietary supplements now include herbs, or other botanicals (except tobacco), and any dietary substance that can be used to supplement the diet.

This has led to many new dietary supplements, for example:

- herbs and other botanicals;
- amino acids;
- extracts from animal glands;

- fibers such as psyllium and guar gum;

- compounds not generally recognized as foods or nutrients such as enzymes and hormone-like compounds.

This new definition has meant that many substances that the FDA [Food and Drug Administration] formerly classified as drugs or unapproved food additives have become readily available as dietary supplements. Thousands of dietary supplements are on the market. Many contain vitamins and minerals to supplement the amounts of these nutrients we get from the foods we eat. There are also many products on the market that contain other substances like high-potency free amino acids, botanicals, enzymes, herbs, animal extracts, bioflavonoids, and synthetically manufactured pro-hormones melatonin and dehydroepiandrosterone (DHEA), which exert drug-like effects on the body.

Supplement Standards/Regulations

The FDA's review of the safety and effectiveness of these products is significantly less than for drugs and foods. Be cautious about using any supplement that claims to treat, prevent, or cure a serious disease. The FDA has approved only a few claims for labeling, based on a review of the scientific evidence (for example, claims about folic acid and a decreased risk of neural tube birth defects). A recent court case prevents the FDA from regulating health claims on dietary supplement labels. Read carefully and think critically about the claims you see on the packages.

Supplement manufacturers do not have to prove that their products are safe! In the past, supplement manufacturers had to prove to the FDA that their products were safe. Under current law, however, it has become the responsibility of the FDA to prove that a supplement is unsafe. With the high number of new supplements coming onto the market and the limited resources of the FDA, it is very likely that a product could cause harm before the FDA can take action. In addition, even after the FDA has declared a supplement unsafe, they then have to prove that the supplement is unsafe in the court of law.

Some dietary supplements may be harmful under some conditions. For example, many herbal products and other "natural" supplements have real and powerful pharmacological effects that can cause harmful reactions in some people or can cause dangerous interactions with prescribed or over-the-counter medicines. It does not necessarily mean that supplements marketed as "natural" are safe and without side effects.

Because of the lack of regulation with dietary supplements, athletes run the risk of consuming a dietary supplement that is contaminated. Steroid contamination, such as nandrolone and testosterone, has been documented. An athlete WILL test positive for drug use if they consume a dietary supplement containing banned substances such as nandrolone and testosterone. Some substances that could be present in the supplements are banned by the NCAA (see the list of banned drug classes at www .ncaa.org/wps/wcm/connect/public/NCAA/Student-Athlete+Experience/ NCAA+banned+drugs+list). Consuming them will jeopardize your eligibility. Visit the Gatorade® Sport Science Institute (at www.gssiweb.com/ Article_List.aspx?topicid=2&subtopicid=111) for more information.

Protein Supplements

The list of protein supplements on the market is never ending. Protein supplements promise anything from increased strength, energy, muscle mass, weight loss, staying fit, and obtaining lean slender bodies. Today you can hardly find a gym where protein supplements are not being used or sold. But are these supplements really beneficial, and who should take them? What are the long-term effects?

For years, research studies have been studying their effects on muscle strength and performance. The results of the different studies are conflicting with little to no data supporting the proclaimed benefits of protein supplements.

Currently, only creatine has been shown to benefit high-intensity, short-duration exercise. However, a few other supplements including amino acids and beta-hydroxy-beta-methylbutyrate (HMB) have shown promise in some studies. More research is necessary to examine their effects on performance and health.

Amino Acids

The athlete's protein source needs to provide the essential amino acids (those not synthesized in the body), since non-essential amino acids can by made by the body when needed. The essential amino acids can easily be obtained from the diet by consuming quality proteins such as egg, chicken, red meats, fish, or milk, etc., thus supplementation is not necessary.

If supplemental amino acids are needed, the key to obtaining benefits from amino acids is the timing of consumption. Amino acids should be consumed either immediately prior to exercise, or during the recovery period one to two hours after exercise. A consumption of 0.1 g of essential amino acids per kilogram of body weight is recommended.

Remember: The amount of protein that the body can utilize is limited. Large protein consumption in one setting that exceeds the body's requirement will be converted into fat. It will NOT increase muscle mass.

HMB

HMB is derived from an amino acid called leucine. HMB is believed to prevent muscle loss with intensive resistive training. Considering muscle breakdown always occurs with exercise, preventing this breakdown preserves and increases muscle mass. However, more research is necessary to verify the effects of this supplement.

Creatine

What Is Creatine?

Discovered in 1832, creatine is a food constituent derived from animals. The compound is primarily found in skeletal muscle and is synthesized in the body and transported to muscle tissues. In muscles, creatine is used in short bouts of intense energy production in the form of creatine-phosphate. The end-product energy release from creatine-phosphate is creatinine, which is excreted by the kidneys in the urine.

Creatine in the Body

Creatine is synthesized in the liver, the kidneys, and the pancreas. After production, it is transported in the blood to body tissues. The creatine transporter is limited in the amount of creatine it can transport. This means that even if a person consumes more creatine, the body has a maximum amount it can use.

Creatine in the Diet

Although creatine is synthesized in the body, it can be obtained from dietary intake and creatine supplementation. A good food source of creatine includes muscle meat, where 1.1 kg (about 2½ pounds) of beef provides 5 g of creatine. A typical American diet, containing some meat, provides approximately 1 g of creatine daily. Creatine obtained from the diet can either be utilized as energy, or be stored in the body. For example, a 70-kg adult man can store approximately 120 g of creatine.

Role in Exercise

Oral creatine supplementation increases muscle creatine-phosphate, which can enhance performance during repeated bouts of high-intensity exercise. The benefit of creatine supplementation for high-intensity and short-duration exercise has been shown to be greater than low-intensity and long-duration exercise.

Creatine Supplementation

Creatine is supplemented to improve muscle power output primarily in high-intensity and short-duration exercise. However, creatine has also been used to prevent breakdown of muscle mass during immobilization. In other words, it may prevent muscle wasting when a person is injured and/or unable to exercise.

Creatine supplementation involves a loading phase and a maintenance phase. For the best results, a loading of about 20 g of creatine monohydrate for four to five days is recommended. Thereafter, to maintain desirable levels of creatine, 3 g of creatine monohydrate per day should be consumed. The response to the supplementation varies depending on individual need. However, the best response will be seen the first three days of ingestion.

Table 10.2. Effects and Benefits of Creatine

Effect of Creatine	Potential Benefit
More power	Perform more exercise repetitions
More strength	Perform more exercise repetitions and enhance activities of daily living performance
More lean mass	Functional recovery
Less oxidative stress	Long-term cellular protection

Side Effects

Scientists are not sure whether long-term creatine supplementation is harmful to humans. Research on long-term safety has been initiated, but currently no severe health implications have been identified. However, water retention and decreased urine production have been reported to cause weight gain with creatine supplementation. Other side effects reported are muscle cramps, headaches, diarrhea, and gastrointestinal pain.

Speculations that creatine supplementation could lead to kidney failure have not been proven. Clinical trials have shown no adverse

Table 10.3. Ergogenic Aids

Ergogenic Aid	Proposed Action	What Research Says	Side Effects
Androstenedione	Steroid hormone that increases testosterone levels	No documented benefits	Major
Caffeine	Increases fat metabolism, thus sparing glucose and glycogen stores; stimulates the central nervous system	Supports	Mild
Carbohydrates	An important energy source for muscles	Supports	Mild at high doses
Creatine	Delays fatigue and improves performance during high, intense bursts of exercise; builds muscle mass	Supports; however, there is limited data on long-term use	Mild
DHEA [dehydro-epiandrosterone]	Increases amount of steroids produced in the body	No benefit in healthy athletes	May be dangerous
HMB	Prevents muscle breakdown, speeds up muscle repair, and increase lean body mass	Limited; some strength benefits	None
Protein	Helps build muscle and improves muscle repair	Supports; high force outputs from their muscles, such as sprinters and weight lifters, need extra protein to ensure muscle maintenance	None
Pycnogenol	Boosts antioxidant levels, enhances recovery	Supports, dietary sources offer same benefit	None
Tryptophan	Increases athletic endurance; decreases pain perception	No definite results; no benefit in trained athletes	Potentially dangerous

Table continues on next page

Table 10.3. *continued*

Ergogenic Aid	Proposed Action	What Research Says	Side Effects
Vitamin B 6 (pyridoxine)	Increases growth of muscle and decreases anxiety	No benefit unless individual has deficiency	Mild at high doses
Vitamin B12 (cobalamin)	Increases growth of muscle	No benefit unless individual has deficiency	None
Vitamin C	Acts as an antioxidant; increases energy production and aerobic reactions	No benefit unless individual has deficiency	Mild at high doses
Vitamin E	Acts as an antioxidant; increases aerobic capacity	No definite results	Mild
Zinc	Increases muscle mass and aerobic capacity	Few studies; mostly negative	Mild

Source: Ahrendt DM. Ergogenic aids: Counseling the athlete. *American Family Physician.* 2001;63:913–22.

effects of low-dose (1.5 g), long-term (one to five years) creatine supplementation on renal function. However, high doses for a prolonged period of time will increase the stress on the kidneys.

Conclusions on Creatine

- Creatine supplementation has only been shown to be beneficial in those sports/exercise of short duration, high intensity.

- Long-term safety of creatine supplementation is unknown.

- Creatine supplements, as other dietary supplements, are not well regulated and could contain contaminants or illegal substances, which could jeopardize an athlete's health and eligibility.

Part Two

Preventing Sports Injuries

Chapter 11

Sports Injury Prevention and First Aid Treatment

Chapter Contents

Section 11.1

Basic Sports Injury Prevention

"Basic Injury Prevention Concepts," by Mary D. Nadelen, MA, ATC. © 2010 American College of Sports Medicine (www.acsm.org). Reprinted with permission of the American College of Sports Medicine, *ACSM Fit Society® Page*, Spring 2010, p. 3.

For any individual who is physically active, there is a possibility of sustaining an injury. While some injuries, such as an ankle sprain or fracture, are difficult to prevent, many other injuries are preventable. By following a few simple guidelines, injuries such as muscle strains, tendonitis, and overuse injuries can be reduced.

Every workout must begin with a warm-up and end with a cool-down. A warm-up is necessary to prepare the body for exercise by increasing heart rate and blood flow to working muscles. The warm-up should start slow and easy and consist of a general cardiovascular exercise such as walking, jogging, or biking. The goal is to break a sweat. After 5 to 10 minutes, the warm-up should focus on muscles and movements more specific to the exercise activity planned. Creating a smooth transition from the warm-up to a specific activity is a great way to prevent injuries. For example, a soccer player could pass, dribble, and shoot a ball; a weightlifter could lift light weights before moving onto greater resistance.

Flexibility is absolutely a part of every good warm-up. Once the muscles are warm, they become more elastic and are ready to be stretched. Whether you choose to perform static stretches (by holding each position for 10–30 seconds) or perform dynamic stretches (by moving the body through a functional range of motion), flexibility prepares the muscles, tendons, and joints for work by allowing them to move freely through a full active range of motion. The more prepared the body is, the less likely it is to get injured.

An area that often gets ignored is the cool-down after activity. Just as the warm-up prepares the body for work, the cool-down brings it back to its normal state. Time spent performing 5 to 10 minutes of low-intensity cardiovascular activity followed by stretching immediately after the workout will decrease muscle soreness and aid in recovery, both helping to prepare the body for the next workout.

Once an exercise program is developed, there are a few things to remember. Start slow: people often jump right into a workout and do too much too fast, creating excessive muscle soreness and tightness. Proper progression is the key to preventing injuries. Slowly increase the amount of time of each workout, the intensity of the workout, and the resistance of the weights. A 5% increase as the exercise becomes too easy is a safe progression. Exercise at a level that is appropriate for your age and your fitness level. A young athlete competing with older children may not be as physically strong, predisposing them to injury. The same can be true for a weekend warrior athlete who jumps into a game with athletes who have trained throughout the week. If equipment is involved in your exercise program, take the time to ensure you have the proper equipment, that it fits correctly, and that it meets safety standards. Too often, old, faulty, or improperly fitted equipment, such as footwear, mouth guards, helmets, goggles, or shin pads, can cause injuries.

One of the best ways to prevent injury is to listen to the warning signs your body gives you. By ignoring little aches and pains in joints and muscles, a more serious injury could develop. Pain is the body's way of telling you something is not right! The common expression "no pain, no gain" creates a large misconception. It is very possible to make cardiovascular and strength gains in your workout routine without causing pain. If your body is tired or too sore from the previous workout, take a day off, cross-train, or work out at a much lower intensity. It is important to add variety to every exercise routine to prevent repetitive, overuse injuries. By switching from running to biking, aerobics to weight lifting, or swimming to spinning, muscles and joints that are worked repetitively during your normal routine will get a break while challenging other parts of the body.

Rest is a critical component to any good workout routine and time spent allowing the body to recover is a great way to prevent injuries. A rest day must occur at least one to two times per week. Even small breaks during a workout are sometimes required to get the most out of the workout and prevent injuries. A healthy, well-balanced diet can aid in injury prevention as well. A poor diet can lead to muscle weakness, decreased muscle strength and endurance. Equally important is maintaining hydration throughout the day, during, and after your workout. A body with adequate fuel (food and water) will stay sharp and keep moving at the intensity you desire.

Following the simple guidelines listed here will help keep you injury-free and focused on your workout goals.

Section 11.2

First Aid for Sports Injuries

"Sports Health and Safety: Treatments for Sports Injuries," Federal
Citizens Information Center (www.pueblo.gsa.gov), April 30, 2010.

Never try to "work-through" the pain of an injury. When you have
pain from a particular movement or activity, STOP! Playing or exercising more only causes more harm. Prompt treatment can often prevent
a minor injury from becoming worse or causing permanent damage.

Seeking Medical Treatment

Some injuries require immediate medical attention. You should call
a health professional if any of the following are true:

- The injury causes severe pain, swelling, or numbness.

- You can't tolerate any weight on the area.

- The pain or dull ache of an old injury is accompanied by
  increased swelling or joint abnormality or instability.

R.I.C.E.

In some instances, injuries can be self-treated. If you don't have any
of the aforementioned symptoms, it may be safe to treat the injury at
home—at least at first. If pain or other symptoms worsen, you should
call your health care provider. Use the R.I.C.E. (Rest, Ice, Compression, and Elevation) method to relieve pain, reduce swelling, and speed
healing. Follow these four steps immediately after the injury occurs
and continue for at least 48 hours:

- **Rest** : Reduce regular exercise or activities as needed.

- **Ice:** Apply an ice pack to the injured area for 20 minutes, four to
  eight times a day. Take the ice off after 20 minutes to avoid cold
  injury. Do not use heat immediately after an injury as this tends
  to increase internal bleeding or swelling. Heat can be used later
  on to relieve muscle tension and promote relaxation.

- **Compression:** Compression of the injured area may help reduce swelling. You can use an elastic wrap, special boot, air cast, or splint.

- **Elevation:** Put the injured area on a pillow at a level above your heart to help decrease swelling.

The R.I.C.E. technique can be helpful for any sports injury but is often just a starting point. Here are some other things your doctor may do to treat your sports injury.

Nonsteroidal anti-inflammatory drugs (NSAIDs): Inflammation causes tissues to become swollen, tender, and painful. To reduce inflammation and pain, your health care provider may suggest that you take an over-the-counter, non-steroidal anti-inflammatory drug such as aspirin, ibuprofen (Advil, Motrin IB, Nuprin), ketoprofen (Actron, Orudis K), or naproxen sodium (Aleve). Another common drug is acetaminophen. It may relieve pain, but it will not reduce swelling. For more severe pain and inflammation, a prescription-strength NSAID may be prescribed.

Immobilization: This involves reducing movement in the area to prevent further damage. Immobilization may reduce pain, swelling, and muscle spasm and can help the healing process begin. Some devises used for immobilization include the following:

- **Slings** are used for arms and shoulders.

- **Splints and casts** support and protect injured bones and soft tissues. Splints generally offer less support and protection than a cast, and therefore may not always be a treatment option.

- **Leg immobilizers** keep the knee from bending after injury or surgery.

Rest: Although it is good to get moving as soon as possible, you must also take time to rest following an injury. All injuries need time to heal; proper rest will help the process.

Conclusion

Most sports injuries can be treated effectively, and most people who suffer injuries can return to a satisfying level of physical activity after appropriate treatment and healing.

Chapter 12

Protective Equipment for Athletes

Chapter Contents

89

Section 12.1

Athletic Shoes

Too many people choose fashion over function when purchasing athletic shoes, not realizing that poor-fitting shoes can lead to pain throughout the body. Because footwear plays such an important role in the function of bones and joints—especially for runners and other athletes—choosing the right shoe can help prevent pain in your back, hips, knees, and feet.

Unfortunately, there is no such thing as the very best athletic shoe—every pair of feet is different, every shoe has different features, and overall comfort is a very personal decision. For this reason, it is recommended that you first determine your foot type: normal, flat, or high-arched.

The Normal Foot

Normal feet have a normal-sized arch and will leave a wet footprint that has a flare, but shows the forefoot and heel connected by a broad band. A normal foot lands on the outside of the heel and rolls slightly inward to absorb shock.

Best shoes: Stability shoes with a slightly curved shape.

The Flat Foot

This type of foot has a low arch and leaves a print that looks like the whole sole of the foot. It usually indicates an over-pronated foot—one that strikes on the outside of the heel and rolls excessively inward (pronates). Over time, this can cause overuse injuries.

Best shoes: Motion-control shoes or high-stability shoes with firm midsoles. These shoes should be fairly resistant to twisting or bending. Stay away from highly cushioned, highly curved shoes, which lack stability features.

The High-Arched Foot

The high-arched foot leaves a print showing a very narrow band—or no band at all—between the forefoot and the heel. A curved, highly arched foot is generally supinated or under-pronated. Because the foot doesn't pronate enough, usually it's not an effective shock absorber.

Best shoes: Cushioned shoes with plenty of flexibility to encourage foot motion. Stay away from motion-control or stability shoes, which reduce foot mobility.

When determining your foot type, consult with your doctor of chiropractic. He or she can help determine your specific foot type, assess your gait, and then suggest the best shoe match.

Shoe Purchasing Tips

Consider the following tips before you purchase your next pair of athletic shoes:

• Match the shoe to the activity. Select a shoe specific for the sport in which you will participate. Running shoes are primarily made to absorb shock as the heel strikes the ground. In contrast, tennis shoes provide more side-to-side stability. Walking shoes allow the foot to roll and push off naturally during walking, and they usually have a fairly rigid arch, a well-cushioned sole, and a stiff heel support for stability.

• If possible, shop at a specialty store. It's best to shop at a store that specializes in athletic shoes. Employees at these stores are often trained to recommend a shoe that best matches your foot type (as mentioned earlier) and stride pattern.

• Shop late in the day. If possible, shop for shoes at the end of the day or after a workout when your feet are generally at their largest. Wear the type of socks you usually wear during exercise, and if you use orthotic devices for postural support, make sure you wear them when trying on shoes.

• Have your feet measured every time. It's important to have the length and width of both feet measured every time you shop for shoes, since foot size often changes with age and most people have one foot that is larger than the other. Also, many podiatrists suggest that you measure your foot while standing in a weight-bearing position because the foot elongates and flattens when you stand, affecting the measurement and the fit of the shoe.

- Make sure the shoe fits correctly. Choose shoes for their fit, not by the size you've worn in the past. The shoe should fit with an index finger's width between the end of the shoe and the longest toe. The toe box should have adequate room and not feel tight. The heel of your foot should fit snugly against the back of the shoe without sliding up or down as you walk or run. If possible, keep the shoe on for 10 minutes to make sure it remains comfortable.

How Long Do Shoes Last?

Once you have purchased a pair of athletic shoes, don't run them into the ground. While estimates vary as to when the best time to replace old shoes is, most experts agree that between 300 and 500 miles is optimal. In fact, most shoes should be replaced even before they begin to show signs of moderate wear. Once shoes show wear, especially in the cushioning layer called the midsole, they also begin to lose their shock absorption. Failure to replace worn shoes is a common cause of injuries like shin splints, heel spurs, and plantar fasciitis.

Section 12.2

Helmets

"Which Helmet for Which Activity?" Consumer Product Safety
Commission (www.cpsc.gov), 2006.

Why are helmets so important?

For many recreational activities, wearing a helmet can reduce the
risk of a serious head injury and even save your life.

How can a helmet protect my head?

During a fall or collision, most of the impact energy is absorbed by
the helmet, rather than your head and brain.

Are all helmets the same?

No. There are different helmets for different activities. Each type
of helmet is made to protect your head from the impacts common to
a particular activity or sport. Be sure to wear a helmet that is appropriate for the particular activity you're involved in. (See the table in
this chapter for guidance). Other helmets may not protect your head
as effectively.

How can I tell which helmet is the right one to use?

Bicycle and motorcycle helmets must comply with mandatory federal safety standards. Many other recreational helmets are subject to
voluntary safety standards.

Helmets certified to a safety standard are designed and tested to
protect the user from serious head injury while wearing the helmet.
For example, all bicycle helmets manufactured after 1999 must meet
the U.S. Consumer Product Safety Commission (CPSC) bicycle helmet
standard. Helmets meeting this standard provide substantial head
protection when the helmet is used properly. The standard requires
that chin straps be strong enough to keep the helmet on the head and
in the proper position during a fall or collision.

Helmets specifically marketed for exclusive use in an activity other than bicycling (for example, go-karting, horseback riding, lacrosse, and skiing) do not have to meet the requirements of the CPSC bicycle helmet standard. However, these helmets should meet other federal and/or voluntary safety standards.

Don't rely on the helmet's name or claims made on the packaging (unless the packaging specifies compliance with an appropriate standard) to determine if the helmet meets the appropriate requirements for your activity. Most helmets that meet a particular standard will

Table 12.1. Which Helmet for Which Activity

1. Activity	2. Helmet Type	3. Applicable Standard(s)
Individual Activities—Wheeled		
Bicycling (including low speed, motor assisted); Roller and Inline Skating—Recreational; Scooter Riding (including low speed, motor assisted)	Bicycle	CPSC, ASTM F1447, Snell B-90/95, Snell N-94†
BMX Cycling	BMX	CPSC, ASTM F2032
Downhill Mountain Bike Racing	Downhill	CPSC, ASTM F1952
Roller and Inline Skating—Aggressive/Trick; Skateboarding	Skateboard	ASTM F1492†, Snell N-94†
Individual Activities—Wheeled Large Motor		
ATV Riding; Dirt-, and Mini-Bike Riding; Motocrossing	Motocross or Motorcycle	DOT FMVSS 218, Snell M-2005
Karting/Go-Karting	Karting or Motorcycle	DOT FMVSS 218, Snell K-98, Snell M-2005
Moped Riding; Powered Scooter Riding	Moped or Motorcycle	DOT FMVSS 218, Snell L-98, Snell M-2005
Individual Activities—Non-Wheeled		
Horseback Riding	Equestrian	ASTM F1163, Snell E-2001
Rock and Wall Climbing	Mountaineering	EN 12492†, Snell N-94†

The federal CPSC Safety Standard for Bicycle Helmets is mandatory for those helmets indicated by CPSC.

† This helmet is designed to withstand more than one moderate impact, but protection is provided for only a limited number of impacts. Replace if visibly damaged (e.g., a cracked shell or crushed liner) and/or when directed by the manufacturer.

‡ Team sport helmets are designed to protect against multiple head impacts typically occurring in the sport (e.g., ball, puck, or stick impacts; player contact; etc.) and, generally, can

contain a special label that indicates compliance (usually found on the liner inside of the helmet).

Are there helmets that I can wear for more than one activity?

Yes, but only a few. You can wear a CPSC-compliant bicycle helmet while bicycling, recreational roller or in-line skating, and riding a nonpowered scooter. Look at the table for other activities that may share a common helmet.

Table 12.1. *continued*

1. Activity	2. Helmet Type	3. Applicable Standard(s)
Team Sport Activities ‡		
Baseball, Softball, and T-Ball	Baseball Batter's	NOCSAE ND022
	Baseball Catcher's	NOCSAE ND024
Football	Football	NOCSAE ND002, ASTM F717
Ice Hockey	Hockey	NOCSAE ND030, ASTM F1045
Lacrosse	Lacrosse	NOCSAE ND041
Winter Activities		
Skiing; Snowboarding	Ski	ASTM F2040, CEN 1077, Snell RS-98 or S-98
Snowmobiling	Snowmobile	DOT FMVSS 218, Snell M-2000

Although a helmet has not yet been designed for the following two activities, until such helmets exist, wearing one of the three listed types of helmets may be preferable to wearing no helmet at all.

Ice Skating; Sledding	Bicycle	CPSC, ASTM F1447, Snell B-90/95 or N-94†
	Skateboard	ASTM F1492†, Snell N-94†
	Ski	ASTM F2040, CEN 1077, Snell RS-98 or S-98

continue to be used after such impacts. Follow manufacturer's recommendations for replacement or reconditioning.

Definitions: ASTM—ASTM International; CEN—European Committee for Standardization; DOT—Dept. of Transportation; EN—Euro-norm or European Standard; NOCSAE—National Operating Committee on Standards in Athletic Equipment; Snell—Snell Memorial Foundation.

Are there any activities for which one shouldn't wear a helmet?

Yes. Make sure your child takes off his/her helmet before playing on playgrounds or climbing trees. If a child wears a helmet during these activities, the helmet's chin strap can get caught on the equipment or tree and pose a risk of strangulation. The helmet itself may present an entrapment hazard.

How can I tell if my helmet fits properly?

A helmet should be both comfortable and snug. Be sure that it is level on your head—not tilted back on the top of the head or pulled too low over your forehead. It should not move in any direction, back-to-front or side-to-side. The chin strap should be securely buckled so that the helmet doesn't move or fall off during a fall or collision.

If you buy a helmet for a child, bring the child with you so that the helmet can be tested for a good fit. Carefully examine the helmet and accompanying instructions and safety literature.

What can I do if I have trouble fitting the helmet?

You may have to apply the foam padding that comes with the helmet and/or adjust the straps. If this doesn't work, consult with the store where you bought the helmet or with the helmet manufacturer. Don't wear a helmet that doesn't fit correctly.

Will I need to replace a helmet after an impact?

That depends on the severity of the impact and whether the helmet can withstand one impact (a single-impact helmet) or more than one impact (a multiple-impact helmet). For example, bicycle helmets are designed to protect against a single severe impact, such as a bicyclist's fall onto the pavement. The foam material in the helmet will crush to absorb the impact energy during a fall or collision and can't protect you again from an additional impact. Even if there are no visible signs of damage to the helmet, you must replace it.

Other helmets are designed to protect against multiple moderate impacts. Two examples are football and ice hockey helmets. These helmets are designed to withstand multiple impacts of the type associated with the respective activities. However, you may still have to replace the helmet after one severe impact, or if it has visible signs of damage, such as a cracked shell or permanent dent in the shell or liner. Consult the manufacturer's instructions for guidance on when the helmet should be replaced.

Where can I find specific information about which helmet to use?

Look at the information in columns 1 to 3 of Table 12.1 and follow these easy steps:

Find the activity of interest in the first column (1).

Read across the row to find the appropriate helmet type for that activity listed in the second column (2).

Once you've found the right helmet, look for a label or other marking stating that it complies with an applicable standard listed in the third column (3).

Section 12.3

Eye Protection

"Sports Eye Safety," © 2009 Prevent Blindness America, "Tips for Buying Sports Eye Protectors" © 2005 Prevent Blindness America, and "Recommended Sports Eye Protectors," © 2005 Prevent Blindness America. All rights reserved. Reprinted with permission. For additional information, visit www.preventblindness.org. Reviewed by David A. Cooke, MD, FACP, August 2011.

Sports Eye Safety

More than 40,000 people a year suffer eye injuries while playing sports.

For all age groups, sports-related eye injuries occur most frequently in baseball, basketball, and racquet sports.

Almost all sports-related eye injuries can be prevented. Whatever your game, whatever your age, you need to protect your eyes!

Take the following steps to avoid sports eye injuries:

- Wear proper safety goggles (lensed polycarbonate protectors) for racquet sports or basketball.

- Use batting helmets with polycarbonate face shields for youth baseball.

- Use helmets and face shields approved by the U.S. Amateur Hockey Association when playing hockey.

- Know that regular glasses don't provide enough protection.

Tips for Buying Sports Eye Protectors

Prevent Blindness America recommends that athletes wear sports eyeguards when participating in sports. Prescription glasses, sunglasses, and even occupational safety glasses do not provide adequate protection. Sports eyeguards come in a variety of shapes and sizes. Eyeguards designed for use in racquet sports are now commonly used for basketball and soccer and in combination with helmets in football, hockey, and baseball. The eyeguards you choose should fit securely and comfortably and allow the use of a helmet if necessary. Expect to spend between $20 and $40 for a pair of regular eyeguards and $60 or more for eyeguards with prescription lenses.

The following guidelines can help you find a pair of eyeguards right for you:

- If you wear prescription glasses, ask your eye doctor to fit you for prescription eyeguards. If you're a monocular athlete (a person with only one eye that sees well), ask your eye doctor what sports you can safely participate in. Monocular athletes should always wear sports eyeguards.

- Buy eyeguards at sports specialty stores or optical stores. At the sports store, ask for a sales representative who's familiar with eye protectors to help you.

- Don't buy sports eyeguards without lenses. Only "lensed" protectors are recommended for sports use. Make sure the lenses either stay in place or pop outward in the event of an accident. Lenses that pop in against your eyes can be very dangerous.

- Fogging of the lenses can be a problem when you're active. Some eyeguards are available with anti-fog coating. Others have side vents for additional ventilation. Try on different types to determine which is most comfortable for you.

- Check the packaging to see if the eye protector you select has been tested for sports use. Also check to see that the eye protector is made of polycarbonate material. Polycarbonate eyeguards are the most impact resistant.

- Sports eyeguards should be padded or cushioned along the brow and bridge of the nose. Padding will prevent the eyeguards from cutting your skin.

- Try on the eye protector to determine if it's the right size. Adjust the strap and make sure it's not too tight or too loose. If you purchased your eyeguards at an optical store, an optical representative can help you adjust the eye protector for a comfortable fit.

Until you get used to wearing a pair of eyeguards, it may feel strange, but bear with it! It's a lot more comfortable than an eye injury.

Recommended Sports Eye Protectors

Baseball

Recommended Protection

- Faceguard (attached to helmet) made of polycarbonate material
- Sports eyeguards

Injuries Prevented

- Scratches on the cornea
- Inflamed iris
- Blood spilling into the eye's anterior chamber
- Traumatic cataract
- Swollen retina

Basketball

Recommended Protection

- Sports eyeguards

Injuries Prevented

- Fracture of the eye socket
- Scratches on the cornea
- Inflamed iris
- Blood spilling into the eye's anterior chamber
- Swollen retina

Soccer

Recommended Protection

- Sports eyeguards

Injuries Prevented

- Inflamed iris
- Blood spilling into the eye's anterior chamber
- Swollen retina

Football

Recommended Protection

- Polycarbonate shield attached to a faceguard
- Sports eyeguards

Injuries Prevented

- Scratches on the cornea
- Inflamed iris
- Blood spilling into the eye's anterior chamber
- Swollen retina

Hockey

Recommended Protection

- Wire or polycarbonate mask
- Sports eyeguards

Injuries Prevented

- Scratches on the cornea
- Inflamed iris
- Blood spilling into the eye's anterior chamber
- Traumatic cataract
- Swollen retina

Section 12.4

Mouth Guards to Prevent Dental Injuries

Anyone who participates in sports, whether for pleasure, in youth or adult leagues, or even on a professional level—knows that losing isn't the worst thing that can happen to a player; sustaining a serious injury is, particularly when that injury is preventable.

That's why it's so important for adults and children who are active in sports to wear protective gear such as helmets, shin guards, knee and elbow pads, and mouth guards. Wearing a mouth guard can prevent serious injury and save a lot of pain. Each year this simple safety measure prevents more than 200,000 oral injuries among athletes.

Mouth Guards Aren't Mandatory in Most Sports. Why Are They Important?

- Facial and head injuries can be sustained in nearly every game, from "contact" sports such as football, soccer, and basketball, to "non-contact" sports like baseball, gymnastics, bicycling, or skateboarding. Damage to the teeth, lips, tongue, and jaws are frequent occurrences in both children and adults. General dentists see more injuries to the mouth as a result of playing sports than from almost any other single cause. A survey conducted by the University of Texas found nearly 5% of male college athletes who played football, basketball, soccer, volleyball, baseball, ice hockey, and lacrosse without wearing a mouth guard sustained some oral injury. That's more than 2,000 injuries in just a single year at the college level alone! It's at the junior high, high school, community, and amateur levels that most injuries occur.

- Although more research is needed, mouth guards may help prevent serious injuries such as concussions. The literature has shown that mouth guards definitely help prevent fractured jaws and teeth, severe cuts to the cheek and tongue (often requiring surgery for repair), and traumatic damage to the roots and bone that hold teeth in place.

- Mouth guards are designed to help cushion the mouth, teeth, and jaw, preventing significant damage where sports injuries are most prevalent. While mouth guards are not required equipment in many sports, wearing one is an important precaution for athletes of any age and ability.

What Should I Know Before Choosing a Mouth Guard?

For a mouth guard to be most effective, it is essential that it fit properly and stay in place during vigorous activity and the various positions the sport requires. Your dentist can determine what appliances (braces, retainers, bridgework, dentures) would be affected by wearing a mouth guard. Because growth spurts occur in the mouth just as they do elsewhere in the body, it's especially important for child's mouth to be evaluated by a dentist before selecting a mouth guard.

Different sports involve different levels of risk and potential injury. With the help of your dentist, you can select the right type of mouth guard for you or your child's sport of choice.

What Are the Different Types of Mouth Guards?

All mouth guards are not created equal. Depending upon the design and materials used, mouthpieces will vary in fit, protection, ease of maintenance, and longevity. Listed here are several types of mouth guards. Consult your dentist before you make a decision.

- **Custom-made:** Formed by your dentist from a cast model of your teeth, these custom-made guards are designed to cover all the teeth and are shown in the literature to be the best type of protection. These mouth guards can cushion falls and blows to the chin. Custom-made mouth guards may be slightly more expensive than commercially produced mouthpieces, but they offer the best possible fit and protection and are the most comfortable.

- **Mouth-formed:** These guards are generally made of acrylic gel or thermoplastic materials shaped to fit the contours of your teeth. They are placed in boiling water then attempted to be formed and molded to the teeth. They are commercially produced and do not offer the same fit and protection as a custom fitted mouth guard made from a model of the mouth.

- **Ready-made stock:** Commercially produced, off-the-shelf mouth guards are the least expensive, but also the least comfortable and the least effective protective mouthpieces. These rubber or polyvinyl pre-formed guards can be purchased at most sporting goods stores. They offer no attempt at fit whatsoever and are not recommended in the dental literature.

What Can I Do to Make My Mouth Guard Last?

Like all sports equipment, proper care will make any mouth guard last longer. Keep your mouthpiece in top shape by rinsing it with soap and water or mouthwash after each use and allowing it to air-dry. With proper care, a mouth guard should last the length of a season. The condition of the mouth guard should be checked before each use, particularly if the athlete has a tendency to chew on it. Mouth guards may be checked by your dentist at your regularly scheduled examinations.

Wearing a Mouth Guard Makes Good Sense

If you or your children participate in sports, make sure that you are informed about the most common injuries that can occur during play and take appropriate steps to be protected. Always wear a properly fitted mouth guard when you play. Do not wear removable appliances (retainers, bridges, or complete or partial dentures) when playing sports.

Staying in shape—and intact—is an integral part of an overall strategy for all sports. Protecting against injuries will keep you in the game. Keep your competitive edge. Protect both your general and oral health for your best performance on and off the field.

Chapter 13

Sport Safety Tips

Chapter Contents

Section 13.1

Baseball

"Safety Tips: Baseball," March 2010, reprinted with permission from www.kidshealth.org. Copyright © 2010 The Nemours Foundation. This information was provided by KidsHealth, one of the largest resources online for medically reviewed health information written for parents, kids, and teens. For more articles like this one, visit www.KidsHealth .org, or www.TeensHealth.org.

There's a reason why baseball has been called our national pastime for decades. It's as American as hot dogs and apple pie. It's been a summer tradition in big cities and little towns across the U.S.A. for generations. It's a great team sport, and it's fun.

Why Is Baseball Safety Important?

Baseball is by no means a dangerous sport. But it can present a very real risk of injuries from things like wild pitches, batted balls, and collisions in the field.

At the high-school level, some pitchers can throw fastballs that reach 80-plus miles per hour, speedy enough to cause painful welts, broken bones, even concussions. Excessive pitching and improper throwing mechanics can lead to major league arm problems, and base runners and fielders frequently collide while running at top speed.

Gear Guidelines

As with all sports, wearing and using the right gear can go a long way toward preventing injuries. The amount of equipment required for baseball isn't on a par with football or hockey, but it is every bit as important. Players need to be sure they always have all the gear required by their league.

Most leagues will insist on the following:

- Batting helmets must be worn whenever a player is at bat, waiting to bat, or running the bases. Some leagues may even require pitchers to wear them. Helmets should always fit properly and be worn correctly. If the helmet has a chin strap, make sure it is fastened, and if the helmet has an eye shield or other faceguard, this should be in good condition, securely attached to the helmet.

- A catcher should always be wearing a helmet, facemask, throat guard, full-length chest protector, athletic supporter with a cup, shin guards, and a catcher's mitt whenever they are catching pitches, whether it's in the game, in the bullpen, or during warm-ups.

- Baseball spikes should have molded plastic cleats rather than metal ones. Most youth leagues don't allow spikes with metal cleats.

- It's possible that your league could have guidelines dictating what kind of bat you can use. Some aluminum bats may be banned for hitting batted balls too hard. Be sure to check your league's policy before choosing a bat.

- All players should wear athletic supporters; most, particularly pitchers and infielders, should wear protective cups. Rules regarding which players must wear cups vary from league to league.

- Additional gear that some players like includes sliding pants, which are meant to go under your baseball pants to protect against scrapes and cuts; batting gloves, which can keep your hands from getting sore while hitting; shin and foot guards, which are designed to protect against balls fouled straight down; and mouthguards.

Breakaway Bases

Base paths are one of the most common places injuries happen. This is especially true when you slide into a traditional stationary base, which puts a rigid obstacle in your path as you slide. Sliding into a fixed base can result in foot, ankle, and lower-leg injuries.

As a result, doctors have started recommending that leagues install breakaway bases in all of their playing fields. These bases, which snap onto grommets on an anchored rubber mat, can be dislodged when a runner slides into one, lessening the chances that a base runner will get injured. During the course of normal base-running, the base is stable and does not detach.

Before You Start the Game

Ideally, you should get plenty of exercise before the season begins and be in the best shape possible before you swing a bat for the first time. This will not only lower your risk of injury, it will also make you a better ballplayer. Be sure to warm up and stretch before a baseball game as you would for any other sport, but remember that in baseball, you have to pay particular attention to your throwing arm. Most arms require plenty of warm-up before they can safely attempt a long, hard throw.

Different people have different preferences when it comes to warming up their arms. Some like to make short throws, while others prefer to start with long, easy tosses. Regardless of how you choose to warm up your arm, the idea is to start with soft throws meant to stretch your muscles and loosen up your joints. As your arm warms up, gradually increase the intensity of your throws until you are throwing as you would during a game situation.

Make sure that all bats, balls, and other equipment used during warm-ups are safely put away before play begins, and always inspect the playing field for holes and debris, especially broken glass.

During Game Play

When you're out in the field, you're going to want to go full speed after every ball hit your way. The problem is that so will your teammates. With your attention focused on the ball, it's easy to lose track of where people are, and painful collisions can and do occur.

Make sure that if there is any doubt as to who should field a ball, one player calls for it as loudly as he or she can to let other players know to back away. Practice doing this with your teammates so you get used to listening for each other's voices.

When you're batting, it's important to stand confidently in the batter's box and not be afraid of the ball. That being said, baseballs are hard objects. Getting hit with a pitch hurts. You'll get a free base if you get plunked, but it probably won't be worth the pain. Know how to safely get out of the way if a pitch is headed toward you. The best way to do this is to duck and turn away from the pitcher, exposing your back and rear end to the pitch instead of your face and midsection.

On the base paths, practice running the bases with your head up, looking out for other players and batted balls, and know how to slide correctly. Many leagues make it illegal for kids to slide headfirst, as this can lead to head injuries and facial cuts.

Excessive Pitching

Pitching, particularly for adolescent arms that are still growing, puts an enormous amount of strain on joints and tendons. Injuries to wrists, elbows, rotator cuffs, ligaments, and tendons can result from excessive pitching but can be largely avoided if players and coaches follow a few simple guidelines:

- Make sure you adhere to your league's rules regarding the maximum number of innings a pitcher is allowed to throw. This will generally range from 4 to 10 innings per week. If you play for more than one team, include all innings pitched each week, not just the ones for each team.

- Most leagues follow rules regarding the number of pitches you can throw in a game. Keep in mind that even major league pitchers have strict pitch counts to keep their arms healthy. Here are the pitch count limits for teens recommended by U.S.A. Little League and the American Sports Medicine Institute:

  - 13–16 years old: 95 pitches a day
  - 17–18 years old: 105 pitches a day

- Pitchers under 14 should limit total pitches to less than 1,000 per season and 3,000 per year.

- All players should take at least three months off per year from overhead sports; in other words, sports that involve a lot of overhead arm movements like baseball or volleyball.

- If pitchers feel persistent pain in their throwing arm, they should not be allowed to pitch again until the pain goes away.

A Few Other Reminders

- Make sure a responsible adult is on hand any time you play a baseball game, whether it's a parent, coach, or umpire. In the event someone gets seriously hurt, you'll want an adult around to take an injured player to the emergency room.

- Make sure first aid is readily available at the fields where you play.

- Steroids or human growth hormones aren't just illegal—they're harmful to your health.

These tips should help you have a great time playing America's pastime. Picture yourself under the lights at Yankee stadium, hitting a home run to win game 7 of the World Series.

Section 13.2

Hockey

With non-stop action and high-speed team play, hockey is one of the most exciting sports. Sometimes called "the fastest game on ice," it's a great way to get exercise, and with youth and adult programs throughout the country, chances are no matter what your age or skill level, there is a league near you to play in.

As fun as it is, though, hockey carries a very real risk of injury. To find out how to stay as safe as possible, follow these tips.

Why Is Hockey Safety Important?

At its highest levels, from high school to college to the NHL, hockey allows "checking," an action that involves a player colliding with an opposing player to stop his forward momentum. This can lead to numerous injuries from players hitting one another or colliding with the ice surface or the boards that line the rink. Even in so-called "no-check" leagues, there will always be a lot of contact. Falls are very common, and ice is just as hard as concrete to land on.

In addition, with every player carrying a stick and wearing sharpened skates, accidents are bound to occur. There's also a good chance that sooner or later you'll get hit by the puck, which is made of hard rubber and can leave a nasty bruise if it catches you in the wrong spot. And, since hockey involves strenuous physical activity, pulled muscles and sprains are a hazard for players who don't warm up and stretch properly.

Gearing Up

Before you start playing hockey, it's very important to get all the right equipment and know how to put it on and use it correctly. Skates and a helmet are a good place to start, but there is a lot more you'll need to wear to keep yourself safe.

Never play a game of hockey without the following:

- **Helmet:** When it comes to preventing serious injuries, this is your most important piece of equipment. Helmets should be certified by the Hockey Equipment Certification Council (HECC) and should include a full facemask with a protective chin cup and a chin strap. Make sure you get a helmet that fits properly, and always keep the chin strap fastened and tightened to ensure that the helmet stays in place.

- **Skates:** As with helmets, be sure to get skates that fit well. You're going to lace them up tight, so the wrong size skates can really hurt your feet. Skates should offer plenty of ankle support and have a steel or hard plastic toe cup. It's also important to keep skates sharp so they perform better and are less likely to get caught in ruts in the ice.

- **Shoulder pads, elbow pads, knee and shin pads:** These are all specific to hockey. Soccer or lacrosse equipment won't give you the protection you need. Lower leg (knee and shin) pads should have a hard plastic exterior and reach the top of your skates.

- **Hockey pants:** Also called breezers, these should reach to your knee and offer padding in the front, rear, and sides of your upper legs and midsection.

- **Gloves:** Another sport-specific item, hockey gloves should allow for mobility while protecting well past your wrist.

- **Athletic supporter and cup:** These are incorporated into most hockey undershorts these days but can also come from other sports.

- **Neck protector:** Although some leagues don't require them, neck protectors are helpful at guarding against wayward hockey sticks and skate blades.

- **Mouthguard:** These not only protect the teeth, but also the lips, cheeks, and tongue, and can help prevent head and neck injuries such as concussions and jaw fractures.

Goalie Gear

Charged with putting their bodies between flying pucks and the goal, hockey goalies need a whole different set of equipment to keep themselves safe. Helmets, skates, neck guards, and athletic protectors and cups are all different for goalies than they are for other positions.

In addition, goalies should always wear:

- **Leg pads:** These should always be the correct length and be thick enough to protect against even the hardest slapshot.

- **Arm pads and chest protector:** Arm pads should reach all the way to your wrist. Chest protectors should wrap slightly around your sides to keep your entire front well armored.

- **Blocker glove:** This glove should allow your fingers to grip the stick easily but be very thick and cover most of your forearm.

- **Catcher glove:** Similar to a first baseman's glove in baseball, catcher gloves should have thick padding over the wrist and palm and should also come well up the forearm.

Before the Puck Is Dropped

Everything you do during a hockey game will be done while you are skating, so be sure you know how to skate well before you play a game. Most rinks offer learn-to-skate classes and open skating sessions when you can practice. Know how to stop, turn, and get up when you fall. It's also helpful to know how to skate, stop, and turn while skating backwards.

Once you feel like you are a good enough skater and you've got the proper equipment and know how to use it, you'll be ready to hit the ice. You may notice that before a game, hockey players generally skate around the rink a few times to warm up. Use this time to loosen up and stretch your muscles.

Important muscle groups to stretch before a game include:

- **Groin:** Unlike walking or running, skating requires you to extend your legs to the side, which can put a lot of pressure on your groin. Stretch out both sides while skating by dragging one foot behind you and getting as low to the ice as you can.

- **Back and torso:** Shooting the puck, which you'll hope to be doing a lot of, subjects your midsection to a strenuous twisting motion that your body isn't used to doing. Trunk twists, while holding your stick behind your shoulders, and toe touches also can be done while skating around the rink.

- **Hamstrings:** Use the side boards of the rink to help you balance while you grab your ankle and pull your bent leg back behind you to stretch your hamstrings.

Keeping It Safe during a Game

There's a reason why tripping, hooking, slashing, high-sticking, and cross-checking bring penalties. Hockey sticks can easily go from being a piece of equipment to being a dangerous weapon. Know all the rules governing the use of your stick and follow them to the letter. You wouldn't want to get hit by someone else's stick, and no one wants to get hit by yours.

Other penalties designed to keep the game safe involve roughing, boarding, and checking from behind. These all have to do with players colliding with one another. If your league allows checking, know the difference between a legal check and an illegal one, and never hit anyone from behind. If you play in a "no-check" league, it means just that: no checking.

As far as fighting is concerned, you may see players in the NHL throw off their gloves and start punching one another, but if you do it, expect to pay a harsh penalty. Almost every youth league will kick players out of the game and suspend them for at least one more game for their first fighting penalty. You won't just be hurting yourself; you'll be letting your team down. Don't do it.

Also, never play a game of hockey without adult supervision. Even if you follow every safety tip, accidents can still happen. There should always be a stocked first-aid kit and a responsible adult on hand in the event of an injury or other emergency. Likewise, be sure to have your games officiated by certified referees who are familiar with the specific rules of your league.

Pond Hockey

Playing a game of hockey with your friends on a frozen pond can be lots of fun, but ponds present their own unique set of safety problems. Be sure to have an adult check the ice to make sure it's thick enough to support your weight before you play, and stay away from any parts of the pond or lake where it looks like the ice might be thin. If a puck goes in a suspect area, just let it go. You can always get another puck. It's not worth the risk of hypothermia or drowning to go after it.

Frozen ponds also go hand in hand with very cold temperatures. Be sure to wear plenty of warm clothing in addition to all your hockey gear anytime you play outdoors, and if you're planning on playing on a sunny day, be sure to use sunscreen on your face. The sun's rays reflecting off ice and snow can be very intense.

Now that you know the best ways to keep yourself safe, get out there and hit the ice. Hockey is a great game that you'll want to play for as many years as you can. Just remember that accidents and injuries can still occur no matter how prepared you are. Follow these tips, though, and you can minimize your risk significantly.

Section 13.3

Football

"Football Injury Prevention," Copyright © 2010 American Orthopaedic Society for Sports Medicine. All rights reserved. Reprinted with permission. This Sports Tip from the American Orthopaedic Society for Sports Medicine provides general information only and is not a substitute for your own good judgment or consultation with a physician. To learn more about orthopaedic sports medicine topics and sports injury prevention, visit www.sportsmed .org or www.StopSportsInjuries.org.

Football is one of the most popular sports played by young athletes, and it leads all other sports in the number of injuries sustained. In 2007, more than 920,000 athletes under the age of 18 were treated in emergency rooms, doctors' offices, and clinics for football-related injuries, according to the U.S. Consumer Product Safety Commission.

What Types of Injuries Are Most Common in Football?

Injuries occur during football games and practice due to the combination of high speeds and full contact. While overuse injuries can occur, traumatic injuries such as concussions are most common. The force applied to either bringing an opponent to the ground or resisting being brought to the ground makes football players prone to injury anywhere on their bodies, regardless of protective equipment.

Common Injuries in Football Players

Traumatic Injuries

Knee injuries in football are the most common, especially those to the anterior or posterior cruciate ligament (ACL/PCL) and to the menisci (cartilage of the knee). These knee injuries can adversely affect a player's long-term involvement in the sport. Football players also have a higher chance of ankle sprains due to the surfaces played on and cutting motions.

Shoulder injuries are also quite common and the labrum (cartilage bumper surrounding the socket part of the shoulder) is particularly susceptible to injury, especially in offensive and defensive linemen. In addition, injuries to the acromioclavicular joint (ACJ) or shoulder are seen in football players.

Concussions

Football players are very susceptible to concussions. A concussion is a change in mental state due to a traumatic impact. Not all those who suffer a concussion will lose consciousness. Some signs that a concussion has been sustained are headache, dizziness, nausea, loss of balance, drowsiness, numbness/tingling, difficulty concentrating, and blurry vision. The athlete should return to play only when clearance is granted by a health care professional.

Overuse Injuries

Low-back pain, or back pain in general, is a fairly common complaint in football players due to overuse. Overuse can also lead to overtraining syndrome, when a player trains beyond the ability for the body to recover. Patellar tendonitis (knee pain) is a common problem that football players develop and can usually be treated by a quadriceps strengthening program.

Heat Injuries

Heat injuries are a major concern for youth football players, especially at the start of training camp. This usually occurs in August when some of the highest temperatures and humidity of the year occur. Intense physical activity can result in excessive sweating that depletes the body of salt and water.

The earliest symptoms are painful cramping of major muscle groups. However, if not treated with body cooling and fluid replacement, this can progress to heat exhaustion and heat stroke—which can even result in death. It is important for football players to be aware of the need for fluid replacement and to inform medical staff of symptoms of heat injury.

How Can Football Injuries Be Prevented?

- Have a pre-season health and wellness evaluation.

- Perform proper warm-up and cool-down routines

- Consistently incorporate strength training and stretching.

- Hydrate adequately to maintain health and minimize cramps.

- Stay active during summer break to prepare for return to sports in the fall.

- Wear properly fitted protective equipment, such as a helmet, pads, and mouthguard.

- Tackle with the head up and do not lead with the helmet.

- Speak with a sports medicine professional or athletic trainer if you have any concerns about injuries or prevention strategies.

Section 13.4

Soccer

"Safety Tips: Soccer," May 2010, reprinted with permission from www.kidshealth.org. Copyright © 2010 The Nemours Foundation. This information was provided by KidsHealth, one of the largest resources online for medically reviewed health information written for parents, kids, and teens. For more articles like this one, visit www.KidsHealth.org, or www.TeensHealth.org.

Soccer is the most popular sport in the world for good reason. It's easy to learn at a young age and a great source of exercise. Plus, it's an exciting, fast-paced game that's lots of fun to play.

But soccer is a contact sport, and injuries are bound to happen. Collisions with other players can cause bruises and even concussions. All the running involved in a soccer game can lead to muscle pulls and strains, and getting hit with a ball or improperly heading one can cause head or neck injuries.

To learn how to keep things as safe as possible while playing soccer, follow these safety tips.

Why Is Soccer Safety Important?

With so many people playing soccer these days, it's only natural that some will end up getting hurt. Fortunately, most soccer injuries are minor, but serious injuries such as broken bones and concussions do happen.

Ankle sprains are the most common soccer injury; other frequent injuries include hamstring pulls or tears, groin pulls, muscle cramps, shin splints, concussions, and pulled or strained calf muscles. In addition, players can get repetitive-stress injuries (RSIs) such as tendonitis or stress fractures from playing too much or playing through pain.

Gear Guidelines

Soccer doesn't require a lot of gear for each player other than shin guards and cleats, but it's a good idea to give some thought to all of these important pieces of equipment before you play:

- **Soccer cleats:** Choose a pair of shoes with molded cleats or ribbed soles. Shoes with screw-in cleats may carry a higher risk of injury, so only use them when you need extra traction, such as on a wet field or a field with tall grass. Make sure your cleats fit properly and are laced up tightly each time you play.

- **Shin guards:** If soccer players get lower leg injuries, it's usually because they weren't protected with adequate shin guards. A good shin guard will mold to the shin, end just below the knee, and fit snugly around the ankle bone. Bring your soccer socks and cleats with you when you buy shin guards to be sure that they'll fit properly.

- **Soccer socks:** These are meant to hold shin guards securely in place and should be worn anytime you practice or play.

- **Other gear:** Mouthguards are a good way to protect your teeth, lips, cheeks, and tongue, and can help prevent head and neck injuries such as concussions and jaw fractures. Mouthguards are recommended for all soccer players. Goalies will want to wear long-sleeved shirts and specialized goalie gloves to protect their hands while stopping shots.

Before You Take the Field

Coming into the soccer season in good shape will not only help you be a better player, it will also go a long way toward preventing injuries.

Start working out and eating right a few months before the season is set to begin. Better yet, get regular exercise and eat a healthy diet year-round, and then you won't need to worry about being in shape for the season.

Here are some other things to bear in mind before you start play:

- Whenever you practice or play, inspect the field to make sure there are no holes or other obstacles, including debris and broken glass. Store extra balls and equipment well off to the sides of the field before you start a game.

- Always warm up and stretch before playing. Do some jumping jacks or run in place for a few minutes to get the blood flowing, and then slowly and gently stretch, paying particular attention to your ankles, calves, knees, and hamstrings. Hold each stretch for at least 30 seconds before moving on to the next one.

- Inspect the goals at each end of the field to make sure they're safe. Goals should be securely anchored to the ground, and goal posts should be well padded to decrease the risk of injuries to goalies and players who collide with the posts. Never climb on a goal or hang from the crossbar. Injuries and even deaths have occurred from nets falling onto players.

- If the field you will be playing on is wet, use synthetic, nonabsorbent balls. Leather balls can become waterlogged and very heavy, increasing the risk of injury.

During Game Play

Know and obey the rules of soccer. Unsafe play is a major cause of injuries and will lead to you getting kicked out of the game. In fact, many leagues will suspend you for additional games if you are a repeat offender.

Keep your head up and be aware of your teammates and opposing players at all times. Collisions are more likely if you go charging blindly down the field and don't pay attention to other players.

Learn and use proper techniques, particularly when it comes to heading the ball. Heading the ball can injure your head and neck if you don't do it properly. If you don't know where other players are, you run the risk of head-to-head collisions if two of you jump to head a ball. And protect your tongue—keep your mouth closed and your tongue away from your teeth while heading a ball.

If you get a cramp or feel pain while playing, ask to come out of the game, and don't start playing again until the pain goes away. Playing through pain might seem like a brave thing to do, but it can increase the severity of an injury and possibly keep you on the sidelines for longer stretches of time.

A Few Other Reminders

- Make sure there is first aid available at the fields where you play and practice, as well as someone who knows how to administer it.

- Be prepared for emergency situations. Have a responsible adult on hand when you play, or have a plan to contact medical personnel so they can quickly treat concussions, fractures, or dislocations.

- Stay hydrated, particularly on hot, sunny days, by drinking plenty of fluids before, during, and after games and practices.

- If you have any piercings or jewelry, be sure to remove them before playing.

- If an opposing player collides with you or does something you disagree with, don't take it personally. Let the referees handle the situation, and never start a fight with another player.

Keep soccer fun. That's why you started playing in the first place, isn't it? Follow some basic precautions and stay aware of what's going on around you, and you should be able to avoid most injuries. And that'll keep you out on the field where you want to be.

Section 13.5

Heading the Ball in Youth Soccer

Soccer has become a popular sport for children and adolescents. A unique feature of soccer is that participants can use their heads to direct the ball. This technique is referred to as "heading." Using improper form and/or technique could result in a concussion, which is any change in the way the brain functions as a result of trauma.

Can heading the soccer ball cause problems with brain function?

Several research studies have looked at this question and the results have been conflicting. At present, there are no studies which show that repeated heading of a soccer ball causes long-term problems with thinking or memory.

Is heading the soccer ball safe for children?

Soccer is a contact sport that carries a risk of head injury and collision. Most head injuries that occur during soccer occur when a player hits his head against the ground or collides with another player. Heading the ball does not seem be a significant cause of acute injury. Most research studies examining the safety of heading have involved collegiate and professional soccer players. We don't have any long-term research studies to show that heading is safe for children. Based on the data that is available, physicians recommend that children who play soccer be taught good heading technique and use a ball that is age-appropriate. Young children may not be have the developmental skills necessary for proper heading which could lead to an increased risk of injuries to the skull, neck, and spine. However, improper heading at any age may expose a player to risk.

At what age should they be allowed to start heading the ball?

There is no consensus in the medical and coaching community about when children should be allowed to begin heading. The American Youth Soccer Organization (AYSO) does not recommend heading below the age of 10.

What are some of the fundamentals of proper heading technique?

- The goal is to contact the ball on the forehead at or near the hairline (the area where you would place your hand to detect a fever).

- The player should be active; the popular coaching adage is "hit the ball; don't let the ball hit you."

- The player's body should have the chin tucked toward the chest.

- The arms are usually placed forward for better balance and to protect the player from other players.

Will wearing protective headgear help prevent concussion?

No studies have proven that headgear reduces concussion rates in soccer players. Laboratory studies using dummies and sensors to monitor force have suggested that headgear may help decrease the risk of head injury as a result of players colliding.

When can a player return to soccer following a head injury?

Every head injury is unique. Children and teens are especially vulnerable to having long-term problems if they return to contact sports too quickly following a head injury. If your child is involved in a collision during soccer and has symptoms of concussion such as headache, memory or concentration difficulty, mood changes, or dizziness, he or she should be evaluated by a physician with experience in treating concussions prior to being allowed to return to play.

Section 13.6

Skateboarding

"Safety Tips: Skateboarding," March 2010, reprinted with permission from www.kidshealth.org. Copyright © 2010 The Nemours Foundation. This information was provided by KidsHealth, one of the largest resources online for medically reviewed health information written for parents, kids, and teens. For more articles like this one, visit www.KidsHealth.org, or www.TeensHealth.org.

There's something undeniably cool about skateboarding, from its rebellious attitude to its larger-than-life stars like Tony Hawk and Shaun White. It's fun, it's hip, it's a way of life. There's a good reason why skateboarding's popularity has soared in the last few decades, and why offshoots like long-boarding and mountain-boarding are becoming more common.

But skateboarding also can be an easy way to hurt yourself, particularly if you skate in the wrong place or don't wear protective gear. Scrapes and bruises are almost a fact of skateboarding life, but broken bones and sprains are also common. To keep it safe while skateboarding, stick to the rules wherever you skate, and follow these safety tips.

Why Is Safety Important?

Believe it or not, more than 25,000 people are treated in hospital emergency rooms for skateboard-related injuries every year. Some of those injuries can be severe, and skateboarders have been killed by head injuries and collisions with cars.

Kids and beginners are the most likely to get hurt. More than half of skateboard injuries happen to people under the age of 15. One-third happen to those who've been skateboarding less than a week.

Experienced skaters get hurt, too. As the difficulty of tricks increases, so does the risk of injury, while things like rocks and poor riding surfaces are always a threat.

Gear Guidelines

It may seem like all you need to start skateboarding is a board and an attitude—until your first wipeout. Asphalt, concrete, wood, and other common riding surfaces have one thing in common: none of them is soft. Helmets are a must for all skateboarders, and all beginners should use pads until they gain more experience.

Here are some of the things you'll need to get started:

- **Skateboard:** Different boards do different things. If you're mountain-boarding, you'll want a big board with knobby tires. In the park, you'll want something considerably smaller. Make sure you have the right board for your activity and that all of its parts are in working order. Check your board for cracks, sharp edges, damaged wheels, and loose parts before you skate.

- **Helmet:** Get a helmet that is specifically meant for skateboarding, not some other activity. Look for a sticker inside the helmet saying it meets the ASTM F1492 skateboard helmet standard. All helmets should have a strong strap and buckle, and the strap should be securely fastened and snug any time you ride.

- **Shoes:** Skateboarding is tough on shoes, not to mention feet and ankles. Spend a little extra money and get a good pair of shoes made with leather or suede. Be sure the soles are made of grippy gum rubber, not regular shoe rubber, and that the shoes fit properly.

- **Pads:** All beginners should start off with at least knee and elbow pads, which are recommended for riders of all levels. These should have a hard plastic shield and should not hinder your movements. Make sure any pads you wear are snug without constricting your circulation.

- **Other gear:** Wrist guards, hip pads, skateboard gloves, and padded jackets and shorts are all available and are a good idea for beginners. Mouthguards are good protection against concussions and broken teeth.

Where to Ride

This may be the single most important decision you make, as far as your safety is concerned. Rough riding surfaces are responsible for more than half of skateboarding injuries.

You'll probably do most of your initial skating in your own driveway, a friend's driveway, or a skate park. Wherever you ride, make sure the area is free of rocks, sticks, and other objects. Look out for potentially dangerous cracks in the surface before you ride, and make sure there is no chance of an encounter with a car.

- **Skate parks:** Obey all the rules governing use of the park, and learn proper park etiquette before you decide to venture into the park's more advanced features. Many skate parks have areas set aside for beginners. Stick to this area or somewhere similarly easy when you get started.

- **Empty pools:** If you're lucky enough to have permission to use an empty pool, familiarize yourself with the pool's surface before you ride. If the pool has fallen into disrepair, it might be more hazard than fun.

- **Trails:** If mountain-boarding is your thing, inspect the trail before you ride it. A surprise encounter with a fallen tree could end badly for you.

The greatest threat to your health while skateboarding is cars. Falls hurt, but they are rarely fatal. Collisions with large objects can kill you. Never ride in the street.

Before You Start

It goes without saying that the better shape you're in, the better you'll be at all athletic activities, not just skateboarding. Eat right and exercise frequently. Warm up and stretch before you skate, especially your back, legs, and ankles.

Make sure the place you plan to skate is dry. Clear the area of anything that might interfere with your wheels.

Before you shove off and start skating, be sure it's your turn and that no one is in the way. Collisions can happen if skaters don't communicate. And never ride with someone else on your skateboard. One rider per board, period.

While Riding

You will fall while skateboarding. That much is a given. So:

- Learning how to fall properly can help reduce your chances of injury. If you start to lose your balance, crouch down so you will not have as far to fall. Try to land on the fleshy parts of your body and roll rather than breaking a fall with your arms and hands.

- Bigger tricks and bigger features equal bigger injuries. Once you've learned a couple of tricks, practice them a lot before you move on to more complicated maneuvers. Leave the gnarly stuff to the experts until you're experienced enough to pull it off safely.

- Know and practice skateboarder etiquette. If you're at a crowded skate park, wait your turn instead of jumping blindly into the bowl. This will not only keep fights from breaking out, it will also help you avoid colliding with another skater.

A Few Other Reminders

- Never hitch a ride from a bicycle, car, truck, bus, or other vehicle.

- Don't take chances. That rail you want to slide might look cool, but is it worth knocking your teeth out? Be aware of all the consequences that could happen if things go wrong.

- Be honest about your abilities. Don't attempt tricks that are too advanced for you. This may well save you some embarrassment as well as an injury or two. Practice what you know until you can do it in your sleep, and then move on to something new.

- Talk to the people at the local skateboard shop when you buy your gear. Not only can they tell you how to get the most out of your gear, they usually also know good, safe places to ride.

Skateboarding is great way to have fun and feel a sense of accomplishment. There's nothing like mastering a new trick to feel a surge of self-confidence and pride. Practice, practice, practice, and before long you'll be the one doing the kick-flips and spins and owning the skate park!

Section 13.7

Biking

"Seven Smart Routes to Bicycle Safety for Adults," National Highway
Traffic Safety Administration (www.nhtsa.gov), May 2007.

Seven Smart Routes to Bicycle Safety

1. Protect your head. Wear a helmet.

Never ride a bicycle without wearing a properly fitted helmet. Helmets are proven to be 85%–88% effective in preventing traumatic brain injury, the primary cause of death and disabling injuries resulting from cycling crashes. Wear a helmet that meets the U.S. Consumer Product Safety Commission (CPSC) standard (see inside of helmet for presence of a label). For more information see the brochure: "Easy Steps to Properly Fit a Bicycle Helmet" in English at www.nhtsa.dot.gov/people/injury/pedbimot/bike/EasyStepsWeb/index.htm and in Spanish at www.nhtsa.dot.gov/people/injury/pedbimot/bike/EasyStepsSpan/index.htm.

2. Assure bicycle readiness. Ensure proper size and function of bicycle.

- Use a bicycle that fits you:
  - Select Size: Stand over the top of your bicycle–there should be one to two inches of clearance between you and the tube (bar) and five inches of clearance if riding a mountain bike.
  - Adjust seat height—with a foot on the pedal, the fully extended leg should have a slight bend.
- Check all parts of the bicycle to make sure they are secure and working well:
  - Handlebars should be firmly in place and turn easily.
  - Wheels must be straight and secure; quick-release wheels must be secured (see your owner's manual).

- Brakes need adjusting by an experienced technician if: you cannot stop quickly, you apply the hand brake levers and they touch the handlebars, or the brake pads are worn unevenly or are separated more than one-eighth of an inch from the rim.

3. Ride wisely. Learn and follow the rules of the road.

Bicyclists are considered vehicles on the road and must follow traffic laws that apply to motor vehicles.

- Always ride with traffic and obey traffic lights, signs, speed limits, and lane markings.

- Know your traffic laws found in the state drivers' licensing handbook.

- Signal in advance of a turn; use correct hand signals so others can anticipate your actions.

- Yield to pedestrians and other vehicles, as appropriate.

- If you choose to ride on a sidewalk, take extra caution at driveways and other intersections.

- Check for traffic by looking left-right-left before entering a street.

- Control your speed by using your brakes. If your bicycle has hand brakes, apply the rear brakes slightly before the front brakes.

4. Be predictable. Act like a driver of a vehicle.

- Older children and adults are safest riding on the road where the behaviors and responsibilities should be the same as all vehicle operators.

- Always ride with the flow of traffic, on the right side of the road, and as far to the right of the road as is practicable and safe. Motorists do not expect to see traffic coming in the opposite direction or on the sidewalk. When motorists don't expect to see you, they may pull across your path or turn into you, causing a crash.

- Ride straight and do not swerve in a lane or in and out of traffic.

5. Be visible. See and be seen at all times.

Always assume you are not seen by others. Cyclists must take responsibility for being visible to motorists, pedestrians, and other cyclists. Follow these tips to enhance your visibility at night and in low-visibility conditions (dawn, dusk, and inclement weather):

- Wear neon and fluorescent colors. Wear special clothing made from reflective materials, for example, retro-reflective vests, jackets, wristbands, and patches for your back, legs and arms, and helmet.

- Install bicycle reflectors on both the front and back of your bicycle. If a carrier is added, make sure the rear reflector is visible. A flashing red light on the rear of the bicycle, backpack, or helmet will increase your visibility to others.

- Be aware of your state or local laws regarding use of lights on bicycles. Many states have laws that require bicyclists to use a white front light at night. Use of lights in low-visibility conditions is also recommended.

Young children should be discouraged from riding at night.

6. "Drive" with care. Share the road.

When you ride, consider yourself the driver of a vehicle and always keep safety in mind.

- Choose to ride in the bike lane, if available. If the roadway or bike lane is wide, ride to the right; if the lane is narrow, you may choose to ride in the middle of the lane just like a motorized vehicle.

- Take extra precautions when riding on a roadway. Bicycles are smaller than motor vehicles and don't protect the operator like a motor vehicle. You should follow these guidelines:

  - Make eye contact, smile, or wave to communicate with motorists. Courtesy and predictability are key to safe cycling.

  - Be considerate and aware of motorists and pedestrians. Learn to anticipate their actions. Remember, pedestrians have the right of way.

  - Ride far enough away from the curb to avoid the unexpected from parked cars (i.e., opening doors or drivers pulling out without checking).

- Keep control of your bicycle: look behind you while maintaining your bicycle in a straight path; be able to ride with one hand on the handlebars and signal a turn. (Practice these skills in a parking lot.)

- Always look over your shoulder and, if possible, signal before changing lanes.

- Make sure that books, clothes, and other items are securely attached to the bicycle or carried in a backpack.

- Use bells, horns, or your voice to alert pedestrians and bicyclists that you are approaching or passing.

7. Stay focused. Stay alert.

- Never wear headphones; they hinder your ability to hear traffic.

- Always look for obstacles in your path (potholes, cracks, expansion joints, railroad tracks, wet leaves, drainage grates, or anything that could make you fall). Before going around any object, scan ahead and behind you for a gap in traffic, signal your intentions to move, then follow through with your intentions.

- Be aware of the traffic around you. Ride defensively.

- Use extra care when riding in wet weather, ice, frost, or snow. Slow your speed and allow extra time and space to stop.

- Use extra care when crossing bridges, which are extra slippery under wet conditions.

- Use caution when crossing a railroad track; cross tracks at a 90-degree angle and proceed slowly.

Section 13.8

Golf

When spring is in the air, golf lovers dust off their clubs and flock
in droves to driving ranges to hit buckets of balls. Or they may simply
race from work directly to the golf course five minutes before tee-time
and start playing without warming up or stretching.

"This is a recipe for injuries," said Dr. Robert G. Davis, orthopaedic
surgeon and sports medicine physician at Beth Israel Deaconess Medical Center in Boston. It's no wonder 60% of all golfers have a major
injury in their careers and 50% of professional golfers miss time each
year due to injuries, he said.

"Many golfers don't bother to warm up because they consider golf
a 'non-athletic sport,'" said Dr. Davis, himself an avid golfer. "Think of
yourself like a pro and take 45 to 60 minutes to warm up." He recommends head-to-toe stretching for 5 to 10 minutes, aerobic activity to
raise the heart rate, and swinging the clubs for about 15–20 minutes,
starting with the short clubs and ending with the longer clubs.

Physical therapists who help golfers prevent injuries and recover
from injuries agree that being in shape, having good body mechanics,
and knowing how to warm up, stretch, and cool down are critical.

"Many golf injuries occur when golfers prep for the season at the
driving range," agreed physical therapist Mark Dynan, supervisor
of Rehabilitation Services at Beth Israel Deaconess Healthcare–
Lexington. "After being sedentary during the winter, you're at the
driving range hitting 75–130 balls for an hour—one after the other,
with no rest in between—bending down repeatedly to move the balls
from the bucket to the tee. Compare this to playing 18 holes—taking
80 to 120 swings over three to four hours, walking between holes, and
resting between putts."

Most golf injuries come from golfing too long or too often, poor mechanics, gripping the club too hard, and poor stance or posture. "See
a physical therapist to learn how to strengthen and stretch muscles
and see a golf instructor to correct technique," Dynan advised. "If you

swing or grip the club incorrectly, it strains your body—particularly your shoulder, back, and elbow."

To avoid having to "rehab" after an injury, Dr. Davis recommends "pre-habilitating" to prevent injuries. Two or three months ahead of golf season, golfers should be strengthening core muscles (abdominals, back, gluteus maximus, and mid-section), work on flexibility, and do exercises designed to help golfers avoid injuries.

The most frequent golf injuries are:

Lower back: This is the most common golf injury because of the twisting and turning in the sport. To shoot straighter and further, you need range of motion and flexibility in your back so that you don't strain the ligaments in the lower back. To reduce pressure from the lower back, hips need to be flexible.

Upper middle back: Between the shoulder blades is often the site of an acute injury in golfers who try to get into the game too quickly. "If people swing improperly they can pull a muscle between the shoulder blade and even fracture a rib," Dr. Davis said.

Shoulder: It's important to strengthen the rotator cuff muscles in the shoulder to keep the ball-and-socket joint operating smoothly.

Elbow: Gripping the club with too much force or swinging too hard can stress tissues that run from the elbow to the wrist. It's called "golfer's elbow" when it's on the inside of the elbow, and "tennis elbow" when it's on the outside; despite the name, golfers can get both conditions. "I see the elbow issue in golfers each week in my practice," Dr. Davis said. You need to strengthen your forearm muscles.

When injuries occur, changes occur in the tendons, chronic inflammation can develop, and pain sets in. Rest, ice packs, nonsteroidal anti-inflammatory agents can help, followed by strengthening exercises and stretching, and gradually returning to the sport.

Dudley Blodget of Winchester, MA, knows firsthand the benefits of working with Dynan on his golf game for many years. He's had golfer's elbow and he's learned how the twisting motion of a golf swing can easily cause muscles to pull and pinch, particularly when you're older. "You're not as flexible at 65 as you were at 18. You have to learn how to adapt your swing to compensate for weakness," Dudley said.

With Dynan's help on flexibility and strength training, Blodget is back playing golf and other sports two to three times a week and exercises on the side. "Mark has helped me stretch and be limber. He's helped me stay in the game," he said.

Section 13.9

Tennis

Tennis, played worldwide, is one of the most popular racket sports. A high number of tournaments for competitive tennis players may lead to overuse injuries, such as "tennis elbow" or wrist injuries. For noncompetitive tennis players, improper or inadequate physical and technique training may be the cause of overuse injuries. Although overuse injuries make up a large chunk of tennis injuries, the good news is that such injuries can be prevented with some changes to technique and training routines.

What Types of Injuries Are Most Common in Tennis?

Two-thirds of tennis injuries are due to overuse and the other one-third is due to a traumatic injury or acute event. Overuse injuries most often affect the shoulders, wrists, and elbows.

What Are Common Injuries and Treatments?

Tennis Elbow

The injury most heard about is "tennis elbow," which is an overuse of the muscles that extend the wrist or bend it backwards. It is also the muscle most used when the tennis ball impacts the racquet. Proper strengthening of this muscle and other muscles around it, along with a regular warm-up routine, will help decrease the likelihood of experiencing tennis elbow. Paying attention to technical components such as grip size and proper technique can also help prevent this condition.

Shoulder Injuries

Shoulder overuse injuries are usually due to poor conditioning and strength of the rotator cuff muscles. The rotator cuff helps to position the shoulder properly in the shoulder socket. When it is fatigued or weak, there is some increased "play" of the ball in the socket, irritating the tissues. The tendon or the bursa can become inflamed and hurt. This usually produces pain with overhead motions such as serving. If the pain persists, it can interfere with sleep and other daily activities.

Flexing and extending the wrist against light resistance with an exercise band three to four times a week may help lessen pain and decrease injuries.

Stress Fractures

Twenty percent of junior players suffer stress fractures, compared to just 7.5% of professional players. Stress fractures are the result of increasing training too rapidly. When the muscles tire, more stress is placed on the bone. If this occurs too quickly, the bone cannot adjust rapidly enough to accommodate the stress and it breaks. These "breaks" are usually cracks in the bone that cause pain rather than an actual break or displacement of the bone. Stress fractures can occur in the leg (tibia or fibula) or in the foot (the navicular or the metatarsals).

These injuries are preventable with proper strength and endurance training prior to extensive tennis playing. Appropriate footwear is also critical to preventing stress fractures.

Muscle Strains

Muscle strains usually occur from quick, sudden moves. A good warm-up followed by proper stretching can help diminish muscle strains. The warm-up should include a slow jog, jumping jacks, or riding a bike at low intensity.

Proper stretching should be slow and deliberate. Do not bounce to stretch; hold the stretch 30 seconds or more. The best stretches are moving stretches, such as swinging your leg as far forward and backward or swinging your arms in circles and across your body. Proper stretching should last at least five minutes.

If you have any concerns about an injury or how to prevent future injuries speak with a sports medicine professional or athletic trainer. The athlete should return to play only when clearance is granted by a health care professional.

Section 13.10

Running

Running is a great form of exercise, recreation, and sport participation for adults, adolescents, and children. Whether alone or in a team environment, running, when done properly, can enhance physical fitness, coordination, sense of accomplishment, and physical and emotional development. However, running under adverse conditions or with inadequate clothing and equipment can cause a variety of injuries and physical stress.

What Are the Signs That I Might Have a Running Injury?

Signs that you may be injured or need to alter or stop your running include:

- pain or discomfort while running;
- pain at rest;
- inability to sleep;
- limping;
- easily experiencing shortness of breath (exercise asthma);
- stiffness;
- headaches during or after running;
- dizziness or lightheaded feeling any time.

What Are Some Common Running Injuries?

Running injuries in kids are relatively common and may include:

- knee injuries (kneecap pain, tendonitis);

- lower leg pain (shin splints, stress fractures, calf problems);
- foot and ankle injuries (ankle sprain, heel pain, plantar fasciitis [bottom of foot pain], toe injuries);
- pelvic and hip injuries (muscle pulls, growth plate stress injuries, tendonitis, groin pain, buttock pain);
- heat injuries (sunburn, dehydration, heat exhaustion, stroke);
- skin injuries (blisters or heat rash).

Why Is It Important to Stop Running If I'm Hurt?

Pushing through pain just makes the problem worse, which will keep you from running for a long time. Stopping when there is a problem and correcting it gets you back running again in the shortest, safest amount of time. Whenever there is a problem, contact your doctor immediately for proper diagnosis and treatment. Most of the time, problems are easily fixed if attended to quickly.

How Can I Prevent Running Injuries?

Planning Goals

- Talk about running with a coach, athletic trainer, knowledgeable adult runner, or running organization.
- Children and parents should consistently discuss the goals of the running program.
- Determine the reason (goal) you are running (e.g., fitness, recreation, training, competition).
- Develop a running plan and strategy that is compatible with your goal and your current level of fitness.
- Set safe, achievable goals and advance slowly and cautiously.

Preparing to Run

- Hydrate (drink water) well in advance.
- Stretch for five minutes before beginning.
- Speed up slowly.

Proper Running Attire

The local running store is a good place to start and ask questions. It's important to remember the following:

- Lightweight, breathable clothing prevents perspiration buildup and allows for better body heat regulation.

- Running hats, head covers, and ear covers shield the sun but allow temperature regulation—they are also excellent for cold weather to avoid frostbite.

- Proper fitting and proper thickness of socks help avoid blisters and irritation.

- Proper shoes with good support arches should fit well and be comfortable.

- Inspect your shoes before running: if they have worn thin or are angled, purchase new shoes.

- Orthotic shoe inserts (commercial off-the-shelf or custom-made) are especially valuable for people with flat feet, high-arched feet, unstable ankles, or foot problems.

Safe Locations and Times to Run

- Flat ground is more gentle on the body than hills.

- Avoid steep hills.

- All-purpose track surfaces (high school track) are ideal—especially for beginners.

- Stay in well-lit areas (e.g., schools, public streets).

- Always run with a partner (preferably a teen or parent).

- A parent should always know:

  - where you are running;

  - when you are running;

  - how far you are running;

  - with whom you are running;

  - when you expect to be back;

  - when you are finished.

- Use a bag to carry a cell phone with you.

- Avoid using headphones, especially if you are running on the street, so you can hear traffic and warning sounds.

Safe Weather Conditions

Children and adolescents cannot tolerate the weather extremes that adults can, making them more susceptible to heat and cold injuries. Prevent heat illnesses (e.g., sunburn, dehydration, exhaustion) or cold injuries (frostbite) by monitoring the weather conditions.

Avoid running if:

- temperatures are over 90 degrees;

- humidity levels are high;

- temperatures are cold or freezing.

Section 13.11

Water Sports

"Take Steps to Stay Safe Around Water," Copyright © 2011 by The American National Red Cross (www.redcross.org). All rights reserved.

Swimming is the most popular summer activity. The best thing you can do to help your family stay safe this summer is to enroll in age-appropriate swim lessons. Contact your local Red Cross chapter to find courses in your area.

Follow these safety tips whenever you are in, on, or around water.

Make Water Safety Your Priority

- Swim in designated areas supervised by lifeguards.

- Always swim with a buddy; do not allow anyone to swim alone. Even at a public pool or a lifeguarded beach, use the buddy system!

- Ensure that everyone in the family learns to swim well. Enroll in age-appropriate Red Cross water orientation and Learn-to-Swim courses.

- Never leave a young child unattended near water and do not trust a child's life to another child; teach children to always ask permission to go near water.

- Have young children or inexperienced swimmers wear U.S. Coast Guard–approved life jackets around water, but do not rely on life jackets alone.

- Establish rules for your family and enforce them without fail. For example, set limits based on each person's ability, do not let anyone play around drains and suction fittings, and do not allow swimmers to hyperventilate before swimming under water or have breath-holding contests.

- Even if you do not plan on swimming, be cautious around natural bodies of water including ocean shoreline, rivers, and lakes. Cold temperatures, currents, and underwater hazards can make a fall into these bodies of water dangerous.

- If you go boating, wear a life jacket! Most boating fatalities occur from drowning.

- Avoid alcohol use. Alcohol impairs judgment, balance, and coordination; affects swimming and diving skills; and reduces the body's ability to stay warm.

Prevent Unsupervised Access to the Water

- Install and use barriers around your home pool or hot tub. Safety covers and pool alarms should be added as additional layers of protection.

- Ensure that pool barriers enclose the entire pool area and are at least four-feet high with gates that are self-closing, self-latching, and open outward and away from the pool. The latch should be high enough to be out of a small child's reach.

- If you have an above-ground or inflatable pool, remove access ladders and secure the safety cover whenever the pool is not in use.

- Remove any structures that provide access to the pool, such as outdoor furniture, climbable trees, decorative walls, and playground equipment.

- Keep toys that are not in use away from the pool and out of sight. Toys can attract young children to the pool.

Maintain Constant Supervision

- Actively supervise children whenever around the water—even if lifeguards are present. Do not just drop your kids off at the public pool or leave them at the beach—designate a responsible adult to supervise.

- Always stay within arm's reach of young children and avoid distractions when supervising children around water.

Know What to Do in an Emergency

- If a child is missing, check the water first. Seconds count in preventing death or disability.

- Know how and when to call 9-1-1 or the local emergency number.

- If you own a home pool or hot tub, have appropriate equipment, such as reaching or throwing equipment, a cell phone, life jackets, and a first aid kit.

- Enroll in Red Cross home pool safety, water safety, first aid, and CPR/AED courses to learn how to prevent and respond to emergencies.

Chapter 14

Winter Sports Safety

Chapter Contents

Section 14.1

Avoiding Winter Sports Injuries through Preparation

"Preparation for Outdoor Winter Activities Prevents Injury,"
© 2011 American Chiropractic Association (www.acatoday.org).
Reprinted with permission.

When snow, ice, and frigid weather blast into town, watch out, says the American Chiropractic Association (ACA). Winter recreational activities and chores can pose problems for the outdoor enthusiast whose body is not in condition. Winter sports like skating, skiing, and sledding can cause painful muscle spasms, strains, or tears if you're not in shape. Even shoveling snow the wrong way, clambering awkwardly over snow banks, slipping on sidewalks, and wearing the wrong kinds of clothing can all pose the potential for spasms, strains, and sprains.

Simply walking outside in the freezing weather without layers of warm clothing can intensify older joint problems and cause a great deal of pain. As muscles and blood vessels contract to conserve the body's heat, the blood supply to extremities is reduced. This lowers the functional capacity of many muscles, particularly among the physically unfit. Preparation for an outdoor winter activity, including conditioning the areas of the body that are most vulnerable, can help avoid injury and costly health care bills.

"Simply put, warming up is essential," says Olympic speedskating gold and silver medalist Derek Parra. "In fact, when pressed for time, it's better to shorten the length of your workout and keep a good warm-up than to skip the warm-up and dive right into the workout. Skipping your warm-up is the best way to get hurt." Parra, who took both the gold and silver medals during the 2002 Winter Olympics in Salt Lake City, Utah, adds that, "You can complete a good warm-up in 15–20 minutes. And believe me, it will make your workout more pleasant and safe."

Derek Parra and the ACA suggest that you start with some light aerobic activity (jogging, biking, fast walking) for about 7–10 minutes. Then follow these tips to help you fight back the winter weather:

- **Skiing:** Do 10 to 15 squats. Stand with your legs shoulder width apart, knees aligned over your feet. Slowly lower your buttocks as you bend your knees over your feet. Stand up straight again.

- **Skating:** Do several lunges. Take a moderately advanced step with one foot. Let your back knee come down to the floor while keeping your shoulders in position over your hips. Repeat the process with your other foot.

- **Sledding/tobogganing:** Do knee-to-chest stretches to fight compression injuries caused by repetitive bouncing over the snow. Either sitting or lying on your back, pull your knees to your chest and hold for up to 30 seconds.

- **Don't forget cool-down stretching for all of these sports:** At the bottom of the sledding hill, for instance, before trudging back up, do some more knees-to-chest stretches, or repetitive squatting movements to restore flexibility.

Shoveling snow can also wreak havoc on the musculoskeletal system. The ACA suggests the following tips for exercise of the snow-shoveling variety:

- If you must shovel snow, be careful. Listen to weather forecasts so you can rise early and have time to shovel before work.

- Layer clothing to keep your muscles warm and flexible.

- Shoveling can strain "de-conditioned" muscles between your shoulders, in your upper back, lower back, buttocks, and legs. So, do some warm-up stretching before you grab that shovel.

- When you do shovel, push the snow straight ahead. Don't try to throw it. Walk it to the snow bank. Avoid sudden twisting and turning motions.

- Bend your knees to lift when shoveling. Let the muscles of your legs and arms do the work, not your back.

- Take frequent rest breaks to take the strain off your muscles. A fatigued body asks for injury.

- Stop if you feel chest pain, or get really tired or have shortness of breath. You may need immediate professional help.

After any of these activities, if you are sore, apply an ice bag to the affected area for 20 minutes, then take it off for a couple of hours. Repeat a couple of times each day over the next day or two.

143

If you continue to feel soreness, pain, or strain after following these tips, it may be time to visit a doctor of chiropractic. "I've always believed in chiropractic care," says Parra. "I've used a lot of other treatments for injuries and pain, but the problem doesn't get fixed until I go to a doctor of chiropractic."

Section 14.2

Skiing and Snowboarding Safety

The popularity of skiing has increased dramatically in the past century. Since its inception in the 1960s, snowboarding has become increasingly popular as well. In fact, almost 40% of all "sliding snow" sports participants today are snowboarders.

Skiing and snowboarding are both wonderful sports. As with most any physical activity, however, there is an element of risk. By following some basic guidelines and learning more about the risks, it is possible to decrease those risks. Remembering the following information can minimize your risks and allow more fun on the slopes.

How Do Skiers Get Hurt?

Many variables affect injury rates in skiers, most commonly ability, age, gender, physical conditioning, and snow conditions. Beginners have three times the injury rate of experts, but their injuries are less severe. Experts have less frequent but more severe injuries (head injuries, fractures, and high-grade ligament sprains). This is probably due to their higher speed on the ski slope. Intermediate skiers fall somewhere in-between.

Another key factor is age. The highest injury rate is among 11- to 13-year-olds. Their ability is intermediate, but their judgment is not as good as adults'. Injures in teenagers (13- to 20-year-olds) are slightly less frequent, but more severe. Many have the skill levels of adults with immature judgment. Finally, children younger than 12 years old have twice the injury rate of adults, but fewer than that of adolescents.

Females have twice the injury rate of males, which is thought to stem from conditioning. One study looking at female ski racers found that their anterior cruciate ligament (ACL) injury rate was six times that of their male counterparts.

Physical conditioning may have a significant impact on injury rates—that is, the better shape a skier is in, the less frequent the injuries. Most studies focus on destination ski resorts, where most skiers are vacationers. Injuries are most likely to occur on:

- the first day of ski week;

- in the early morning when the skier is not warmed up;

- in the late morning and late in the day when fatigue sets in; and

- at the end of the week when the cumulative effects of the vacation make the skier tired.

Snow conditions affect injury patterns, as well. Hard pack snow generally yields high-speed and impact injuries. Powder and heavy snow is associated with more torsional or twisting injuries. Quick changes in snow conditions, such as hitting the line between groomed and ungroomed snow, may cause a fall that leads to an injury.

Equipment-Related Injuries

Skis have a rigid coupling with the foot that increases the forces to the leg and knee. These forces are often greater than our bodies can absorb. This boot-binding interface is the most common cause of equipment-related injury. The modern bindings, which release in a multidirectional pattern, have decreased the incidence of fractures by more than 80%. Unfortunately, knee ligament sprains have not decreased and have actually increased over the last 20 to 30 years. Bindings are continuing to improve every year. If you have only one piece of equipment that is new, it should be your ski binding.

To improve the safety of your skiing, your bindings should be no more than three to four years old. The release properties should be tested each year in a certified shop. You can also perform a self-release test each day of skiing by kicking out of your bindings. It is also very important to make sure that you have no dirt or grit in your binding or in the boot/binding interface.

Boots are less important in the prevention of injuries, though you should be mindful of their proper fit and the amount of external wear on your boots. When buying boots, be sure to get a proper fit from a knowledgeable salesperson. Check that the toe and heel of your boots have little external wear and are clean. This will allow proper release from the binding.

Proper ski length may also affect injury rate. Shorter skis are easier to turn and control but may be less stable at high speeds. Newer skis have more sidecut (the curve on the sides of your ski). This helps skiers of all ability levels carve turns more easily. Some research suggests that this feature may cause more twisting injuries to the knee. Regardless, it is important to keep your ski edges in good condition to allow for proper carving of a turn and to control your speed, especially on hard pack or icy conditions.

Ski poles can influence thumb and hand injuries. When a skier falls on an outstretched hand that is holding a ski pole, the pole can cause a tear of the ulnar collateral ligament of the thumb. This is one of the most common injuries in skiing. The best way to prevent this injury is to drop your pole when you fall. It is important to not wear your ski pole straps. This allows the pole to fall away when you drop it. In deep powder snow this may not be as important.

Ski clothing, goggles, and headgear are important as well. It is important to dress in layers to allow for adjustment to changing weather conditions. Goggles and sunglasses will protect your eyes from UV [ultraviolet] radiation, wind, snow, and other hazards you may find on the slope. One important trend is the use of helmets on the ski mountain, which is analogous to biking helmets. After all, most of us would not go biking without a helmet, particularly at speeds in excess of 30 miles per hour. Head injuries are the most common cause of death from skiing collisions. Many of these may be prevented by wearing a helmet.

ACL Injuries

One of the most common injuries in skiing is the ACL tear. Some experts say that incidence of this injury has tripled over the last 20 years. Vermont Safety Research has instituted a program to prevent ACL injuries in ski professionals. Their techniques, which have been shown to significantly reduce the ACL injury rate, are available from http://www.vermontskisafety.com/.

Snowboarding Injury Trends

Snowboarding has a slightly higher potential for upper extremity injuries, but it may be safer on the knees. There is an increased rate of foot and ankle injuries associated with snowboarding. The lead foot has twice the number of injuries than the back foot. One study showed that the hybrid or "mid-stiffness" boots were the safest style of boots. There may be more high-energy injuries such as femur fractures, high-speed injuries, and injuries caused by getting "big air."

General Injury Prevention

- Prepare for the season and get in shape.

- Get your equipment checked at a certified shop.

- Self-release your bindings each day you ski.

- Warm up and stretch before skiing.

- Don't ski while intoxicated.

- Wear a helmet.

Section 14.3

Helmets for Winter Sports

Outdoor winter sports and activities are popular in the United States and around the world. Many involve speed and the adrenaline rush that goes along with it. Unfortunately, the faster you go, the higher your risk of injury. Head injury is common in the higher speed winter sports, including skiing, snowboarding, and snowmobiling. There is mounting evidence that head injury is increasingly common among sledders as well, especially in young children.

Skiers and snowboarders often move at speeds much higher than the average bicyclist, yet more people wear helmets while biking.

Skiing and Snowboarding

Many studies have been published reporting the incidence of injuries while skiing and snowboarding. Collisions resulting in serious head injury are the leading cause of death. Most collisions are with fixed objects (such as trees) or with other people on the hill. Collisions with other people are often more serious than with fixed objects. Data suggest that head and brain injuries in skiing are increasing.

One study found the risk of death in skiers and snowboarders was twice as high for males as females and nearly three times as high for skiers/boarders 35 years of age or younger compared to those over 35 years old. In a study of helmet use in young skiers and snowboarders, researchers found a 43% decrease in head, neck, and face injuries in people who wore a helmet compared to those who did not.

Snowmobiling

The snowmobile was originally developed as a means of transporting people and supplies in remote northern regions. Today snowmobiling is very popular, with more than two million people of all ages snowmobiling in North America alone. Modern snowmobiles with engines over 1200 cc can attain speeds well over 100 miles per hour; however, as the speed increases so does the risk. Many states allow children as young as eight years old to operate snowmobiles and most have no helmet laws. Many states have no speed limit and use the term "reasonable and prudent" as their guideline.

Blunt trauma is the main cause of death related to snowmobile use. Even though many snowmobile riders wear a helmet, head injury is the leading cause of death from blunt trauma. In the majority of snowmobile deaths, head and neck injury is the predominant cause of death. Poor judgment, high speeds, and alcohol are often involved in injuries. Speed limits, helmet laws, and age restrictions may improve the safety of this activity.

Sledding and Tobogganing

Sledding and tobogganing are enjoyable winter recreational activities that, too, have their share of injuries, especially among young children. The highest numbers of injuries occur in children 5–14 years old and the injuries are most often caused by falls or collisions. Sledding and tobogganing are mainly enjoyed by very young children, which may explain the higher rate of injury. Older sledders (those 20 years of age and older) who are injured often have poorer outcomes from their injuries than younger sledders. Older sledders who sustain injuries also tend to require hospitalization more frequently than persons injured in other types of sports and recreational activities.

The American Academy of Orthopaedic Surgeons has recommended the use of helmets to improve sledding safety, among other guidelines. Riders should always sit on sleds and toboggans facing forward and upright, and always should go downhill feet first.

Use Your Head—Wear a Helmet

Owners and operators of snow sports resorts have not yet mandated helmet use for skiers and snowboarders. Instead, they take the position that the decision to wear a helmet should be a matter of individual choice. Participants—especially parents—should educate themselves about the benefits and limitations of available helmets and make the choice that is right for them (and their families). The "Lids on Kids" helmet education campaign sponsored by the skiing and snowboarding industry is an excellent source of helmet information (see www .lidsonkids.org).

Conclusion

Perhaps the best advice for skiers and snowboarders is this: *"If you are going to wear a helmet, ski and ride as if you aren't wearing one. Don't alter your behavior, take more risks, or ski or ride faster because you're outfitted in a helmet. Make sure that you remain in control and ski and ride responsibly."*

It makes sense to wear a helmet while participating in alpine and winter activities. The new designs are light and warm. Wear a helmet and encourage your family and friends to do the same the next time they participate in the "speed" winter activities.

Chapter 15

Resistance Training Safety

Chapter Contents

Section 15.1

Resistance Training and Injury Prevention

© 2007 American College of Sports Medicine (www.acsm.org). Reprinted with permission of the American College of Sports Medicine, "ACSM Current Comment: Resistance Training and Injury Prevention," written for the American College of Sports Medicine by Jay Hoffman, Ph.D., FACSM.

The benefits of resistance training in both competitive and recreational athletes have been well documented over the past 20 years. Improvements in muscle strength and power, increase in muscle size, and improvement in sports performance are common benefits resulting from resistance training programs. In addition, resistance training has also been suggested to reduce the risk for musculoskeletal injuries, or perhaps reduce the severity of such injury. Although studies reporting the direct effect of resistance training on injury rate reduction are limited, the physiological adaptations seen consequent to resistance training on bone, connective tissue, and muscle does imply enhanced protection against injury for individuals who participate in such a training program.

Effect on Bone

Because bone is living tissue, it has the ability to remodel and adapt to the physical stresses imposed on it. Individuals who are physically active have been shown to have greater bone mineral density than sedentary individuals. In general, physically active persons are at a reduced risk for osteoporosis, fracture, or other ailments related to bone deterioration. Although bone will respond to many types of training programs, especially those with high strain such as jumping or running, it does appear that resistance training provides the greatest osteogenic (increase in bone mineral density) effect. Resistance training is beneficial for increasing bone strength, and muscular strength also appears to be positively related to bone mineral content and bone strength. As lower-body strength levels increase, the incidence of stress fracture is reduced. Thus muscular strength improves bone strength as well. However, it is not clear whether the relative improvements in bone and muscle strength during a resistance training program are similar.

152

Effect on Connective Tissue

Connective tissue provides the support or framework of the body. It consists of cells and fibers imbedded in a gel-like material containing tissue fluids and various metabolites. The primary fiber of connective tissue is collagen. Although to date there has been little research conducted on the direct effect of resistance training on connective tissue adaptations, what studies there are have reported increases in both the size and strength of ligaments and tendons. Increases in the size of connective tissues are thought to be the result of an increase in the collagen content within the connective tissue sheaths. Although collagen content increases with training, comparisons between untrained individuals and body builders suggest that the increase in collagen content is proportional to the increase in muscle. Body builders seem to have greater absolute collagen content, but relative values are similar to untrained controls. Thus, increases in muscle mass are likely met by increases in the size and strength of the connective tissue.

Effect on Muscle

Decreases in muscle mass (sarcopenia) and subsequent reductions in muscle strength as one ages not only results in a loss of functional ability, but also increases the risk for falls and fractures. Resistance training programs for an aging population have the same benefits for increase in both strength and muscle size as such programs do for the younger and more active population. As functional ability is maintained or improved, the risk for injury is significantly reduced. Resistance training also has an important role in reducing the risk for musculoskeletal injuries related to muscle imbalance, expressed as either an agonist to antagonist ratio (i.e., knee flexors/knee extensors) or as a bilateral comparison (i.e., right and left knee flexors). Correction of the existing imbalance through a resistance training program is important to reducing the individual's risk for muscle injury.

Resistance training programs also have a positive effect on reducing low back injuries. Whether this reduced risk is related to increased strength in the lumbar extensors or to stronger lumbar vertebrae is not known. However, the benefits of resistance training on reducing back injuries and associated expenses are well acknowledged.

Reducing the incidence of injury by engaging in a resistance training program is as beneficial for the noncompetitive beginner as it is for the professional athlete. The most important step, after medical clearance, is to locate a qualified individual (exercise scientist/physiologist or sport trainer) to develop a safe and effective resistance training program.

Section 15.2

Overuse Injuries in Resistance Training

© 2007 American College of Sports Medicine (www.acsm.org). Reprinted with permission of the American College of Sports Medicine, "ACSM Current Comment: Overtraining with Resistance Exercise," written for the American College of Sports Medicine by Andrew C. Fry, Ph.D.

One of the fastest growing and most popular types of exercise in recent years is resistance exercise, whether used for the purpose of general fitness, rehabilitation, or athletic performance. Resistance exercise comes in many different forms, each of which can produce distinctly different responses (e.g., increased size, strength, power, contraction velocity, muscular endurance, etc.). Each individual training session can be described by the five acute training variables: choice of exercise, order of exercise, exercise volume (sets x repetitions), load or intensity (percent repetition maximum), and rest (between sets). Each of these variables present numerous possible combinations resulting in literally thousands of possible single-session protocols. Over a longer training period or cycle, the training variables can be altered to provide the individual with the necessary variability for long-term improvement. Such variety in the long-term program is called periodization, and helps to ensure that the body is continually being presented with a stress that permits both progress and adequate recovery. Often associated with training programs for advanced athletes, such training variety is also critical for the individual who is embarking on a lifetime exercise program for general fitness. This variation of the resistance exercise prescription also avoids the monotony that can occur when the identical exercise protocol is performed each session with little or no variation.

One common problem when prescribing resistance exercise is determining the appropriate combination of training volume and intensity. Excessive volume or intensity may produce less than optimal results, and may actually create a situation where performance is impaired. If physical performance is depressed for extended periods of time, and requires long recovery periods, overtraining has occurred. This situation may result in a decreased desire to exercise, and can also increase the risk of illness or injury. Such a situation can be avoided through proper prescription of volume and intensity. It must be noted that increasing training volume or intensity is not necessarily bad. There may even be phases of training where an individual experiences short-term performance decrements that are easily recovered from with several days of decreased exercise stress. This is called overreaching, and when carefully prescribed can contribute to long-term progress.

The typical overtraining scenario, however, occurs when either training volume or intensity is excessive for too long. It is also important to note that training volume and intensity are inversely related. In other words, when training volume is greatest, intensity must be relatively low, and vice versa. Unfortunately, many individuals prescribing resistance exercise programs fail to realize this, and simply follow the axiom that "more is better" for both volume and intensity. The net result is that performance is either impaired or at best is less than optimal.

One type of overtraining can occur when training volume is excessive for prolonged periods. This can occur by increasing training frequency, adding exercises, or performing more exercise sets. It appears that this type of overtraining manifests many signs/symptoms similar to those seen with overtraining with endurance exercise. Two hormones often impacted by overtraining are testosterone and cortisol, and overtraining due to high training volumes often results in a decrease in the ratio between resting concentrations of these hormones (testosterone/cortisol). While this ratio may not be directly responsible for the performance decrements observed, it has been repeatedly shown that this ratio decreases as training volume increases. It also appears that the use and mobilization of free fatty acid, which expends more fat by using energy in the metabolic cycle, increases during high volume phases of resistance exercise. This may contribute in part to decreases in body fat with this type of training stress. Although it has been theorized that the sympathetic nervous system may become exhausted with this type of training (the parasympathetic overtraining syndrome), this has yet to be demonstrated with resistance exercise.

At the other end of the training spectrum is the effect of excessive training intensity; that is, using too heavy a resistance for extended periods of time. This scenario seems to present a physiologically different profile than high volume overtraining. The limited data available indicate that the testosterone/cortisol ratio is not altered with this type of overtraining, even when strength performance is dramatically impaired. Exercise-induced concentrations of catecholamines, on the other hand, are markedly elevated with this type of overtraining. This suggests a sympathetic overtraining syndrome where increases

155

in sympathetic activity in the nervous system may be an attempt to compensate for decreases in muscle strength capabilities.

It is believed that most real-life overtraining scenarios are due to a combination of excessive volume and intensity. Furthermore, many exercise programs include not only resistance exercise, but also some form of exercise for cardiovascular fitness. Such a combination presents a very complex setting from a physiological standpoint. The few data available on this type of training suggest that both the resistance exercise and the cardiovascular exercise components may have to be modified somewhat to allow the individual to tolerate such combination training.

Performance decrements may also occur through pathological mechanisms such as joint overuse. When this occurs, strength and power decrements may be due to afferent inhibition from the affected joints rather than due to decreases in muscular capabilities. Perhaps the most intriguing area of research is the evaluation of psychological states accompanying overtraining. Although most data on the psychology of overtraining are from other types of exercise, it appears that a decreased desire to train often occurs with resistance exercise overtraining. Furthermore, measures of self-efficacy (confidence in performance) appear to be adversely affected with some forms of resistance exercise overtraining.

Numerous signs and symptoms of overtraining have been suggested. It should be noted that not all of these symptoms will be present, and that the presence of some of these symptoms does not automatically mean an individual is overtrained. The ultimate determination of overtraining is whether performance is impaired or plateaued. Listed here are some frequently cited signs of overtraining:

Performance

- Decreased performance (strength, power, muscle endurance, cardiovascular endurance)
- Decreased training tolerance and increased recovery requirements
- Decreased motor coordination
- Increased technical faults

Physiology

- Altered resting heart rate (HR), blood pressure, and respiration patterns
- Decreased body fat and post-exercise body weight

- Increased VO$_2$ [volume of oxygen], VE [ventilation, the amount of air moved in and out of the lungs], and HR during submaximal work
- Decreased lactate response
- Increased basal metabolic rate
- Chronic fatigue
- Sleep and eating disorders
- Menstrual disruptions
- Headaches, gastrointestinal distress
- Muscle soreness and damage
- Joint aches and pains

Physiological

- Depression and apathy
- Decreased self-esteem
- Decreased ability to concentrate
- Decreased self-efficacy
- Sensitive to stress

Immunological

- Increased occurrence of illness
- Decreased rate of healing
- Impaired immune function (neutrophils, lymphocytes, mitogen responses, eosinophils)

Biochemical

- Hypothalamic dysfunction
- Increased serum cortisol and SHBG [sex hormone binding globulin]
- Decreased serum total and free testosterone, testosterone/cortisol ratio
- Decreased muscle glycogen
- Decreased serum hemoglobin, iron, and ferritin
- Negative N$_2$ balance

The majority of these signs and symptoms are derived from endurance exercise overtraining research. Not all of these signs and symptoms have been linked with resistance exercise overtraining, due partly to a lack of relevant research on the topic, and to the fact that resistance exercise presents different physiological stress compared to endurance exercise.

- If overtraining from resistance exercise has occurred, several simple steps can be taken, including:
  - one or more recovery days should be added to each training week;
  - periodized training programs can provide the necessary training variety to avoid overtraining;
  - avoid monotonous training;
  - check that training volume and training intensity are inversely related;
  - avoid too great a relative intensity (percent 1RM [one rep max]) for extended periods;
  - avoid too great a training volume (number of sessions, exercises, sets and reps) for extended periods;
  - avoid performing every set of every exercise of every session to absolute failure, with no variation;
  - avoid incorrect exercise selection (overuse of certain muscles or joints);
  - avoid excessive use of eccentric muscle actions;
  - take into account the cumulative training stresses from other forms of exercise (i.e., cardiovascular training, sport-specific training, etc.).

Overtraining is of growing concern; more research is necessary for full understanding. It is clear that the exercise prescription is critically important to avoid a problem. Periodized training allows variation and is important for best results. Periodization includes phases of high training stress and planned periods for recovery and restoration. This applies to elite athletes as well as to individuals exercising for general health and fitness.

Chapter 16

Outdoor Sports Safety in Weather Conditions

Chapter Contents

Section 16.1

Safety in the Heat

Introduction

As the temperature and humidity rise, so does the incidence of heat-related illnesses to which anyone is susceptible. When exercising outside, an individual's body temperature begins to rise due to the combination of increased air temperature and increased metabolism, while high humidity prevents the body's cooling mechanism, evaporation of perspiration, from working effectively.

If you intend to exercise outside this summer, please take precautions to avoid heat-related illnesses and be aware of the signs and treatment of the following conditions.

Heat Cramps

Heat cramps are involuntary muscle spasms caused by dehydration, electrolyte loss, and inadequate blood flow to muscles. They usually occur in the quadriceps, hamstrings, and calves.

When heat cramps occur, discontinue activity, slowly stretch the affected area, and drink cool water. When the spasms subside, activity can be resumed. If the spasms do not improve within five minutes, they may be caused by another injury. See a physician.

Heat Exhaustion

Heat exhaustion is a shock-like condition that occurs when excessive sweating causes dehydration and electrolyte loss. A person with heat exhaustion may have a headache, nausea, dizziness, chills, fatigue, and extreme thirst. Signs of heat exhaustion are:

- pale, cool, and clammy skin;
- a rapid, weak pulse;

- loss of coordination;

- dilated pupils;

- profuse sweating (most important).

Take the following steps when signs of heat exhaustion occur:

- Rest in a cool, shaded area.

- Drink cool water.

- Apply ice to the neck, back, or stomach to help cool the body.

- Monitor breathing and heart rate; rescue breathing or CPR [cardiopulmonary resuscitation] may be necessary.

- If the condition does not improve (or worsens), call 9-1-1.

Activity may not be resumed the same day and not until fluid loss is replaced.

Heatstroke

Heatstroke is a life-threatening condition in which the body stops sweating and body temperature rises dangerously high. It occurs when the body's temperature control center malfunctions due to dehydration. A person with heatstroke may feel extremely hot, nauseated, confused, irritable, and fatigued. Signs of heatstroke are:

- hot, dry, flushed skin (most important);

- very high body temperature (>103° F);

- lack of sweat;

- rapid pulse;

- rapid breathing;

- constricted pupils;

- vomiting or diarrhea;

- seizures, unconsciousness, cardiac arrest (possibly).

Take the following steps when signs of heat exhaustion occur:

- Call 9-1-1.

- Rest in a cool, shaded area.

- Remove excess clothing.

- Cool the body with cool, wet towels or by pouring cool water over the individual.

- Apply ice packs to the armpits, neck, back, stomach, and groin.

- Monitor breathing and heart rate; rescue breathing or CPR may be necessary.

- Drink cool water.

Activity may not be resumed until a physician's release is obtained.

Prevention

Simple steps can be taken to prevent heat-related illnesses. When exercising in high heat and humidity, rest for 10 minutes every hour and change wet clothes frequently. Exercise in the evening or early morning if possible. Wear light-colored clothing.

If you are out of shape, working out extremely hard, or heavily muscled, take a water break every 15 to 20 minutes. Most importantly, replace body fluids and electrolytes lost through sweat by eating a healthy diet and drinking plenty of water.

Fluid Replacement for Exercise in Heat

Second only to spinal injuries, heat causes more deaths in high school/college football than any other factor. The number of heat-related injuries are common in summer and early fall sports. Most of these injuries can be avoided by following some simple guidelines when beginning workouts:

- All athletes should weigh themselves before and after practice. A loss of more than 2% of body weight between workouts is a sign of dehydration, which compromises physical performance. Losses greater than 3% body weight increase an athlete's risk of heat illness.

- Some athletes sweat more than others. These athletes need to consume more fluids than those who sweat less. Athletes who sweat heavily may need electrolyte replacement. Salt is abundant in the normal diet. The addition of calcium and potassium may be necessary. Milk and dairy products and green leafy vegetables are excellent calcium sources. Fruits (bananas, apricots, and dates) are excellent sources of potassium.

- Athletes need to pre-hydrate before exercise and re-hydrate during and after exercise. Athletes should consume about 20 ounces of fluid two to three hours before exercise. Most should be during meals and rest. During exercise, they should re-hydrate every 10 to 15 minutes with 8 to 10 ounces of fluid and continue to re-hydrate after practice until body weight is within 1% of pre-exercise norms.

- Sports drinks do little during exercise but may help after exercise. The electrolytes and carbohydrates they contain do little to help the athlete except in intense, sustained training (more than one hour). After exercise, these drinks may be beneficial in performance recovery. Sports drinks, fruit juice, and CHO [carbohydrate] gels should contain 6% sugar or less. Greater concentrations may delay fluid absorption, thus increasing dehydration. Soda, alcohol, and caffeine should be avoided altogether when dehydration is a factor.

- Children are not small adults. Children use more energy during exercise but have less blood/plasma volume to absorb and dissipate heat. Smaller skin area and fewer sweat glands further delay evaporation and cooling. Childhood fat also affects heat dissipation; fat acts as insulation. Overweight or obese athletes need to be closely monitored in the heat.

Section 16.2

Cold Weather Safety

Introduction

When exercising in cold weather, preventing cold-related injuries, such as "frostnip," frostbite, and hypothermia, is a major concern.

Another problem for athletes exercising outdoors for long periods is dehydration—even in cold weather. Fluid loss can also be monitored and avoided. With proper precautions, many training regimens can be maintained regardless of inclement weather.

Frostnip and Frostbite

Frostnip injuries to toes, fingers, ears, nose, and cheeks can occur in cold weather. Frostnip is the freezing of superficial tissue. The skin has a white, waxy appearance. This can be treated immediately by the contact of warm skin to the frozen part. The color change will be almost immediate. Do not rub.

Frostbite is a deeper, significantly more serious deep freezing of tissue. This requires skilled treatment to prevent permanent damage. *Seek medical attention.*

Hypothermia

Hypothermia is the cooling of core temperature. This is not a local cooling danger, but a cooling of the entire body. It brings a number of physiological risks, including cardiac arrhythmia, ataxia, and confusion.

Hypothermia is usually presented as uncoordinated movement, stumbling, slurred speech, and often inability to continue. The result can be cardiac arrhythmia and death. Care requires the immediate removal from the cold environment, and especially protection from any wind and/or rain. *Seek medical attention immediately.*

Clothing Selection for Exercise in the Cold

Cold-related injuries are avoidable with proper clothing selection. Clothing reduces airflow near the skin to reduce heat loss. Layering of clothing allows more exact alteration of insulation relative to changing exercise levels.

First layer: Select a material with a high wicking ability and low vapor retention for next to the skin, such as CoolMax or polypropylene. The high wicking ability moves sweat away before the cooling effect of evaporation occurs.

Second layer: The next layer should be thicker material for insulation. Synthetic fabrics such as fleece are ideal for this. These come in various thicknesses.

Third layer: Finally, wear an outer layer to block wind or rain as appropriate. Windproof and breathable fabrics are ideal. Cold rain can be more chilling than much colder dry temperatures. The face can be protected with a hood which extends forward of the face, but be careful of the limitations this puts on peripheral vision.

Keeping the trunk, legs, and arms warm with adequate clothing helps to keep toes and fingers warm. Remember that track shoes are usually designed for cooling, not insulation. Extra protection may be needed for the feet if running or cycling. Consult the running and cycling experts for good gear suggestions.

Thirst and Cold Weather

Exercising or playing sports in cold weather tends to make people less thirsty than at higher temperatures. Therefore, many of us are not concerned with fluid intake when the temperature is cold. Unfortunately, thirst is not a good indicator of body fluid needs. Dehydration can be a serious problem in cold weather if fluid consumption is not adequately maintained. Even a 1% to 2% loss in water can negatively influence athletic performance.

Cold weather usually involves dry air, which makes it more difficult to notice fluid loss. Unlike a hot and humid environment, where sweat visibly drips off the body, in a cold environment sweat can evaporate so quickly that you are unaware how rapidly fluid loss is occurring. Along with evaporation, cold weather also creates a loss of fluid through expired air. When cold air is inhaled it becomes saturated with water vapor from the respiratory tract and is then exhaled out of the body.

When it is cold enough that you can "see your breath," what you're really seeing is water escaping from your body. This can account for a fluid loss of 0.2–1.5 liters per day. These values increase with activity intensity.

Conclusion

A lot of people perform activities in the cold, whether working, playing football, jogging, or just walking. With proper clothing and fluid intake, most training regimens can be maintained in cold weather with excellent results.

Section 16.3

Lightning Safety

This section excerpted from "Lightning Risk Reduction Outdoors" and "Lightning Kills—Play It Safe," undated documents produced by the National Oceanic and Atmospheric Administration National Weather Service, available online at www.lightningsafety.noaa.gov/outdoors.htm and www .lightningsafety.noaa.gov/sports.htm.

Lightning Risk Reduction Outdoors

Definitions

Safe buildings: A safe building is one that is fully enclosed with a roof, walls, and floor, and has plumbing or wiring. Examples include a home, school, church, hotel, office building, or shopping center. Once inside, stay away from showers, sinks, bathtubs, and electronic equipment such as TVs, radios, corded telephones, and computers.

Unsafe buildings include car ports, open garages, covered patios, picnic shelters, beach pavilions, golf shelters, tents of any kinds, baseball dugouts, sheds, and greenhouses.

Safe vehicles: A safe vehicle is any fully enclosed metal-topped vehicle such as a hard-topped car, minivan, bus, truck, etc. While inside a safe vehicle, do not use electronic devices such as radio communications during a thunderstorm. If you drive into a thunderstorm, slow down and use extra caution. If possible, pull off the road into a safe area. Do not leave the vehicle during a thunderstorm.

Unsafe vehicles include convertibles, golf carts, riding mowers, open cab construction equipment, and boats without cabins.

Lightning Risk Reduction When a Safe Location Is Nearby

Run to a safe building or vehicle when you first hear thunder, see lightning, or observe dark threatening clouds developing overhead. Stay inside until 30 minutes after you hear the last clap of thunder.

Do not shelter under trees. You are *not safe* anywhere outside.

Plan ahead! Your best source of up-to-date weather information is a NOAA (National Oceanic and Atmospheric Administration) Weather Radio (NWR). Portable weather radios are handy for outdoor activities. If you don't have NWR, stay up to date via Internet, TV, local radio, or cell phone. If you are in a group, make sure all leaders or members of the group have a lightning safety plan and are ready to use it.

Outdoor Lightning Risk Reduction When a Safe Location Is Not Nearby

Remember, there is NO safe place outside in a thunderstorm. If you absolutely can't get to safety, this section may help you slightly lessen the threat of being struck by lightning while outside. Don't kid yourself—you are *not* safe outside.

Being stranded outdoors when lightning is striking nearby is a harrowing experience. Your first and only truly safe choice is to get to a safe building or vehicle. If you cannot get to a safe vehicle or building, follow these last-resort tips. They will not prevent you from being struck by lightning but may slightly lessen the odds.

- Know the weather patterns of the area. For example, in mountainous areas, thunderstorms typically develop in the early afternoon, so plan to hike early in the day and be down the mountain by noon.

- Listen to the weather forecast for the outdoor area you plan to visit. If there is a high chance of thunderstorms, stay inside.

These actions may slightly reduce your risk of being struck by lightning:

- If camping, hiking, etc., far from a safe vehicle or building, avoid open fields, the top of a hill, or a ridge top.

167

- Stay away from tall, isolated trees or other tall objects. If you are in a forest, stay near a lower stand of trees.

- Stay away from water, wet items (such as ropes), and metal objects (such as fences and poles). Water and metal are excellent conductors of electricity. The current from a lightning flash will easily travel for long distances.

Lightning Kills—Play It Safe

It's a common situation—a thunderstorm is approaching or nearby. Are conditions safe, or is it time to head for safety? Not wanting to appear overly cautious, many people wait far too long before reacting to this potentially deadly weather threat.

Each year across the United States, thunderstorms produce an estimated 25 million cloud-to-ground flashes of lightning—each one of those flashes is a potential killer. Based on cases documented by the National Weather Service over the past 30 years, an average of 55 people are killed by lightning each year and hundreds more are injured, some suffering devastating neurological injuries that persist for the rest of their lives. A growing percentage of those struck are involved in outside recreational activities.

Officials responsible for sports events and other outdoor activities often lack an adequate knowledge of thunderstorms and lightning to make educated decisions on when to seek safety. Without knowledge, officials base their decisions on personal experience and, sometimes, on the desire to complete the activity. Due to the nature of lightning, however, personal experience can be misleading. While many people routinely put their lives in jeopardy when thunderstorms are nearby, few are actually struck by lightning. This results in a false sense of safety. Unfortunately, this false sense of safety has resulted in numerous lightning deaths and injuries during the past several decades because people made decisions that unknowingly put their lives or the lives of others at risk.

For organized outdoor activities, the National Weather Service recommends that organizers have a lightning safety plan, and that they follow the plan without exception. The plan should give clear and specific safety guidelines in order to eliminate errors in judgment. These guidelines should answer the questions that follow in this section.

In addition, prior to an activity or event, organizers should listen to the latest forecast to determine the likelihood of thunderstorms. A NOAA Weather Radio is a good source of up-to-date weather information. If thunderstorms are forecast, organizers should consider canceling or postponing the activity or event. In some cases, the event can be moved indoors. Once people start to arrive at an event, the guidelines in the lightning safety plan should be followed. The following is some information to consider when making a lightning safety plan.

When should activities be stopped?

The sooner that activities are stopped and people get to a safe place, the greater the level of safety. In general, a significant lightning threat extends outward from the base of a thunderstorm cloud about 6 to 10 miles. Therefore, people should move to a safe place when a thunderstorm is 6 to 10 miles away. Also, the plan's guidelines should account for the time it will take for everyone to get to safety. Here are some criteria that could be used to halt activities.

- **If you see lightning:** The ability to see lightning varies depending on the time of day, weather conditions, and obstructions such as trees, mountains, etc. In clear air, and especially at night, lightning can be seen from storms more than 10 miles away provided that obstructions don't limit the view of the thunderstorm.

- **If you hear thunder:** Thunder can usually be heard for a distance of about 10 miles provided that there is no background noise. Traffic, wind, and precipitation may limit the ability to hear thunder to less than 10 miles. If you hear thunder, though, it's a safe bet that the storm is within 10 miles.

- **If the sky looks threatening:** Thunderstorms can develop directly overhead and some storms may develop lightning just as they move into an area.

Where should people go for safe shelter?

There is no place outside that is safe in or near a thunderstorm. Consequently, people need to stop what they are doing and get to a safe place immediately. Small outdoor buildings including dugouts, rain shelters, sheds, etc., are *not safe*.

Substantial buildings with wiring and plumbing provide the greatest amount of protection. Office buildings, schools, and homes are examples of buildings that would offer good protection. Once inside, stay away from windows and doors and anything that conducts electricity such as corded phones, wiring, plumbing, and anything connected to these.

In the absence of a substantial building, a hard-topped metal vehicle with the windows closed provides good protection. Occupants should avoid contact with metal in the vehicle and, to the extent possible, move away from windows.

When should activities be resumed?

Because electrical charges can linger in clouds after a thunderstorm has passed, experts agree that people should wait at least 30 minutes after the storm before resuming activities.

Who should monitor the weather and who is responsible to make the decision to stop activities?

Lightning safety plans should specify that someone be designated to monitor the weather for lightning. The "lightning monitor" should not be the coach, umpire, or referee, as they are not able to devote the attention needed to adequately monitor conditions. The "lightning monitor" must know the plan's guidelines and be empowered to assure that those guidelines are followed.

What should be done if someone is struck by lightning?

Most victims can survive a lightning strike; however, medical attention may be needed immediately—have someone call for medical help. Victims do not carry an electrical charge and should be attended to at once. In many cases, the victim's heart and/or breathing may have stopped and CPR and/or an automated external defibrillator (AED) may be needed to revive them. The victim should continue to be monitored until medical help arrives; heart and/or respiratory problems could persist, or the victim could go into shock. If possible, move the victim to a safer place away from the threat of another lightning strike.

Part Three

Head and Facial Injuries

Chapter 17

Sports-Related Head Injuries

Chapter Contents

Section 17.1

Traumatic Brain Injuries (TBI)

This section excerpted from "Traumatic Brain Injury: Hope through
Research," National Institute of Neurological Disorders and Stroke
(www.ninds.nih.gov), April 15, 2011.

What is a traumatic brain injury (TBI)?

TBI, a form of acquired brain injury, occurs when a sudden trauma
causes damage to the brain. The damage can be focal—confined to
one area of the brain—or diffuse—involving more than one area of
the brain. TBI can result from a closed head injury or a penetrating
head injury. A closed injury occurs when the head suddenly and vio-
lently hits an object but the object does not break through the skull. A
penetrating injury occurs when an object pierces the skull and enters
brain tissue.

What are the signs and symptoms of TBI?

Symptoms of a TBI can be mild, moderate, or severe, depending on
the extent of the damage to the brain. Some symptoms are evident
immediately, while others do not surface until several days or weeks
after the injury. A person with a mild TBI may remain conscious or
may experience a loss of consciousness for a few seconds or minutes.
The person may also feel dazed or not like himself for several days
or weeks after the initial injury. Other symptoms of mild TBI include
headache, confusion, lightheadedness, dizziness, blurred vision or tired
eyes, ringing in the ears, bad taste in the mouth, fatigue or lethargy,
a change in sleep patterns, behavioral or mood changes, and trouble
with memory, concentration, attention, or thinking.

A person with a moderate or severe TBI may show these same
symptoms, but may also have a headache that gets worse or does
not go away, repeated vomiting or nausea, convulsions or seizures,
inability to awaken from sleep, dilation of one or both pupils of the
eyes, slurred speech, weakness or numbness in the extremities, loss
of coordination, and/or increased confusion, restlessness, or agitation.

Small children with moderate to severe TBI may show some of these signs as well as signs specific to young children, such as persistent crying, inability to be consoled, and/or refusal to nurse or eat. Anyone with signs of moderate or severe TBI should receive medical attention as soon as possible.

What are the different types of TBI?

Concussion is the most minor and the most common type of TBI. Technically, a concussion is a short loss of consciousness in response to a head injury, but in common language the term has come to mean any minor injury to the head or brain.

Other injuries are more severe. As the first line of defense, the skull is particularly vulnerable to injury. Skull fractures occur when the bone of the skull cracks or breaks. A *depressed skull fracture* occurs when pieces of the broken skull press into the tissue of the brain. A *penetrating skull fracture* occurs when something pierces the skull, such as a bullet, leaving a distinct and localized injury to brain tissue.

Skull fractures can cause bruising of brain tissue called a *contusion*. A contusion is a distinct area of swollen brain tissue mixed with blood released from broken blood vessels. A contusion can also occur in response to shaking of the brain back and forth within the confines of the skull, an injury called *contrecoup*. In addition, contrecoup can cause *diffuse axonal injury*, also called *shearing*, which involves damage to individual nerve cells (neurons) and loss of connections among neurons. This can lead to a breakdown of overall communication among neurons in the brain.

Damage to a major blood vessel in the head can cause a *hematoma*, or heavy bleeding into or around the brain. Three types of hematomas can cause brain damage. An epidural hematoma involves bleeding into the area between the skull and the dura. With a subdural hematoma, bleeding is confined to the area between the dura and the arachnoid membrane. Bleeding within the brain itself is called intracerebral hematoma.

Another insult to the brain that can cause injury is *anoxia*. Anoxia is a condition in which there is an absence of oxygen supply to an organ's tissues, even if there is adequate blood flow to the tissue. *Hypoxia* refers to a decrease in oxygen supply rather than a complete absence of oxygen. Without oxygen, the cells of the brain die within several minutes. This type of injury is often seen in near-drowning victims, in heart attack patients, or in people who suffer significant blood loss from other injuries that increase blood flow to the brain.

What medical care should a TBI patient receive?

Medical care usually begins when paramedics or emergency medical technicians arrive on the scene of an accident or when a TBI patient arrives at the emergency department of a hospital. Because little can be done to reverse the initial brain damage caused by trauma, medical personnel try to stabilize the patient and focus on preventing further injury. Primary concerns include insuring proper oxygen supply to the brain and the rest of the body, maintaining adequate blood flow, and controlling blood pressure. Emergency medical personnel may have to open the patient's airway or perform other procedures to make sure the patient is breathing. They may also perform CPR [cardiopulmonary resuscitation] to help the heart pump blood to the body, and they may treat other injuries to control or stop bleeding. Because many head-injured patients may also have spinal cord injuries, medical professionals take great care in moving and transporting the patient.

As soon as medical personnel have stabilized the head-injured patient, they assess the patient's condition by measuring vital signs and reflexes and by performing a neurological examination. They check the patient's temperature, blood pressure, pulse, breathing rate, and pupil size in response to light. They assess the patient's level of consciousness and neurological functioning using the Glasgow Coma Scale, a standardized, 15-point test that uses three measures—eye opening, best verbal response, and best motor response—to determine the severity of the patient's brain injury.

How does a TBI affect consciousness?

A TBI can cause problems with arousal, consciousness, awareness, alertness, and responsiveness. Generally, there are five abnormal states of consciousness that can result from a TBI: stupor, coma, persistent vegetative state, locked-in syndrome, and brain death.

Stupor is a state in which the patient is unresponsive but can be aroused briefly by a strong stimulus, such as sharp pain. *Coma* is a state in which the patient is totally unconscious, unresponsive, unaware, and unarousable. Patients in a coma do not respond to external stimuli, such as pain or light, and do not have sleep-wake cycles. Coma generally is of short duration, lasting a few days to a few weeks. After this time, some patients gradually come out of the coma, some progress to a vegetative state, and others die.

Patients in a *vegetative state* are unconscious and unaware of their surroundings, but they continue to have a sleep-wake cycle and can have periods of alertness.

176

Many patients emerge from a vegetative state within a few weeks, but those who do not recover within 30 days are said to be in a *persistent vegetative state (PVS)*. The chances of recovery depend on the extent of injury to the brain and the patient's age, with younger patients having a better chance of recovery than older patients. The longer a patient is in a PVS, the more severe the resulting disabilities will be.

Locked-in syndrome is a condition in which a patient is aware and awake, but cannot move or communicate due to complete paralysis of the body. The majority of locked-in syndrome patients do not regain motor control, but several devices are available to help patients communicate.

With the development over the last half-century of assistive devices that can artificially maintain blood flow and breathing, the term *brain death* has come into use. Brain death is the lack of measurable brain function due to diffuse damage to the cerebral hemispheres and the brainstem, with loss of any integrated activity among distinct areas of the brain. Brain death is irreversible. Removal of assistive devices will result in immediate cardiac arrest and cessation of breathing.

What disabilities can result from a TBI?

Disabilities resulting from a TBI depend upon the severity of the injury, the location of the injury, and the age and general health of the patient. Some common disabilities include problems with cognition (thinking, memory, and reasoning), sensory processing (sight, hearing, touch, taste, and smell), communication (expression and understanding), and behavior or mental health (depression, anxiety, personality changes, aggression, acting out, and social inappropriateness).

Within days to weeks of the head injury, approximately 40% of TBI patients develop a host of troubling symptoms collectively called postconcussion syndrome (PCS). A patient need not have suffered a concussion or loss of consciousness to develop the syndrome, and many patients with mild TBI suffer from PCS. Symptoms include headache, dizziness, vertigo (a sensation of spinning around or of objects spinning around the patient), memory problems, trouble concentrating, sleeping problems, restlessness, irritability, apathy, depression, and anxiety. These symptoms may last for a few weeks after the head injury.

What kinds of rehabilitation should a TBI patient receive?

Rehabilitation is an important part of the recovery process for a TBI patient. During the acute stage, moderately to severely injured patients may receive treatment and care in an intensive care unit of a hospital. Once stable, the patient may be transferred to a subacute unit of the medical center or to an independent rehabilitation hospital. At this point, patients follow many diverse paths toward recovery because there are a wide variety of options for rehabilitation.

Testing by a trained neuropsychologist can assess the individual's cognitive, language, behavioral, motor, and executive functions and provide information regarding the need for rehabilitative services.

Section 17.2

Concussions

This section excerpted from "Concussion in Sports," December 8, 2009, and "Concussion: What Can I Do to Help Feel Better after a Concussion?" March 8, 2010, Centers for Disease Control and Prevention (www.cdc.gov).

Concussion in Sports

- A concussion is a brain injury and all are serious.

- Most concussions occur without loss of consciousness.

- Recognition and proper response to concussions when they first occur can help prevent further injury or even death.

A concussion is a type of traumatic brain injury, or TBI, caused by a bump, blow, or jolt to the head that can change the way your brain normally works. Concussions can also occur from a blow to the body that causes the head to move rapidly back and forth. Even a "ding," "getting your bell rung," or what seems to be mild bump or blow to the head can be serious.

Concussions can occur in any sport or recreation activity. So, all coaches, parents, and athletes need to learn concussion signs and symptoms and what to do if a concussion occurs.

Recognizing a Possible Concussion

To help recognize a concussion, you should watch for the following two things among your athletes:

- a forceful bump, blow, or jolt to the head or body that results in rapid movement of the head *and*
- any change in the athlete's behavior, thinking, or physical functioning.

Athletes who experience any of the signs and symptoms listed here after a bump, blow, or jolt to the head or body should be kept out of play the day of the injury and until a health care professional, experienced in evaluating for concussion, says they are symptom-free and it's okay to return to play.

Signs Observed by Coaching Staff

- Appears dazed or stunned
- Is confused about assignment or position
- Forgets an instruction
- Is unsure of game, score, or opponent
- Moves clumsily
- Answers questions slowly
- Loses consciousness (even briefly)
- Shows mood, behavior, or personality changes
- Can't recall events prior to hit or fall
- Can't recall events after hit or fall

Symptoms Reported by Athlete

- Headache or "pressure" in head
- Nausea or vomiting
- Balance problems or dizziness
- Double or blurry vision
- Sensitivity to light
- Sensitivity to noise
- Feeling sluggish, hazy, foggy, or groggy
- Concentration or memory problems

179

- Confusion

- Does not "feel right" or is "feeling down"

Remember, you can't see a concussion and some athletes may not experience and/or report symptoms until hours or days after the injury. Most people with a concussion will recover quickly and fully. But for some people, signs and symptoms of concussion can last for days, weeks, or longer.

If a Concussion Occurs

If you suspect that an athlete has a concussion, implement your four-step action plan:

1. Remove the athlete from play. Look for signs and symptoms of a concussion if your athlete has experienced a bump or blow to the head or body. When in doubt, keep the athlete out of play.

2. Ensure that the athlete is evaluated by a health care professional experienced in evaluating for concussion. Do not try to judge the severity of the injury yourself. Health care professionals have a number of methods that they can use to assess the severity of concussions. As a coach, recording the following information can help health care professionals in assessing the athlete after the injury:

   - Cause of the injury and force of the hit or blow to the head or body

   - Any loss of consciousness (passed out/knocked out) and, if so, for how long

   - Any memory loss immediately following the injury

   - Any seizures immediately following the injury

   - Number of previous concussions (if any)

3. Inform the athlete's parents or guardians about the possible concussion and give them a fact sheet on concussion. Make sure they know that the athlete should be seen by a health care professional experienced in evaluating for concussion.

4. Keep the athlete out of play the day of the injury and until a health care professional, experienced in evaluating for concussion, says they are symptom-free and it's okay to return to play. A repeat concussion that occurs before the brain recovers

from the first—usually within a short period of time (hours, days, or weeks)—can slow recovery or increase the likelihood of having long-term problems. In rare cases, repeat concussions can result in edema (brain swelling), permanent brain damage, and even death.

Preventing Concussions

As a coach or parent, you play a key role in preventing concussions and responding properly when they occur. Here are some steps you can take to help prevent concussions and ensure the best outcome for your athletes, the team, league, or school.

Check with your league, school, or district about concussion policies. Concussion policy statements can be developed to include a commitment to safety, a brief description about concussion, and information on when athletes can safely return to play. Parents and athletes should sign the concussion policy statement at the beginning of each sports season.

Involve and get support from other parents and/or league or school officials to help ensure that the concussion policy is in place before the first practice.

Create a concussion action plan. To ensure that concussions are identified early and managed correctly, have an action plan in place before the season starts. This plan can be included in your school or district's concussion policy.

Educate athletes and other parents or coaches about concussion. Before the first practice, talk to athletes and parents, and other coaches and school officials, about the dangers of concussion and potential long-term consequences of concussion. Explain your concerns about concussion and your expectations of safe play. Show the videos and pass out the concussion fact sheets for athletes and for parents at the beginning of the season and again if a concussion occurs. Remind athletes to tell coaching staff right away if they suspect they have a concussion or that a teammate has a concussion.

Monitor the health of your athletes. Make sure to ask if an athlete has ever had a concussion and insist that your athletes are medically evaluated and are in good condition to participate. Some schools and leagues conduct preseason baseline testing (also known as neurocognitive tests) to assess brain function—learning and memory skills, ability to pay attention or concentrate, and how quickly someone can think and solve problems. These tests can be used again during the season if an athlete has a concussion to help identify the effects of the injury. Prior to the first practice, determine whether your school or league would consider conducting baseline testing.

Prevention during the Season: Practices and Games

Make safety a priority. Insist that safety comes first.

- Teach and practice safe playing techniques.

- Encourage athletes to follow the rules of play and to practice good sportsmanship at all times.

- Make sure athletes wear the right protective equipment for their activity (such as helmets, padding, shin guards, and eye and mouth guards). Protective equipment should fit properly, be well maintained, and be worn consistently and correctly.

Teach athletes it's not smart to play with a concussion. Rest is key after a concussion. Sometimes athletes, parents, and other school or league officials wrongly believe that it shows strength and courage to play injured. Discourage others from pressuring injured athletes to play. Don't let your athlete convince you that they're "just fine."

Prevent long-term problems. If an athlete has a concussion, their brain needs time to heal. Don't let them return to play the day of the injury and until a health care professional, experienced in evaluating for concussion, says they are symptom-free and it's okay to return to play. A repeat concussion that occurs before the brain recovers from the first—usually within a short time period (hours, days, weeks)—can slow recovery or increase the chances for long-term problems.

Work closely with league or school officials. Be sure that appropriate individuals are available for injury assessment and referrals for further medical care. Enlist health care professionals (including school nurses) to monitor any changes in the athlete's behavior that could indicate that they have a concussion. Ask athletes or parents to report concussions that occurred during any sport or recreation activity. This will help in monitoring injured athletes who participate in multiple sports throughout the year.

Postseason Prevention

Keep track of concussion. Coaches should work with other school or league officials to review injuries that occurred during the season. Discuss with others any needs for better concussion prevention or response preparations.

Review your concussion policy and action plan. Discuss any need for improvements in your concussion policy or action plan with appropriate health care professionals and school and league officials.

What Can I Do to Help Feel Better after a Concussion?

Although most people recover fully after a concussion, how quickly they improve depends on many factors. These factors include how severe their concussion was, their age, how healthy they were before the concussion, and how they take care of themselves after the injury.

Some people who have had a concussion find that at first it is hard to do their daily activities, their job, to get along with everyone at home, or to relax.

Rest is very important after a concussion because it helps the brain to heal. Ignoring your symptoms and trying to "tough it out" often makes symptoms worse. Be patient because healing takes time. Only when your symptoms have reduced significantly, in consultation with your health care professional, should you slowly and gradually return to your daily activities, such as work or school. If your symptoms come back or you get new symptoms as you become more active, this is a sign that you are pushing yourself too hard. Stop these activities and take more time to rest and recover. As the days go by, you can expect to gradually feel better.

Getting Better: Tips for Adults

- Get plenty of sleep at night, and rest during the day.

- Avoid activities that are physically demanding (e.g., heavy housecleaning, weightlifting/working out) or require a lot of concentration (e.g., balancing your checkbook). They can make your symptoms worse and slow your recovery.

- Avoid activities, such as contact or recreational sports, that could lead to another concussion. (It is best to avoid roller coasters or other high-speed rides that can make your symptoms worse or even cause a concussion.)

- When your health care professional says you are well enough, return to your normal activities gradually, not all at once.

- Because your ability to react may be slower after a concussion, ask your health care professional when you can safely drive a car, ride a bike, or operate heavy equipment.

- Talk with your health care professional about when you can return to work. Ask about how you can help your employer understand what has happened to you.

- Consider talking with your employer about returning to work gradually and about changing your work activities or schedule until you recover (e.g., work half-days).

- Take only those drugs that your health care professional has approved.

- Do not drink alcoholic beverages until your health care professional says you are well enough. Alcohol and other drugs may slow your recovery and put you at risk of further injury.

- Write down the things that may be harder than usual for you to remember.

- If you're easily distracted, try to do one thing at a time. For example, don't try to watch TV while fixing dinner.

- Consult with family members or close friends when making important decisions.

- Do not neglect your basic needs, such as eating well and getting enough rest.

- Avoid sustained computer use, including computer/video games, early in the recovery process.

- Some people report that flying in airplanes makes their symptoms worse shortly after a concussion.

Getting Better: Tips for Children

Parents and caregivers of children who have had a concussion can help them recover by taking an active role in their recovery:

- Have the child get plenty of rest. Keep a regular sleep schedule, including no late nights and no sleepovers.

- Make sure the child avoids high-risk/high-speed activities such as riding a bicycle, playing sports, climbing playground equipment, or roller coasters or rides that could result in another bump, blow, or jolt to the head or body. Children should not return to these types of activities until their health care professional says they are well enough.

- Give the child only those drugs that are approved by the pediatrician or family physician.

- Talk with their health care professional about when the child should return to school and other activities and how the parent or caregiver can help the child deal with the challenges that the child may face. For example, your child may need to spend fewer hours at school, rest often, or require more time to take tests.

- Share information about concussion with parents, siblings, teachers, counselors, babysitters, coaches, and others who interact with the child to help them understand what has happened and how to meet the child's needs.

Help Prevent Long-Term Problems

If you already had a medical condition at the time of your concussion (such as chronic headaches), it may take longer for you to recover from the concussion. Anxiety and depression may also make it harder to adjust to the symptoms of a concussion. While you are healing, you should be very careful to avoid doing anything that could cause a bump, blow, or jolt to the head or body. On rare occasions, receiving another concussion before the brain has healed can result in brain swelling, permanent brain damage, and even death, particularly among children and teens.

After you have recovered from your concussion, you should protect yourself from having another one. People who have had repeated concussions may have serious long-term problems, including chronic difficulty with concentration, memory, headache, and occasionally, physical skills, such as keeping one's balance.

Chapter 18

Sports Injuries to the Face

Chapter Contents

Section 18.1

Jaw Injuries

A broken jaw is a break in the jaw bone. A dislocated jaw means the lower part of the jaw has moved out of its normal position at one or both joints where the jaw bone connects to the skull (temporomandibular joints [TMJs]).

Considerations

A broken or dislocated jaw usually heals completely after treatment. However, the jaw may become dislocated again in the future.
Complications may include:

- airway blockage;

- bleeding;

- breathing blood or food into the lungs;

- difficulty eating (temporary);

- difficulty talking (temporary);

- infection of the jaw or face;

- jaw joint (TMJ) pain and other problems;

- problems aligning the teeth.

Causes

The most common cause of a broken or dislocated jaw is injury to the face. This may be due to:

- assault;

- industrial accident;

- motor vehicle accident;
- recreational or sports injury.

Symptoms

Symptoms of a dislocated jaw include:

- bite that feels "off" or crooked;
- difficulty speaking;
- drooling because of inability to close the mouth;
- inability to close the mouth;
- jaw that may protrude forward;
- pain in the face or jaw, located in front of the ear on the affected side, and gets worse with movement;
- teeth that do not line up properly.

Symptoms of a fractured (broken) jaw include:

- bleeding from the mouth;
- difficulty opening the mouth widely;
- facial bruising;
- facial swelling;
- jaw stiffness;
- jaw tenderness or pain, worse with biting or chewing;
- loose or damaged teeth;
- lump or abnormal appearance of the cheek or jaw;
- numbness of the face (particularly the lower lip);
- very limited movement of the jaw (with severe fracture).

First Aid

A broken or dislocated jaw requires immediate medical attention because of the risk of breathing problems or significant bleeding. Call your local emergency number (such as 911) or local hospital for further advice.

Hold the jaw gently in place with your hands while traveling to the emergency room. A bandage may also be wrapped over the top of the head and under the jaw. However, such a bandage should be easily removable in case you need to vomit.

If breathing problems or heavy bleeding occurs, or if there is severe facial swelling, a tube may be placed into your airways to help you breathe.

Dislocated Jaw

If the jaw is dislocated, the health care provider may be able to place it back into the correct position using the thumbs. Numbing medications (anesthetics) and muscle relaxants may be needed to relax the strong jaw muscles.

The jaw may need to be stabilized. This usually involves bandaging the jaw to keep the mouth from opening widely. In some cases, surgery may be needed to do this, particularly if repeated jaw dislocations occur.

After dislocating your jaw, you should not open your mouth widely for at least six weeks. Support your jaw with one or both hands when yawning and sneezing.

Fractured Jaw

Temporarily bandaging the jaw (around the top of the head) to prevent it from moving may help reduce pain.

The specific treatment for a fractured jaw depends on how badly the bone is broken. If you have a minor fracture, you may only need pain medicines and to follow a soft or liquid diet for a while.

Surgery is often needed for moderate to severe fractures. The jaw may be wired to the teeth of the opposite jaw to improve stability. Jaw wires are usually left in place for six to eight weeks. Small rubber bands (elastics) are used to hold the teeth together. After a few weeks, some of the elastics are removed to allow motion and reduce joint stiffness.

If the jaw is wired, you can only drink liquids or eat very soft foods. Have blunt scissors readily available to cut the elastics in the event of vomiting or choking. If the wires must be cut, consult a health care provider promptly so they can be replaced.

DO NOT

Do NOT attempt to correct the position of the jaw.

When to Contact a Medical Professional

A broken or dislocated jaw requires immediate medical attention. Emergency symptoms include difficulty breathing or heavy bleeding.

Prevention

Safe practices in work, sports, and recreation, such as wearing a proper helmet when playing football, may prevent some accidental injuries to the face or jaw.

Section 18.2

Eye Injuries

Introduction

While eye injuries in sports are not common, they can be serious when they occur.

While the risk of eye injury is related to sport, most injuries can be prevented with protective eyewear.

Injuries to the eye range from foreign bodies (dirt, sand, etc.) to orbital fractures. These injuries have increased in past years due to the popularity of baseball and softball. Foreign bodies and abrasions (scratches) to the eyes are among the more common injuries during athletics.

Athletes often say they "feel something in their eye." It is important to know that foreign bodies in the eye and abrasion injuries produce the same symptoms. These symptoms include pain, increased tearing, and the sensation of something in the eye. Do not rub the eye, as this will make matters worse. Have the athlete close the eye until the initial pain subsides. Most of the time the increased tearing will "wash out" the foreign object. Rinsing with water may also help remove the foreign object.

If you try to wash out the object and it does not come out, do not try to remove it by using your fingernail, Q-tip, or other small object. Cover the eye and take the athlete to the doctor or emergency room to have the object removed. Sometimes these objects can become imbedded in the eye and attempts to remove them can make matters worse.

If you do remove the object and the athlete still complains of "something in there," there may be an abrasion of the eye. In this case, the athlete needs to see a doctor. This injury can also occur from getting "a finger in the eye."

Even though the eye is well protected within the eye socket, it can be bruised during sports. The injury can be as mild as a bruise or as severe as an orbital fracture.

Most of the injuries to the eye are of the mild type, commonly, the "dreaded" black eye. A blow to this area can cause damage to the tissue surrounding the eye causing the black eye. Use ice after a black eye to help control swelling and pain in the area. Don't blow your nose following a black eye as this will cause increased swelling.

Symptoms that indicate a serious eye injury include: blurred vision that does not clear when blinking, loss of part or all vision in the affected eye, a sharp stabbing or throbbing pain in the eye, or double vision. A bubbling sensation or crackling sounds in the soft tissues near the nose or over the cheek may indicate an orbital floor fracture. *If any these symptoms occur, the athlete should cover the eye and be taken to the emergency room.*

Eye injuries should be taken seriously. Athletes should not return to sports until pain-free full vision is obtained. If a physician saw

Table 18.1. Sports Eye Injuries in the U.S.

Sport	Percent
Baseball	27
Racquet sports	20
Basketball	20
Football and soccer	7
Ice hockey	4

Modern Principles of Athletic Training, 9th Edition by Daniel Arnheim and William Prentice.

the athlete, a medical clearance must be obtained to return to activity. Eye injuries are not very commonplace, but can be serious if left untreated.

Section 18.3

Cauliflower Ear

"What Is Cauliflower Ear?," September 2010, reprinted with permission from www.kidshealth.org. Copyright © 2010 The Nemours Foundation. This information was provided by KidsHealth, one of the largest resources online for medically reviewed health information written for parents, kids, and teens. For more articles like this one, visit www.KidsHealth.org, or www.TeensHealth.org.

Have you ever seen someone whose ear looks bumpy and lumpy? The person might have cauliflower ear.

Cauliflower ear occurs after someone gets a hit or repeated hits to the ear. Wrestlers and boxers are more likely to have cauliflower ear because their ears may be hit while they're in a match. These blows can damage the shape and structure of the outside of the ear.

For cauliflower ear to form, the ear has to be struck hard enough for a large blood clot (lump of blood) to develop under the skin. Another way cauliflower ear can happen is when the ear's skin is stripped away from the cartilage, the flexible material that gives a normal ear its shape.

This cartilage needs oxygen and nutrients carried by the flow of blood. A tear, severe bruise, or blood clot can block the blood flow. If that happens, the cartilage can die. Without cartilage to keep its firm, rounded shape, the ear shrivels a bit and the cauliflower look begins to appear. Once this happens, the person's ear may look like this permanently.

You may be wondering if there's any way to prevent cauliflower ear. Wearing the right headgear when playing sports—especially contact sports—is a must. Helmets not only can save you from developing cauliflower ear but protect you from serious head injury as well. Always wear a helmet if you are biking, blading, riding your scooter, or playing any sport where helmets or other forms of headgear are recommended or required (like football, baseball, hockey, boxing, or wrestling).

If someone receives a sharp blow to the ear, there are ways to prevent cauliflower ear. A doctor can drain the blood from the ear through a cut and then reconnect skin to the cartilage by applying a tight bandage. Sometimes stitches are needed to sew the ear if the skin is badly ripped. The doctor may sometimes give the patient antibiotics to prevent an infection. If it's caught and treated early enough, a person usually will not get cauliflower ear.

With a little protection, you can make sure that the only cauliflower you see is on your dinner plate!

Part Four

Back, Neck,
and Spine Injuries

Chapter 19

Lower Back Pain in Athletes

If you have lower back pain, you are not alone. Nearly everyone at some point has back pain that interferes with work, routine daily activities, or recreation. Americans spend at least $50 billion each year on low back pain, the most common cause of job-related disability and a leading contributor to missed work. Back pain is the second most common neurological ailment in the United States—only headache is more common. Fortunately, most occurrences of low back pain go away within a few days. Others take much longer to resolve or lead to more serious conditions.

Acute or short-term low back pain generally lasts from a few days to a few weeks. Most acute back pain is mechanical in nature—the result of trauma to the lower back or a disorder such as arthritis. Pain from trauma may be caused by a sports injury, work around the house or in the garden, or a sudden jolt such as a car accident or other stress on spinal bones and tissues. Symptoms may range from muscle ache to shooting or stabbing pain, limited flexibility and/or range of motion, or an inability to stand straight. Occasionally, pain felt in one part of the body may "radiate" from a disorder or injury elsewhere in the body. Some acute pain syndromes can become more serious if left untreated.

Chronic back pain is measured by duration—pain that persists for more than three months is considered chronic. It is often progressive, and the cause can be difficult to determine.

This chapter excerpted from "Low Back Pain Fact Sheet," National Institute of Neurological Disorders and Stroke (www.ninds.nih.gov), April 20, 2011.

What structures make up the back?

The back is an intricate structure of bones, muscles, and other tissues that form the posterior part of the body's trunk, from the neck to the pelvis. The centerpiece is the spinal column, which not only supports the upper body's weight but houses and protects the spinal cord—the delicate nervous system structure that carries signals that control the body's movements and convey its sensations. Stacked on top of one another are more than 30 bones—the vertebrae—that form the spinal column, also known as the spine. Each of these bones contains a roundish hole that, when stacked in register with all the others, creates a channel that surrounds the spinal cord. The spinal cord descends from the base of the brain and extends in the adult to just below the rib cage. Small nerves ("roots") enter and emerge from the spinal cord through spaces between the vertebrae. Because the bones of the spinal column continue growing long after the spinal cord reaches its full length in early childhood, the nerve roots to the lower back and legs extend many inches down the spinal column before exiting. This large bundle of nerve roots was dubbed by early anatomists as the cauda equina, or horse's tail. The spaces between the vertebrae are maintained by round, spongy pads of cartilage called intervertebral discs that allow for flexibility in the lower back and act much like shock absorbers throughout the spinal column to cushion the bones as the body moves. Bands of tissue known as ligaments and tendons hold the vertebrae in place and attach the muscles to the spinal column.

The lumbar region of the back, where most back pain is felt, supports the weight of the upper body.

What causes lower back pain?

As people age, bone strength and muscle elasticity and tone tend to decrease. The discs begin to lose fluid and flexibility, which decreases their ability to cushion the vertebrae.

Pain can occur when, for example, someone lifts something too heavy or overstretches, causing a sprain, strain, or spasm in one of the muscles or ligaments in the back. If the spine becomes overly strained or compressed, a disc may rupture or bulge outward. This rupture may put pressure on one of the more than 50 nerves rooted to the spinal cord. When these nerve roots become compressed or irritated, back pain results.

Low back pain may reflect nerve or muscle irritation or bone lesions. Most low back pain follows injury or trauma to the back, but pain may also be caused by degenerative conditions such as arthritis or disc disease, osteoporosis or other bone diseases, viral infections, irritation to joints and discs, or congenital abnormalities in the spine. Obesity, smoking, weight gain during pregnancy, stress, poor physical condition, posture inappropriate for the activity being performed, and poor sleeping position also may contribute to low back pain. Additionally, scar tissue created when the injured back heals itself does not have the strength or flexibility of normal tissue. Buildup of scar tissue from repeated injuries eventually weakens the back and can lead to more serious injury.

Occasionally, low back pain may indicate a more serious medical problem. Pain accompanied by fever or loss of bowel or bladder control, pain when coughing, and progressive weakness in the legs may indicate a pinched nerve or other serious condition. People with these symptoms should contact a doctor immediately to help prevent permanent damage.

Who is most likely to develop low back pain?

Nearly everyone has low back pain sometime. Men and women are equally affected. It occurs most often between ages 30 and 50, due in part to the aging process but also as a result of sedentary lifestyles with too little (sometimes punctuated by too much) exercise. The risk of experiencing low back pain from disc disease or spinal degeneration increases with age.

Low back pain unrelated to injury or other known cause is unusual in preteen children. However, a backpack overloaded with schoolbooks and supplies can quickly strain the back and cause muscle fatigue.

What conditions are associated with low back pain?

Conditions that may cause low back pain and require treatment by a physician or other health specialist include the following:

Bulging disc (also called protruding, herniated, or ruptured disc) involves the intervertebral discs. As discs degenerate and weaken, cartilage can bulge or be pushed into the space containing the spinal cord or a nerve root, causing pain. Studies have shown that most herniated discs occur in the lower, lumbar portion of the spinal column.

Sciatica is a condition in which a herniated or ruptured disc presses on the sciatic nerve, the large nerve that extends down the spinal column to its exit point in the pelvis and carries nerve fibers to the leg. This compression causes shock-like or burning low back pain combined with pain through the buttocks and down one leg to below the knee, occasionally reaching the foot.

Spinal degeneration from disc wear and tear can lead to a narrowing of the spinal canal. A person with spinal degeneration may experience stiffness in the back upon awakening or may feel pain after walking or standing for a long time.

Osteoporosis is a metabolic bone disease marked by progressive decrease in bone density and strength. Fracture of brittle, porous bones in the spine and hips results when the body fails to produce new bone and/or absorbs too much existing bone. Women are four times more likely than men to develop osteoporosis.

Fibromyalgia is a chronic disorder characterized by widespread musculoskeletal pain, fatigue, and multiple "tender points," particularly in the neck, spine, shoulders, and hips. Additional symptoms may include sleep disturbances, morning stiffness, and anxiety.

Spondylitis refers to chronic back pain and stiffness caused by a severe infection to or inflammation of the spinal joints. Other painful inflammations in the lower back include osteomyelitis (infection in the bones of the spine) and sacroiliitis (inflammation in the sacroiliac joints).

How is low back pain diagnosed?

A thorough medical history and physical exam can usually identify any dangerous conditions or family history that may be associated with the pain. The patient describes the onset, site, and severity of the pain; duration of symptoms and any limitations in movement; and history of previous episodes or any health conditions that might be related to the pain. The physician will examine the back and conduct neurological tests to determine the cause of pain and appropriate treatment. Blood tests may also be ordered. Imaging tests may be necessary to diagnose tumors or other possible sources of the pain.

A variety of diagnostic methods are available to confirm the cause of low back pain:

X-ray imaging includes conventional and enhanced methods that can help diagnose the cause and site of back pain. A conventional X-ray, often the first imaging technique used, looks for broken bones or an injured vertebra.

Discography involves the injection of a special contrast dye into a spinal disc thought to be causing low back pain. The dye outlines the damaged areas on X-rays taken following the injection.

Computerized tomography (CT) is a quick and painless process used when disc rupture, spinal stenosis, or damage to vertebrae is suspected as a cause of low back pain. X-rays are passed through the body at various angles and are detected by a computerized scanner to produce two-dimensional slices of internal structures of the back.

Magnetic resonance imaging (MRI) is used to evaluate the lumbar region for bone degeneration or injury or disease in tissues and nerves, muscles, ligaments, and blood vessels. A computer processes the results into either a three-dimensional picture or a two-dimensional "slice" of the tissue being scanned and differentiates between bone, soft tissues, and fluid-filled spaces by their water content and structural properties.

Electrodiagnostic procedures include electromyography (EMG), nerve conduction studies, and evoked potential (EP) studies. EMG assesses the electrical activity in a nerve and can detect if muscle weakness results from injury or a problem with the nerves that control the muscles. With nerve conduction studies the doctor uses two sets of electrodes that are placed on the skin over the muscles so the doctor can determine if there is nerve damage. EP tests also involve two sets of electrodes—one set to stimulate a sensory nerve and the other on the scalp to record the speed of nerve signal transmissions to the brain.

Bone scans are used to diagnose and monitor infection, fracture, or disorders in the bone. Scanner-generated images are sent to a computer to identify specific areas of irregular bone metabolism or abnormal blood flow, as well as to measure levels of joint disease.

Thermography involves the use of infrared sensing devices to measure small temperature changes between the two sides of the body or the temperature of a specific organ. Thermography may be used to detect the presence or absence of nerve root compression.

Ultrasound imaging, also called ultrasound scanning or sonography, uses high-frequency sound waves to obtain images inside the body. Ultrasound imaging can show tears in ligaments, muscles, tendons, and other soft tissue masses in the back.

How is back pain treated?

Most low back pain can be treated without surgery. Treatment involves using analgesics, reducing inflammation, restoring proper function and strength to the back, and preventing recurrence of the injury. Most patients with back pain recover without residual functional loss. Patients should contact a doctor if there is not a noticeable reduction in pain and inflammation after 72 hours of self-care.

Ice and heat (the use of cold and hot compresses) have never been scientifically proven to quickly resolve low back injury, but compresses may help reduce pain and inflammation and allow greater mobility for some individuals. As soon as possible following trauma, patients should apply a cold pack or a cold compress (such as a bag of ice or bag of frozen vegetables wrapped in a towel) to the tender spot several times a day for up to 20 minutes. After two to three days of cold treatment, they should then apply heat (such as a heating lamp or hot pad) for brief periods to relax muscles and increase blood flow. Warm baths may also help relax muscles. Patients should avoid sleeping on a heating pad, which can cause burns and lead to additional tissue damage.

Bed rest of one to two days at most may be beneficial. A 1996 Finnish study found that persons who continued their activities without bed rest following onset of low back pain appeared to have better back flexibility than those who rested in bed for a week. Other studies suggest that bed rest alone may make back pain worse and can lead to secondary complications. Patients should resume activities as soon as possible. At night or during rest, patients should lie on one side, with a pillow between the knees.

Exercise may be the most effective way to speed recovery from low back pain and help strengthen back and abdominal muscles. Doctors and physical therapists can provide a list of gentle exercises that help keep muscles moving and speed the recovery process. A routine of back-healthy activities may include stretching exercises, swimming, walking, and movement therapy to improve coordination and develop proper posture and muscle balance. Any mild discomfort felt at the start of these exercises should disappear as muscles become stronger. But if pain is more than mild and lasts more than 15 minutes during exercise, patients should stop exercising and contact a doctor.

Medications are often used to treat acute and chronic low back pain. Effective pain relief may involve a combination of prescription drugs and over-the-counter remedies. Patients should always check with a doctor before taking drugs for pain relief. Certain medicines, even those sold over the counter, are unsafe during pregnancy, may conflict with other medications, may cause side effects, or may lead to liver damage.

- **Over-the-counter analgesics**, including nonsteroidal anti-inflammatory drugs (aspirin, naproxen, and ibuprofen), are taken orally to reduce stiffness, swelling, and inflammation and to ease mild to moderate low back pain. Counter-irritants applied topically to the skin stimulate the nerve endings in the skin to provide feelings of warmth or cold and dull the sense of pain. Topical analgesics can also reduce inflammation and stimulate blood flow.

- **Anticonvulsants**—drugs primarily used to treat seizures—may be useful in treating certain types of nerve pain and may also be prescribed with analgesics.

- **Some antidepressants**, particularly tricyclic antidepressants such as amitriptyline and desipramine, have been shown to relieve pain (independent of their effect on depression) and assist with sleep.

- **Opioids** such as codeine, oxycodone, hydrocodone, and morphine are often prescribed to manage severe acute and chronic back pain but should be used only for a short period of time and under a physician's supervision.

Spinal manipulation is literally a "hands-on" approach in which professionally licensed specialists (doctors of chiropractic care) use leverage and a series of exercises to adjust spinal structures and restore back mobility.

When back pain does not respond to more conventional approaches, patients may consider alternative options, such as acupuncture, biofeedback, interventional therapy, traction, transcutaneous electrical nerve stimulation (TENS), and ultrasound.

In the most serious cases, when the condition does not respond to other therapies, surgery may relieve pain caused by back problems or serious musculoskeletal injuries. Some surgical procedures may be performed in a doctor's office under local anesthesia, while others require hospitalization. It may be months following surgery before the patient is fully healed, and he or she may suffer permanent loss of flexibility. Since invasive back surgery is not always successful, it should be performed only in patients with progressive neurological disease or damage to the peripheral nerves.

Can back pain be prevented?

Recurring back pain resulting from improper body mechanics or other nontraumatic causes is often preventable. A combination of exercises that don't jolt or strain the back, maintaining correct posture, and lifting objects properly can help prevent injuries.

Many work-related injuries are caused or aggravated by stressors such as heavy lifting, contact stress (repeated or constant contact between soft body tissue and a hard or sharp object, such as resting a wrist against the edge of a hard desk or repeated tasks using a hammering motion), vibration, repetitive motion, and awkward posture. Applying ergonomic principles—designing furniture and tools to protect the body from injury—at home and in the workplace can greatly reduce the risk of back injury and help maintain a healthy back.

The use of wide elastic belts that can be tightened to "pull in" lumbar and abdominal muscles to prevent low back pain remains controversial. A landmark study of the use of lumbar support or abdominal support belts worn by persons who lift or move merchandise found no evidence that the belts reduce back injury or back pain.

What activities can promote a healthier back?

Following any period of prolonged inactivity, begin a program of regular low-impact exercises. Speed walking, swimming, or stationary bike riding 30 minutes a day can increase muscle strength and flexibility. Yoga can also help stretch and strengthen muscles and improve posture. Ask your physician or orthopedist for a list of low-impact exercises appropriate for your age and designed to strengthen lower back and abdominal muscles.

- Always stretch before exercise or other strenuous physical activity.

- Don't slouch when standing or sitting. When standing, keep your weight balanced on your feet. Your back supports weight most easily when curvature is reduced.

- At home or work, make sure your work surface is at a comfortable height for you.

- Sit in a chair with good lumbar support and proper position and height for the task. Keep your shoulders back. Switch sitting positions often and periodically walk around the office or gently stretch muscles to relieve tension. A pillow or rolled-up towel placed behind the small of your back can provide some lumbar support. If you must sit for a long period of time, rest your feet on a low stool or a stack of books.

- Wear comfortable, low-heeled shoes.

- Sleep on your side to reduce any curve in your spine. Always sleep on a firm surface.

- Don't try to lift objects too heavy for you. Lift with your knees, pull in your stomach muscles, and keep your head down and in line with your straight back. Keep the object close to your body. Do not twist when lifting.

- Maintain proper nutrition and diet to reduce and prevent excessive weight, especially weight around the waistline that taxes lower back muscles. A diet with sufficient daily intake of calcium, phosphorus, and vitamin D helps to promote new bone growth.

- If you smoke, quit. Smoking reduces blood flow to the lower spine and causes the spinal discs to degenerate.

Chapter 20

Spondylolysis and Spondylolisthesis

Overview

Spondylolysis (spon-dee-low-lye-sis) and spondylolisthesis (spon-dee-low-lis-thee-sis) are conditions that affect the moveable joints of the spine that help keep the vertebrae aligned one on top of the other. Spondylolysis is actually a weakness or stress fracture in one of the bony bridges that connects the upper and lower facet joints. This fracture can happen at any level of the spine but usually occurs at the fourth (L4) or fifth (L5) lumbar vertebra. This weakness can cause the vertebrae to slip forward out of their normal position, a condition called spondylolisthesis. Treatment options include physical therapy to strengthen the muscles surrounding the area. Sometimes the patient is placed in a brace. In severe cases, surgery is also an option.

Anatomy of the Facet Joints

Your spine is made of 24 moveable bones called vertebrae that provide the main support for your body, allowing you to bend and twist. Each of the vertebrae are separated and cushioned by a gel-like disc, keeping them from rubbing together. The vertebrae are connected and held to each other by ligaments and joints, called facet joints.

The upper facet joint (superior facet) and the lower (inferior facet) are connected by a narrow bridge called the pars interarticularis, which literally means the "piece between the articulations." The inferior facet of one vertebra fits perfectly into the superior facet of the one below it—overlapping like shingles—beginning with the vertebra at the base of your skull and ending at your tailbone.

What Are Spondylolysis and Spondylolisthesis?

Spondylolysis and spondylolisthesis are separate, yet related conditions. Spondylolysis usually comes first, though not always. The term comes from "spondylo," which means "spine," and "lysis," which means to divide. Spondylolysis is a breakdown or fracture of the narrow bridge between the upper and lower facets, called the pars interarticularis. It can occur on one side (unilateral) or both sides (bilateral) and at any level of the spine, but most often at the fourth or fifth lumbar vertebra. If spondylolysis is present, then you have the potential to develop spondylolisthesis.

The term spondylolysis is misleading. There may be no crack in the bone because that bone could just be cartilage that never formed into bone. This shows up as a hole or gap on an X-ray. Or it could be that the back part of the vertebra broke off and tried to heal itself with scar tissue sometime in childhood.

Spondylolisthesis is the actual slipping forward of the vertebral body (the term "listhesis" means "to slip forward"). It occurs when the pars interarticularis separates and allows the vertebral body to move forward out of position causing pinched nerves and pain. Spondylolisthesis usually occurs between the fourth and fifth lumber vertebra or at the last lumbar vertebra and the sacrum. This is where your spine curves into its most pronounced *S* shape and where the stress is heaviest.

Slippage is measured on a scale from grade 1 slippage (25%) to grade 4 (100%). The more the lower back curves in (swayback or lordosis), the steeper the grade.

What Are the Symptoms?

Mild cases of spondylolysis and spondylolisthesis usually cause minimal pain. In fact, the conditions are often found by accident when a person has a pre-employment exam or an X-ray of the back for an unrelated reason.

When spondylolysis and spondylolisthesis do cause pain, you may experience low back pain, stiffness, and muscle spasms. You may also have sciatica (pain radiating down one or both legs), or numbness, though this is not common. Leg pain will usually be worse when you stand or walk.

The amount of pain you have depends on how fast your vertebrae are slipping. If you have very subtle symptoms, you may only feel tightness in your hamstrings or find that you can no longer touch your toes, but not feel any nerve pain.

What Are the Causes?

Spondylolisthesis is most often caused by spondylolysis. The cause of spondylolysis is not as clearly defined. Most believe it is due to a genetic weakness of the pars interarticularis. Both spondylolysis and spondylolisthesis can be present at birth or occur through injury. Repeated stress fractures caused by hyperextension of the back (as in gymnastics and football) and traumatic fractures are also causes. The most common cause in adults is degenerative arthritis.

Who Is Affected?

Those who play sports, especially gymnasts and football players, are more likely to have spondylolisthesis. The condition most often affects people over 40 years of age. About 5% of Americans have this structural deficiency and don't know it. Just because it appears on an X-ray doesn't mean you'll have pain.

How Is a Diagnosis Made?

When you first have pain, consult your family doctor. They will take a complete medical history to understand your symptoms, any prior injuries or conditions, and determine if any lifestyle habits are causing the pain. Next a physical exam is performed to determine the source of the pain and test for muscle weakness or numbness.

- **X-ray** test uses X-rays to view the bony vertebrae in your spine and can tell your doctor if any of them are too close together or whether you have arthritic changes, bone spurs, fractures, or any slippage of the vertebrae.

- **Magnetic resonance imaging (MRI)** scan is a noninvasive test that uses a magnetic field and radiofrequency waves to give a detailed view of the soft tissues of your spine. Unlike an X-ray, nerves and discs are clearly visible. It allows your doctor to view your spine three-dimensionally in slices, as if it were sliced layer-by-layer like a loaf of bread with a picture taken of each slice. The pictures can be taken from the side or from the top as a cross-section. It may or may not be performed with a dye (contrast agent) injected into your bloodstream. An MRI can tell your doctor where your spine is damaged and if there is any nerve compression. It can also detect bony overgrowth, spinal cord tumors, or abscesses.

- **Computed tomography (CT)** scan is a safe, noninvasive test that uses an X-ray beam and a computer to make two-dimensional images of your spine. Similar to an MRI, it allows your doctor to view your spine in slices, as if it were sliced layer-by-layer with a picture taken of each slice. It may or may not be performed with a dye (contrast agent) injected into your bloodstream.

- **Single photon emission computed tomography (SPECT)** scan is a sensitive diagnostic tool used to analyze blood flow to an organ which may help determine how that organ is functioning. It involves the injection of a small amount of radioactive substance into a vein. As the substance is circulated in the blood, it is absorbed by the tissues and then gives off energy. This energy is captured by a special camera that transfers the information to a computer. There the information is converted into a three-dimensional picture. This picture can detect stress fractures, spondylolysis, infection, and tumors by the differences in how the radioactive substance is absorbed by normal healthy tissue vs. diseased tissue.

What Treatments Are Available?

First, athletic activity should be stopped to allow the fracture to heal. Conservative nonsurgical treatment is the first step and may include medication, rest, physical therapy, home exercises, hydrotherapy, a brace, and pain management. Periodic X-rays will allow the doctor to watch the degree of slippage. Surgery may be needed if slippage continues or if your pain is not relieved by conservative treatment.

Nonsurgical Treatments

Self care and braces: Using correct posture and keeping your spine in alignment are the most important things you can do for your back.

The lower back (lumbar curve) bears most of your weight, so proper alignment of this section can prevent further slippage and injury to your spinal nerves and discs. You may need to make adjustments to your daily standing, sitting, and sleeping habits. You may also need to learn proper ways to lift and bend. You may need to wear a back brace for a short period of time while you strengthen the abdominal and lower back muscles. The brace may decrease muscle spasm and pain as well as help immobilize your spine and help the healing process. Your doctor may refer you to an orthotist who specializes in custom-made braces.

Physical therapy: The goal of physical therapy is to help you return to full activity as soon as possible. Exercise is very helpful for pain and it can help you heal faster. Physical therapists can instruct you on proper lifting and walking techniques, and they'll work with you to strengthen your abdominal muscles and lower back. They'll also encourage you to increase the flexibility of your spine and legs.

Medications: Your doctor may prescribe pain relievers, nonsteroidal anti-inflammatory medications (NSAIDs), and steroids. Sometimes muscle relaxers are prescribed for muscle spasms.

- **Nonsteroidal anti-inflammatory drugs (NSAIDs)**, such as aspirin, naproxen (Aleve, Naprosyn), and ibuprofen (Motrin, Nuprin, Advil), are used to reduce inflammation and relieve pain.

- **Analgesics**, such as acetaminophen (Tylenol), can relieve pain but don't have the anti-inflammatory effects of NSAIDs. Long-term use of analgesics and NSAIDs may cause stomach ulcers as well as kidney and liver problems.

- **Steroids** can be used to reduce the swelling and inflammation of the nerves. They are taken orally (as a Medrol dose pack) in a tapering dosage over a five-day period. They have the advantage of providing pain relief within a 24-hour period.

- **Epidural steroid injections:** This minimally invasive procedure involves an injection of corticosteroid and an analgesic-numbing agent into the epidural space of the spine to reduce the swelling and inflammation of the nerves. About 50% of patients will notice relief after an epidural injection, although the results tend to be temporary. If the injections are helpful, they can be done up to three times a year.

- **Facet injections:** This minimally invasive procedure involves an injection of corticosteroid and an analgesic-numbing agent to the painful facet joint, either inside the joint capsule or in the tissue surrounding the joint capsule.

Holistic therapy: Some patients want to try holistic therapies such as acupuncture, acupressure, nutritional supplements, and biofeedback. The effectiveness of these treatments for spondylolysis and spondylolisthesis may aid you in learning coping mechanisms for managing pain as well as improving your overall health.

Surgical Treatments

If slippage continues or if your pain doesn't respond to conservative treatment, surgery may be necessary. Surgery can address both the instability of the spine and compression of the nerve roots. The surgeon may first perform a lumbar laminectomy to relieve pressure on the nerve root. Then a bone graft will be used to fuse the loose vertebrae and keep them from sliding out of place. In some cases metal plates, hooks, rods, and screws may be used to support the fusion. It may take a while for the two pieces of bone to grow together, so you should avoid extremes of motion while healing.

Fusion is successful in over 90% of cases because it stops the instable motion and keeps your spinal canal from narrowing further.

Chapter 21

Cervical Fractures (Broken Neck)

Overview

A cervical fracture means that a bone is broken in the cervical (neck) region of the spine. A cervical dislocation means that a ligament injury in the neck has occurred, and two (or more) of the adjoining spine bones have become abnormally separated from each other, causing instability. Patients can have a cervical fracture or dislocation, or both. Fractures and dislocations of the cervical spine are not uncommon, and account for almost half of all spinal column injuries that occur every year. According to a study published by Lasfargues in 1995, over 25,000 cervical fractures occur each year in the United States. The majority of fractures and dislocations of the spinal column occur in the cervical spine because it is the most mobile portion of the spinal column and, understandably, the most vulnerable to injury. Although the lumbar (low back) region is most commonly injured during daily laborious, low-energy activities, the neck is most likely to be injured during high-energy trauma such as motor vehicle accidents.

Cervical fractures and dislocations are typically classified according to their region/location and injury/fracture pattern. Because of the unique anatomy of the spine in the region close to the head, cervical injuries are categorized as occipital-cervical (occiput-C2) and subaxial

---

cervical spine (C3-C7) injuries. Within each of these categories, injuries are further stratified according to the specific location of injury and injury/fracture pattern.

Occipital-Cervical Spine (Occiput-C2)

- Atlanto-occipital dislocation (AOD)
- Occipital condyle fracture
- Atlanto-axial instability
- Atlanto-axial rotatory subluxation
- Atlas fractures (C1)
- Odontoid fractures (C2 dens)
- Traumatic spondylolisthesis of the axis (C2)
- Axis fractures (C2 vertebral body)

Subaxial Cervical Spine (C3-C7)

- Distraction-flexion (facet fracture/dislocation)
- Vertical compression (burst fracture)
- Compression-flexion (teardrop fracture)
- Compression-extension
- Distraction-extension
- Lateral flexion

Causes

The most common causes of cervical fractures and dislocations are motor vehicle accidents, falls, violence, and sports activities. The abrupt impact and/or twisting of the neck that occurs in a millisecond during the trauma can cause the spine bones to crack or the ligaments to rupture, or both. The initial trauma or event may cause a cervical fracture and/or instability, which may also cause damage to the spinal cord and neurologic structures. The resultant spinal cord injury and neurologic deficit, if it occurs, is the most devastating aspect of a cervical injury, primarily because it is often irreversible and permanent. The majority of spinal column and spinal cord injuries occur in males between the ages of 15 and 24 years old.

Symptoms

Patients with cervical fractures typically have significant, localized neck pain and stiffness. However, patients with other injuries may complain of pain in other areas and not notice the severity of neck pain. Patients who have neurologic compression or irritation may have numbness or weakness in the arms and/or legs. There may or may not be associated radiating pain symptoms. Upper cervical spine fractures and spinal cord injuries can affect the neurologic control of breathing, and patients may complain of difficulty breathing or the inability to take a deep breath.

Physical Findings

The physical findings for patients with cervical fractures are variable. Patients will typically demonstrate profound tenderness and spasm, with significantly decreased neck range of motion. There is often visible swelling and ecchymosis (bruising) over the fracture site in the back of the neck. If the fracture/dislocation is severe, there will be a visible and palpable "step-off," meaning the bones are not lined up properly, which can be seen and felt by the examiner. If the spinal nerves are severely compressed, there may be significant weakness and numbness in the arms and/or legs. Patients will have complete loss of strength and sensation in the setting of a complete spinal cord injury. Deep tendon reflexes may be diminished or absent. Pulses and vascularity of the arms and legs should be normal.

Imaging Studies

Plain X-rays of the cervical spine are essential to adequately evaluate a cervical fracture and dislocation. It is sometimes difficult to see a non-displaced or minimally displaced fracture or instability; therefore, a computed tomography (CT) scan is usually ordered. A CT scan is the best test to verify that a fracture is or is not present. If no fracture is identified, but a patient has neck pain and was involved in large trauma or accident, flexion/extension X-rays are often obtained to verify that there if no evidence of ligamentous instability. A magnetic resonance imaging (MRI) test is useful to evaluate the severity of nerve compression or spinal cord injury but is less accurate at detecting a fracture than a CT scan. A MRI test should generally always be obtained before performing a reduction procedure (closed or operative) in neurologically intact patients with a cervical fracture/dislocation.

215

Laboratory Tests

There are no laboratory tests used to diagnose a cervical fracture. Occasionally, specific tests are ordered to rule out infection or other metabolic conditions that may be suspected as an underlying cause.

Diagnosis

Cervical spine fractures and dislocations should always be suspected when a patient has been involved in a trauma or accident, especially those patients with neck pain. The diagnosis can be complicated when the symptoms or physical findings are atypical. Some patients with other fractures or injuries will complain about pain in other locations, but not complain of neck pain.

At times, patients may downplay the severity of the motor vehicle accident or trauma. These scenarios may sway the clinician away from ordering cervical X-rays and imaging studies, which are crucial in the diagnosis of cervical injuries. It is important for the clinician to conduct a thorough history and clinical examination (especially inspection and palpation of the spine) prior to formulating a diagnosis so as not to misdiagnose this condition. Any patient involved in a severe accident or trauma, especially those patients with neck pain, should be carefully evaluated with X-rays (and additional imaging studies if necessary) to accurately diagnose a cervical injury.

Treatment Options

The treatment options for patients with a cervical fracture and/or dislocation are limited and can be categorized as conservative (nonoperative) and surgical (operative). Initial treatment of severe cervical fractures and dislocations may involve skeletal traction and closed reduction, with metal pins placed in the skull connected to a pulley, rope, and weights. Nonoperative treatments include brace (orthotic) treatment and medications. There are a wide range of cervical orthoses that range from soft collars to hard plastic cervical-thoracic orthoses to halo vest immobilization (using pins anchored into the skull stabilized by a padded plastic vest). Surgical treatments frequently involve posterior (back of the neck incision) cervical fusion (mending the spine bones together) and instrumentation (small metal screws and rods stabilizing the spine). Other options include anterior (front of the neck incision) decompression and fusion, with or without instrumentation (metal plate and screws). Severely unstable fractures may require anterior and posterior neck surgery. The overall goals of treatment are to preserve or improve neurologic function, provide stability, and decrease pain. If these goals can be accomplished with conservative (nonoperative) means, then that is generally preferred. However, because many cervical fractures and dislocations are highly unstable and will not adequately heal on their own, surgical stabilization is routinely performed. Surgical decompression (removal of bone fragments off of the spinal cord) may also be necessary to maximize a patient's chances for neurologic improvement and recovery from a spinal cord injury.

Chapter 22

Spinal Cord Injuries

Spinal cord injury/dysfunction (SCI/D) is damage to the spinal cord that results in a loss of function such as mobility or feeling. Frequent causes of damage are trauma (car accident, gunshot, falls, etc.) or disease (polio, spina bifida, multiple sclerosis, transverse myelitis, etc.)

The spinal cord does not have to be severed for a loss of functioning to occur. In fact, in most people with SCI/D, the spinal cord is intact, but the damage to it results in loss of functioning. SCI is very different from back injuries such as ruptured disks, spinal stenosis, or pinched nerves.

A person can "break their back or neck" yet not sustain a spinal cord injury if only the bones around the spinal cord (the vertebrae) are damaged but the spinal cord is not affected. In these situations, the individual may not experience paralysis after the bones are stabilized.

What are the spinal cord and the vertebra?

The spinal cord is the major "bundle of nerves" that carries nerve impulses to and from the brain to the rest of the body. The brain and the spinal cord constitute the central nervous system. Motor and sensory nerves outside the central nervous system constitute the peripheral nervous system. Another diffuse system of nerves that control involuntary functions such as blood pressure and temperature regulation is the sympathetic and parasympathetic nervous systems.

The spinal cord is surrounded and protected by rings of bone called vertebra. These bones constitute the spinal column (back bones). In general, the higher in the spinal column the injury occurs, the more dysfunction a person will experience. The vertebra are named according to their location.

The eight vertebra in the neck are called the cervical vertebra. The top vertebra is called C-1, the next is C-2, etc. Cervical SCIs usually cause loss of function in the arms and legs, resulting in quadriplegia or tetraplegia. The 12 vertebra in the chest are called the thoracic vertebra. The first thoracic vertebra, T-1, is the vertebra where the top rib attaches. Injuries in the thoracic region usually affect the chest and the legs and result in paraplegia.

The lumbar vertebra are in the lower back between where the ribs attach and the pelvis (hip bone) is. The sacral vertebra run from the pelvis to the end of the spinal column. Injuries to the five lumbar vertebra (L-1 thru L-5) and similarly to the five sacral vertebra (S-1 thru S-5) generally result in some loss of functioning in the hips and legs.

What are the effects of SCI?

The effects of SCI depend on the type of injury and the level of the injury. SCI can be divided into two types of injury—complete and incomplete. A complete injury means that there is no motor or sensory function preserved in the S4 and S5 area, or anal area. Therefore there is no function below the level of the injury; no sensation and no voluntary movement. Both sides of the body are generally equally affected. An incomplete injury means that there is some functioning below the primary level of the injury. A person with an incomplete injury may be able to move one limb more than another, may be able to feel parts of the body that cannot be moved, or may have more functioning on one side of the body than the other. Incomplete injuries are becoming more common. Factors contributing to this include positive prevention promotion such as the use of seatbelts and no diving in shallow water or while drinking, highly trained first responders, better diagnostic capabilities, and a more thorough understanding of the initial injury.

The level of injury is very helpful in predicting what parts of the body might be affected by paralysis and loss of function. Remember that in incomplete injuries there will be some variation in these prognoses. Cervical (neck) injuries usually result in quadriplegia/tetraplegia. Injuries above the C-4 level may require a ventilator for the person to breathe. C-5 injuries often result in shoulder and biceps control; however, the person will have no control at the wrist or hand. C-6 injuries generally yield wrist control, but no hand function. Individuals with C-7 and T-1 injuries can straighten their arms but still may have agility problems with the hand and fingers.

Injuries at the thoracic level and below result in paraplegia; the hands are not affected. At T-1 to T-8 there is poor trunk control due to the lack of abdominal muscle function. At lower T-injuries (T-9 to T-12), the abdominal muscles are functional, thereby enabling good trunk control. Sitting balance is very good at this injury level. Lumbar and sacral injuries yield decreasing control of the hip flexors and legs.

Besides a loss of sensation or motor functioning, individuals with SCI also experience other changes. For example, they may experience alterations of the bowel, bladder, and sexual functioning. Persons with very high injuries (C-1, C-2) can experience a loss of many involuntary functions including the ability to breathe, necessitating breathing aids such as mechanical ventilators or diaphragmatic pacemakers. Other effects of SCI may include low blood pressure, inability to regulate blood pressure effectively, reduced control of body temperature, inability to sweat below the level of injury, and chronic pain.

How many people have SCI?

Who are they? Approximately 232,000 to 316,000 people live with SCI in the U.S. There are about 12,000 new SCIs every year; the majority of them (80.7%) involve males and most are between the ages of 16–30. These injuries result from motor vehicle accidents (40.4%), violence (15%), or falls (27.9%). Quadriplegia is slightly more common than paraplegia.

Is there a cure for SCI?

Currently there is no "cure" for SCI. There are many researchers studying this problem and there have been many advances in the laboratory. Many of the most exciting advances have resulted in a decrease in damage at the time of the injury. Steroid drugs such as methylprednisolone reduce swelling, which is a common cause of secondary damage at the time of injury. There are also a variety of SCI clinical trials in various stages of completion offering hope for improved function for new as well as chronically injured individuals.

Do people with SCI ever get better?

When a SCI occurs, there is swelling at the site of the injury. This causes changes in virtually every system in the body. The good news is, though, after an injury that dramatically and instantly changes one's life, people typically begin to improve. After days or weeks, the swelling begins to go down and people may regain some function or sensation.

With many injuries, especially incomplete injuries, the individual may recover some function as late as 18 to 24 months after the injury. In rare cases, people with SCI will regain some function years after the injury. However, only a very small fraction of individuals sustaining SCIs recover all functioning. Over time, following appropriate SCI rehabilitation, individuals with spinal cord injury learn to adapt and live with a newly functioning body. They are able to successfully reintegrate back into their communities and regain an improved quality of life and increased independence.

Does everyone who sustains SCI use a wheelchair?

No. Wheelchairs are a tool for mobility. High cervical level injuries usually require that the individual use a sophisticated and expensive power wheelchair. Persons with low cervical level injuries and below generally can use a manual chair. Advantages of high-quality manual chairs are that they cost and weigh less than power chairs, disassemble into smaller pieces, and enable more diverse activities. However, for the person who needs a power chair for mobility, the independence afforded by them is limitless. Some people are able to use braces and crutches for ambulation. These methods of mobility do not mean that the person will never use a wheelchair. Many people who use braces still find wheelchairs more useful for longer distances. However, the therapeutic and activity benefits allowed by standing or walking briefly may make braces a reasonable alternative for some people.

Of course, people who use wheelchairs aren't always in them. They drive, swim, fly planes, ski, scuba dive, cycle with family, and do many activities out of their chair. If you hang around people who use wheelchairs long enough, you may see them sitting in the grass pulling weeds, sitting on your couch, or playing on the floor with children or pets. And of course, people who use wheelchairs don't sleep in their chairs, they transfer into a bed. No one is "wheelchair bound"! Their chair is used for the mobility they require.

Do people with SCI have jobs?

Well of course they do! People with SCI have the same desires as other people; these include a desire to work and be productive. The Americans with Disabilities Act (ADA) promotes the inclusion of people with SCI for full participation in day-to-day society. Nevertheless, unemployment among persons living with SCI remains high. By 20 years post-injury, 35.2% of those living with SCI are employed according to the UAB [University of Alabama at Birmingham] National SCI Statistical Center. Of course, people with disabilities may need some changes/accommodations to make their workplace more accessible, but surveys indicate that the cost of making accommodations to the workplace in 70% of cases is $500 or less.

Can people with SCI have sex, children?

Since a spinal cord injury affects virtually every system of the body, many people who sustain SCI have serious concerns about how their injuries will affect their ability to participate in and enjoy a sexual relationship. Injury to the spinal cord will therefore have some effect on one's sexual functioning. The extent to which sexual functioning may be impaired will depend on the level and severity of the injury. However, there are many therapies that allow people with SCI to lead an active and satisfying sex life. Fertility is also frequently affected in men with SCI. Methods similar to those used for non-disabled men with fertility issues have allowed many men with SCI to father their own children.

The fertility of women with SCI may be affected in the first months after injury. However, most women regain the ability to become pregnant after SCI and are able to carry babies to full term. However, it is important that she consult and be managed by a physician experienced in SCI and pregnancy. Of course, adoption is another option.

What do I say when I meet a person with SCI?

"Hi."

A person living with a SCI is no different than a non-disabled individual with few exceptions. Although disabled individuals do some things differently than non-disabled individuals, the result is the same. People with SCI have the same hopes, interests, and desires as other people. They have a wide range of interests, abilities, likes, and dislikes, just as you. People with disabilities are "people first"; please try to remember that always when you interact with someone with a disability. Always speak in your usual tone of voice directly to the person with the disability and not their companion, aide, or interpreter. If the person does use a wheelchair for mobility, be respectful of the wheelchair by not touching or leaning on the chair, as it is part of their personal space. By all means, if the individual appears to need help, offer your assistance but accept their response. However, do not always assume they need your help. Individuals with disabilities live with them every day and they want to remain independent as possible.

The most important thing to remember is: Life does not end with spinal cord injury.

Chapter 23

Spinal Fractures

Chapter Contents

Section 23.1

Compression Fractures of the Spine

Overview

The spine is made up of strong bones called vertebrae, but they can break just like any other bone in the body. When they do, the result is called a vertebral compression fracture, because the main section of each vertebra collapses in height. These fractures usually occur in the lower thoracic spine (the middle portion of the spine).

A disease that causes the thinning of bones with reduction in bone mass due to the depletion of calcium and bone protein is osteoporosis. The effects of this disease frequently result in compression fractures. It often afflicts older women.

Causes

Compression fractures of the spine generally occur from too much pressure on a vertebra. The fracture occurs when the vertebra breaks, or collapses, causing it to become wedge shaped. The bone tissue on the inside of the vertebra is crushed, or compressed.

There are several causes of compression fractures. If the vertebra is too weak to hold normal pressure, it may take very little pressure to cause it to collapse. Most healthy bones can withstand pressure and the spine is able to absorb the shock. However, if the forces are too high, one or more vertebrae may fracture.

Spinal compression fractures are the most common type of fracture caused by osteoporosis. In fact, 40% of all women will have at least one by the time they turn 80 years old. This type of vertebral fracture causes loss of body height and a humped back (kyphosis), especially in elderly women.

Compression fractures due to trauma can come from a fall, a forceful jump, a car accident, or any event that stresses the spine past its breaking point.

Yet another cause of spinal compression fractures is cancer that spreads to the spine weakening the supportive structure.

Symptoms

If the fracture is caused by a sudden, forceful injury, patients will probably feel severe pain in their back, legs, and arms. They might also feel weakness or numbness if the fracture injures the nerves of the spine. Should the bone collapse be gradual, such as a fracture from bone thinning, the pain will usually be milder. There might not be any pain at all until the bone actually breaks.

If the compression fracture is caused by osteoporosis, initially the patient may not feel any pain. Over time, symptoms may include muscle fatigue and soreness at the site of the fracture.

In very severe compression fractures, parts of the vertebra may actually put pressure on the spinal cord. Fortunately this does not happen often.

Diagnosis

In order to diagnose a compression fracture, doctors must first obtain a patient's complete history and conduct a physical exam. These tests may be recommended:

- An X-ray of the spine.

- A CT [computed tomography] scan to make sure that the broken bone is stable and that the nerves are not in danger. The CT scan will be combined with a myelogram if there are any concerns about the spinal cord.

- An MRI [magnetic resonance imaging] may be recommended if there is a chance that nerves are hurt in the fracture or if there is some question about what is causing the pain.

- A bone scan may be ordered to help determine if the fracture is the result of osteoporosis.

- A neurological exam may also be conducted to help determine whether nerve damage has occurred.

Treatment Options

Most compression fractures respond well to conservative therapies such as pain medications, decreasing activity, and bracing. Doctors are also using minimally invasive procedures called vertebroplasty and kyphoplasty. Vertebral fractures usually take about three months to fully heal. X-rays may be taken monthly to check on the healing progress. Surgery for compression fractures is rarely needed.

Pain Medication

Mild pain medications may be prescribed. While pain medications will not help the fracture to heal, they can help control soreness and discomfort.

External Back and Neck Bracing

Another common form of treatment for some types of vertebral compression fractures is a back support (called an orthosis). The brace supports the back and helps restricts movement.

Minimally Invasive Methods

Today doctors may recommend vertebroplasty or kyphoplasty—minimally invasive procedures specifically designed to treat spinal compression fractures.

- In vertebroplasty, special cement is injected into the broken vertebra to improve its strength and ease pain.

- In kyphoplasty, a tube with a deflated balloon is slipped inside the broken bone. The balloon is then inflated to help restore the height of the broken vertebra. Bone cement is injected into the space formed by the balloon to hold the vertebra at its corrected height.

Section 23.2

Tailbone Injuries

Introduction

Coccydynia is an uncommon painful condition that originates from the coccyx, the tailbone at the end of the spine. Trauma and falls are the most frequent causes of coccydynia. In the vast majority of cases, nonsurgical treatment, such as medications and physical therapy, work well to ease symptoms.

Anatomy

The spine is composed of a series of bones called vertebrae. Joints that allow movement while providing stability connect the vertebrae. The end of the spine, the coccyx, has three to five small bones.

The coccyx bones align in a curve like a small tail. Some of the coccyx bones may be fused together. However, fewer than 10% of people have a completely fused coccyx.

Muscles, ligaments, and tendons attach to the coccyx. It plays a role in weight bearing when seated.

Causes

Coccydynia is caused by trauma to the coccyx, such as from a fall, injury during childbirth, or prolonged sitting. Trauma can cause ligament inflammation or injure the coccyx where it attaches to the spine. In some cases, the cause is unknown.

Symptoms

The primary symptom of coccydynia is pain. You may experience increased sensitivity to pressure, especially when sitting and leaning backwards. The area around your tailbone may ache. Coccydynia can

229

cause pain that shoots down the legs. It can also contribute to pain during sexual intercourse or bowel movements.

Diagnosis

A doctor can diagnose coccydynia by reviewing your medical history and examining you. You should tell your doctor if you have fallen or given birth recently. Imaging tests, such as X-ray or MRI, may be used to rule out other sources of pain. Electromyography (EMG) and nerve conduction studies may be used to assess nerve function.

Treatment

Coccydynia is typically first treated with non-steroidal anti-inflammatory medications. Your doctor may recommend that you sit on a donut-shaped pillow to help relieve tailbone pressure. It may take several weeks or months for the pain to decrease.

For persistent or severe pain, your doctor may prescribe pain medications. Local medication injections are used to place numbing and anti-inflammatory medications near the source (joint or bursa) of the pain. Nerve blocks are used to interrupt a nerve's ability to transmit pain signals.

Your doctor may gently move (manipulate) the coccyx after you receive a pain relieving injection. You may be referred to physical therapy for gentle stretching. Ultrasound therapy may be used, which soothes pain with warmth.

If treatments fail to relieve symptoms, surgery may be used to remove a portion of the coccyx (coccygectomy). The short outpatient surgery is successful for relieving symptoms for most people. However, surgery is very rarely used.

Chapter 24

Herniated Discs

When people say they have a "slipped" or "ruptured" disk in their neck or lower back, what they are actually describing is a herniated disk—a common source of pain in the neck, lower back, arms, or legs.

Anatomy

Disks are soft, rubbery pads found between the hard bones (vertebrae) that make up the spinal column. The spinal canal is a hollow space in the middle of the spinal column that contains the spinal cord and other nerve roots. The disks between the vertebrae allow the back to flex or bend. Disks also act as shock absorbers.

Disks in the lumbar spine (low back) are composed of a thick outer ring of cartilage (annulus) and an inner gel-like substance (nucleus). In the cervical spine (neck), the disks are similar but smaller in size.

Cause

A disk herniates or ruptures when part of the center nucleus pushes through the outer edge of the disk and back toward the spinal canal. This puts pressure on the nerves. Spinal nerves are very sensitive to even slight amounts of pressure, which can result in pain, numbness, or weakness in one or both legs.

Risk Factors/Prevention

In children and young adults, disks have high water content. As people age, the water content in the disks decreases and the disks become less flexible. The disks begin to shrink and the spaces between the vertebrae get narrower. Conditions that can weaken the disk include:

- improper lifting;

- smoking;

- excessive body weight that places added stress on the disks (in the lower back);

- sudden pressure (which may be slight);

- repetitive strenuous activities.

Symptoms

Lower Back

Low back pain affects four out of five people. Pain alone is not enough to recognize a herniated disk. See your doctor if back pain results from a fall or a blow to your back. The most common symptom of a herniated disk is sciatica—a sharp, often shooting pain that extends from the buttocks down the back of one leg. It is caused by pressure on the spinal nerve. Other symptoms include:

- weakness in one leg;

- tingling (a "pins-and-needles" sensation) or numbness in one leg or buttock;

- loss of bladder or bowel control (if you also have significant weakness in both legs, you could have a serious problem and should seek immediate attention);

- a burning pain centered in the neck.

Neck

As with pain in the lower back, neck pain is also common. When pressure is placed on a nerve in the neck, it causes pain in the muscles between your neck and shoulder (trapezius muscles). The pain may shoot down the arm. The pain may also cause headaches in the back of the head. Other symptoms include:

- weakness in one arm;

- tingling (a "pins-and-needles" sensation) or numbness in one arm;

- loss of bladder or bowel control (if you also have significant weakness in both arms or legs, you could have a serious problem and should seek immediate attention);

- burning pain in the shoulders, neck, or arm.

Diagnosis

To diagnose a herniated disk, your doctor will ask for your complete medical history. Tell him or her if you have neck/back pain with gradually increasing arm/leg pain. Tell the doctor if you were injured.

A physical examination will help determine which nerve roots are affected (and how seriously).

A simple X-ray may show evidence of disk or degenerative spine changes.

MRI (magnetic resonance imaging) or CT (computed tomography) (imaging tests to confirm which disk is injured) or electromyography (a test that measures nerve impulses to the muscles) may be recommended if the pain continues.

Treatment

Nonsurgical Treatment

Nonsurgical treatment is effective in treating the symptoms of herniated disks in more than 90% of patients. Most neck or back pain will resolve gradually with simple measures.

- Rest and over-the-counter pain relievers may be all that is needed.

- Muscle relaxers, analgesics, and anti-inflammatory medications are also helpful.

- Cold compresses or ice can also be applied several times a day for no more than 20 minutes at a time.

- After any spasms settle, gentle heat applications may be used.

Any physical activity should be slow and controlled, especially bending forward and lifting. This can help ensure that symptoms do not return—as can taking short walks and avoiding sitting for long periods.

For the lower back, exercises may also be helpful in strengthening the back and abdominal muscles. For the neck, exercises or traction may also be helpful. To help avoid future episodes of pain, it is essential that you learn how to properly stand, sit, and lift.

If these nonsurgical treatment measures fail, epidural injections of a cortisone-like drug may lessen nerve irritation and allow more effective participation in physical therapy. These injections are given on an outpatient basis over a period of weeks.

Surgical Treatment

Surgery may be required if a disk fragment lodges in the spinal canal and presses on a nerve, causing significant loss of function. Surgical options in the lower back include microdiskectomy or laminectomy, depending on the size and position of the disk herniation.

In the neck, an anterior cervical diskectomy and fusion are usually recommended. This involves removing the entire disk to take the pressure off the spinal cord and nerve roots. Bone is placed in the disk space and a metal plate may be used to stabilize the spine.

For some patients, a smaller surgery may be performed on the back of the neck that does not require fusing the bones together.

Each of these surgical procedures is performed with the patient under general anesthesia. They may be performed on an outpatient basis or require an overnight hospital stay. You should be able to return to work in two to six weeks after surgery.

Chapter 25

Spinal Nerve Injuries

Chapter Contents

Section 25.1

Stingers

"Stingers and Burners," by Kurt E. Jacobson, M.D., *Hughston Health Alert*, Spring 2000. © 2000 Hughston Sports Medicine Foundation, Inc. All rights reserved. Reprinted with permission. Reviewed by David A. Cooke, MD, FACP, September 2011.

Few sports injuries are as eye-opening for the athlete as a "stinger" or "burner." This intense neurologic (nerve) event occurs most commonly in football players. It also can occur in people who participate in wrestling, cycling, gymnastics, snow skiing, martial arts, or other sports. This section discusses the condition in football players and highlights several key points.

What is a stinger or burner?

A stinger or burner is an intensely painful nerve injury. The nerves that give feeling to the arms and hands originate from the cervical (neck) spinal cord. As these nerves leave the neck, they form the brachial plexus. They weave together then branch as they pass under the clavicle (collar bone) on the way to the shoulder.

Nerve injury often happens when the athlete makes a hard hit using his shoulder. The direct blow to the top of the shoulder drives it down and causes the neck to bend toward the opposite side. This motion severely stretches or compresses the nerves and triggers an intense discharge of electricity. For a few seconds, the electricity shoots down the nerves to the tip of the fingers.

After this intense electrical discharge, the nerves' motor fibers that allow movement in the arm do not function well. The dysfunction is evident by weakness in the arm. The weakness often involves the muscles that allow the athlete to lift the arm away from the body, to bend the elbow, and to grip. Symptoms also include sensations of tingling and of burning or stinging pain in the arm and hand. The extent of the damage varies considerably. The pain usually lasts only a few minutes, but the weakness can last weeks, months, or years. Rarely, the injury may cause permanent damage.

Treatment of a stinger or burner usually begins as soon as the player runs off the field with the limp arm hanging by his side. The certified athletic trainer, physical therapist, or team doctor carefully examines the cervical spine, evaluates nerve function in the neck and upper back, tests muscle strength, and tests reflexes. If the athletic trainer, physical therapist, or doctor suspects that the athlete has a spinal cord injury, he or she treats the condition as a medical emergency with full spinal precautions.

How do I know it's a stinger and not something else?

Stingers or burners produce symptoms in only one arm. Injuries that can accompany a stinger include fractures, dislocations, or damage to the ligaments (tissue connecting two bones) of the cervical spine. Therefore, when treating an athlete who has a stinger, the doctor takes appropriate precautions to protect the spine.

A spinal cord injury usually causes symptoms involving more than just one arm and possibly the legs. This injury must be treated as a medical emergency. A contusion (bruise) to the spinal cord in the neck during athletic competition can lead to temporary quadriparesis, producing symptoms of pain and tingling in both arms and both legs. Certain athletes may be more prone to this injury because the space in their necks through which the spinal cord travels is narrow (see "Congenital Spinal Stenosis" at http://www.hughston.com/hha/a_12_2_2 .htm). Other injuries to the spinal cord can cause lasting, serious nerve damage. The health care provider always treats neck injuries with full precautions until serious injuries are ruled out.

When can the injured athlete go back in the game?

If the certified athletic trainer, physical therapist, or team doctor determines that the athlete's sense of feeling, strength, neck motion, and reflexes have returned to normal, the athlete may be able to return to the game. All protective gear should be inspected to ensure it fits properly and is in good condition. Additional shoulder pads or a neck roll may be added. Do not attach restraining straps or other similar devices to the helmet because they can lead to more severe injuries. The athlete should be examined frequently during the game for further problems including recurrence of symptoms.

How should the athlete be treated following the game?

After the game, the athlete should be re-examined in the locker room and, if necessary, at his doctor's office. An athlete who has a stiff neck following a stinger is more prone to further, more serious injury and needs a thorough evaluation of the neck, shoulder, and nerves by an orthopedic doctor. An athlete who has had a stinger cannot return to play until the health care provider notes that he has no pain or tenderness and that he exhibits full range of motion and strength in the neck, shoulder, and arm.

How do we prevent these injuries?

Preventing recurrent stingers is important. Subsequent injuries tend to be increasingly severe and can damage the nerve permanently. Athletes, coaches, officials, athletic trainers, and parents need to ensure that athletes follow these three minimal guidelines. First, use proper technique in tackling as mandated by the 1979 football rule outlawing spearing or head tackling. Second, make sure that the shoulder pads and neck roll, if used, fit properly and are in good condition. Third, before the season begins, participate in an exercise program to develop full range of motion and protective strength of the neck and shoulder muscles.

Section 25.2

Sciatica

Sciatica refers to pain, weakness, numbness, or tingling in the leg. It is caused by injury to or pressure on the sciatic nerve. Sciatica is a symptom of another medical problem, not a medical condition on its own.

Causes

Sciatica occurs when there is pressure or damage to the sciatic nerve. This nerve starts in the lower spine and runs down the back of each leg. This nerve controls the muscles of the back of the knee and lower leg and provides sensation to the back of the thigh, part of the lower leg, and the sole of the foot.

Common causes of sciatica include:

- slipped disk;
- piriformis syndrome (a pain disorder involving the narrow muscle in the buttocks);
- pelvic injury or fracture;
- tumors.

Symptoms

Sciatica pain can vary widely. It may feel like a mild tingling, dull ache, or a burning sensation. In some cases, the pain is severe enough to make a person unable to move.

The pain most often occurs on one side. Some people have sharp pain in one part of the leg or hip and numbness in other parts. The pain or numbness may also be felt on the back of the calf or on the sole of the foot. The affected leg may feel weak.

The pain often starts slowly. Sciatica pain may get worse:

- after standing or sitting,

- at night;

- when sneezing, coughing, or laughing;

- when bending backwards or walking more than a few yards, especially if caused by spinal stenosis.

Exams and Tests

The health care provider will perform a physical exam. This may show:

- weakness of knee bending or foot movement;

- difficulty bending the foot inward or down;

- abnormal or weak reflexes;

- pain when lifting the leg straight up off the examining table.

Tests determine the suspected causes. They are often not needed unless pain is severe or long lasting. They may include:

- blood tests;

- X-rays;

- MRIs [magnetic resonance imaging] or other imaging tests.

Treatment

Because sciatica is a symptom of another medical condition, the underlying cause should be identified and treated.

In some cases, no treatment is required and recovery occurs on its own.

Conservative treatment is best in many cases. Your doctor may recommend the following steps to calm your symptoms and reduce inflammation.

- Apply heat or ice to the painful area. Try ice for the first 48–72 hours, then use heat after that.

- Take over-the-counter pain relievers such as ibuprofen (Advil, Motrin IB) or acetaminophen (Tylenol).

Bed rest is not recommended. Reduce your activity for the first couple of days. Then, slowly start your usual activities after that. Avoid heavy lifting or twisting of your back for the first six weeks after the pain begins. You should start exercising again after two to three weeks. This should include exercises to strengthen your abdomen and improve flexibility of your spine.

If at-home measures do not help, your doctor may recommend injections to reduce inflammation around the nerve. Other medicines may be prescribed to help reduce the stabbing pains associated with sciatica.

Physical therapy exercises may also be recommended. Additional treatments depend on the condition that is causing the sciatica.

Nerve pain is very difficult to treat. If you have ongoing problems with pain, you may want to see a neurologist or a pain specialist to ensure that you have access to the widest range of treatment options.

Outlook (Prognosis)

Often, sciatica will get better on its own. However, is it common for it to return.

When to Contact a Medical Professional

Call your doctor right away if you have:

- unexplained fever with back pain;

- back pain after a severe blow or fall;

- redness or swelling on the back or spine;

- pain traveling down your legs below the knee;

- weakness or numbness in your buttocks, thigh, leg, or pelvis;

- burning with urination or blood in your urine;

- pain that is worse when you lie down, or awakens you at night;

- severe pain and you cannot get comfortable;

- loss of control of urine or stool (incontinence).

Also call if:

- you have been losing weight unintentionally;

- you use steroids or intravenous drugs;

- you have had back pain before but this episode is different and feels worse;

- this episode of back pain has lasted longer than four weeks.

Prevention

Prevention varies depending on the cause of the nerve damage. Avoid prolonged sitting or lying with pressure on the buttocks.

Part Five

Shoulder and
Upper Arm Injuries

Chapter 26

Common Shoulder Problems

What are the most common shoulder problems?

The most movable joint in the body, the shoulder is also one of the most potentially unstable joints. As a result, it is the site of many common problems. They include sprains, strains, dislocations, separations, tendonitis, bursitis, torn rotator cuffs, frozen shoulder, fractures, and arthritis.

How common are shoulder problems?

According to the Centers for Disease Control and Prevention, nearly 1.5 million people in the United States visited an emergency room in 2006 for shoulder problems.

What are the structures of the shoulder and how does it function?

The shoulder joint is composed of three bones: the clavicle (collarbone), the scapula (shoulder blade), and the humerus (upper arm bone). Two joints facilitate shoulder movement. The acromioclavicular (AC) joint is located between the acromion (part of the scapula that forms the highest point of the shoulder) and the clavicle. The glenohumeral

This chapter excerpted from "Questions and Answers about Shoulder Problems," National Institute of Arthritis and Musculoskeletal and Skin Diseases (www.niams.nih.gov), May 2010.

joint, commonly called the shoulder joint, is a ball-and-socket-type joint that helps move the shoulder forward and backward and allows the arm to rotate in a circular fashion or hinge out and up away from the body. (The "ball," or humerus, is the top, rounded portion of the upper arm bone; the "socket," or glenoid, is a dish-shaped part of the outer edge of the scapula into which the ball fits.) The capsule is a soft tissue envelope that encircles the glenohumeral joint. It is lined by a thin, smooth synovial membrane.

In contrast to the hip joint, which more closely approximates a true ball-and-socket joint, the shoulder joint can be compared to a golf ball and tee, in which the ball can easily slip off the flat tee. Because the bones provide little inherent stability to the shoulder joint, it is highly dependent on surrounding soft tissues such as capsule ligaments and the muscles surrounding the rotator cuff to hold the ball in place. Whereas the hip joint is inherently quite stable because of the encircling bony anatomy, it also is relatively immobile. The shoulder, on the other hand, is relatively unstable but highly mobile, allowing an individual to place the hand in numerous positions. It is, in fact, one of the most mobile joints in the human body.

The bones of the shoulder are held in place by muscles, tendons, and ligaments. Tendons are tough cords of tissue that attach the shoulder muscles to bone and assist the muscles in moving the shoulder. Ligaments attach shoulder bones to each other, providing stability.

What are the origins and causes of shoulder problems?

The shoulder is easily injured because the ball of the upper arm is larger than the shoulder socket that holds it. To remain stable, the shoulder must be anchored by its muscles, tendons, and ligaments.

Although the shoulder is easily injured during sporting activities and manual labor, the primary source of shoulder problems appears to be the natural age-related degeneration of the surrounding soft tissues such as those found in the rotator cuff. The incidence of rotator cuff problems rises dramatically as a function of age and is generally seen among individuals who are more than 60 years old. Often, the dominant and nondominant arm will be affected to a similar degree. Overuse of the shoulder can lead to more rapid age-related deterioration.

How are shoulder problems diagnosed?

As with any medical issue, a shoulder problem is generally diagnosed using a three-part process:

- **Medical history:** The patient tells the doctor about any injury or other condition that might be causing the pain.

- **Physical examination:** The doctor examines the patient to feel for injury and to discover the limits of movement, location of pain, and extent of joint instability.

- **Tests:** The doctor may order one or more tests, such as X-ray, arthrogram, ultrasound, or magnetic resonance imaging (MRI), to make a specific diagnosis.

What should I know about specific shoulder problems, including their symptoms and treatment?

The symptoms of shoulder problems, as well as their diagnosis and treatment, vary widely, depending on the specific problem. Here are some of the most common shoulder problems.

Dislocation: The shoulder joint is the most frequently dislocated major joint of the body. In a typical case of a dislocated shoulder, either a strong force pulls the shoulder outward (abduction) or extreme rotation of the joint pops the ball of the humerus out of the shoulder socket. Dislocation commonly occurs when there is a backward pull on the arm that either catches the muscles unprepared to resist or overwhelms the muscles. When a shoulder dislocates frequently, the condition is referred to as shoulder instability. A partial dislocation in which the upper arm bone is partially in and partially out of the socket is called a subluxation.

Separation: A shoulder separation occurs where the collarbone (clavicle) meets the shoulder blade (scapula). When ligaments that hold the joint together are partially or completely torn, the outer end of the clavicle may slip out of place, preventing it from properly meeting the scapula. Most often, the injury is caused by a blow to the shoulder or by falling on an outstretched hand.

Rotator cuff tendonitis and bursitis: These conditions are closely related and may occur alone or in combination.

Tendonitis is inflammation (redness, soreness, and swelling) of a tendon. In tendonitis of the shoulder, the rotator cuff and/or biceps tendon become inflamed, usually as a result of being pinched by surrounding structures. The injury may vary from mild inflammation to involvement of most of the rotator cuff. Squeezing of the rotator cuff is called impingement syndrome.

Bursitis, or inflammation of the bursa sacs that protect the shoulder, may accompany tendonitis and impingement syndrome. Inflammation caused by a disease such as rheumatoid arthritis may cause rotator cuff tendonitis and bursitis. Sports involving overuse of the shoulder and occupations requiring frequent overhead reaching are other potential causes of irritation to the rotator cuff or bursa and may lead to inflammation and impingement.

If the rotator cuff and bursa are irritated, inflamed, and swollen, they may become squeezed between the head of the humerus and the acromion. Repeated motion involving the arms, or the effects of the aging process on shoulder movement over many years, may also irritate and wear down the tendons, muscles, and surrounding structures.

Torn rotator cuff: Rotator cuff tendons often become inflamed from overuse, aging, or a fall on an outstretched hand or another traumatic cause. Sports or occupations requiring repetitive overhead motion or heavy lifting can also place a significant strain on rotator cuff muscles and tendons. Over time, as a function of aging, tendons become weaker and degenerate. Eventually, this degeneration can lead to complete tears of both muscles and tendons. These tears are surprisingly common. Fortunately, these tears do not lead to any pain or disability in most people. However, some individuals can develop very significant pain as a result of these tears and may require treatment.

Frozen shoulder (adhesive capsulitis): As the name implies, movement of the shoulder is severely restricted in people with a "frozen shoulder." This condition, which doctors call adhesive capsulitis, is frequently caused by injury that leads to lack of use due to pain. Rheumatic disease progression and recent shoulder surgery can also cause frozen shoulder. Intermittent periods of use may cause inflammation. Adhesions (abnormal bands of tissue) grow between the joint surfaces, restricting motion. There is also a lack of synovial fluid, which normally lubricates the gap between the arm bone and socket to help the shoulder joint move. It is this restricted space between the capsule and ball of the humerus that distinguishes adhesive capsulitis from a less complicated painful, stiff shoulder.

Fracture: A fracture involves a partial or total crack through a bone. The break in a bone usually occurs as a result of an impact injury, such as a fall or blow to the shoulder. A fracture usually involves the clavicle or the neck (area below the ball) of the humerus.

What does it mean to treat shoulder injuries with RICE (rest, ice, compression, and elevation)?

- **Rest:** Reduce or stop using the injured area for 48 hours.

- **Ice:** Put an ice pack on the injured area for 20 minutes at a time, four to eight times per day. Use a cold pack, ice bag, or a plastic bag filled with crushed ice that has been wrapped in a towel.

- **Compression:** Compress the area with bandages, such as an elastic wrap, to help stabilize the shoulder. This may help reduce the swelling.

- **Elevation:** Keep the injured area elevated above the level of the heart. Use a pillow to help elevate the injury.

- If pain and stiffness persist, see a doctor.

Chapter 27

Problems with Shoulder Motion Loss

Chapter Contents

Section 27.1

Shoulder Impingement

What is shoulder impingement?

Impingement refers to mechanical compression and/or wear of the rotator cuff tendons. The rotator cuff is actually a series of four muscles connecting the scapula (shoulder blade) to the humeral head (upper part of the shoulder joint). The rotator cuff is important in maintaining the humeral head within the glenoid (socket) during normal shoulder function and also contributes to shoulder strength during activity. Normally, the rotator cuff glides smoothly between the undersurface of the acromion, the bone at the point of the shoulder and the humeral head.

How does shoulder impingement occur?

Any process which compromises this normal gliding function may lead to mechanical impingement. Common causes include weakening and degeneration within the tendon due to aging, the formation of bone spurs and/or inflammatory tissue within the space above the rotator cuff (subacromial space), and overuse injuries. Overuse activities that can lead to impingement are most commonly seen in tennis players, pitchers, and swimmers.

How is shoulder impingement diagnosed?

The diagnosis of shoulder impingement can usually be made with a careful history and physical exam. Patients with impingement most commonly complain of pain in the shoulder, which is worse with overhead activity and sometimes severe enough to cause awakening in the night. Manipulation of the shoulder in a specific way by your doctor will usually reproduce the symptoms and confirm the diagnosis. X-rays are also helpful in evaluating the presence of bone spurs and/or the narrowing of the subacromial space. MRI (magnetic resonance imaging), a test that allows visualization of the rotator cuff, is usually not necessary in cases of shoulder impingement, but may be used to rule out more serious diagnoses.

How is shoulder impingement treated?

The first step in treating shoulder impingement is eliminating any identifiable cause or contributing factor. This may mean temporarily avoiding activities like tennis, pitching, or swimming. A nonsteroidal anti-inflammatory medication may also be recommended by your doctor. The mainstay of treatment involves exercises to restore normal flexibility and strength to the shoulder girdle, including strengthening both the rotator cuff muscles and the muscles responsible for normal movement of the shoulder blade. This program of instruction and exercise demonstration may be initiated and carried out either by the doctor, certified athletic trainer, or a skilled physical therapist. Occasionally, an injection of cortisone may be helpful in treating this condition.

Is surgery necessary?

Surgery is not necessary in most cases of shoulder impingement. But if symptoms persist despite adequate nonsurgical treatment, surgical intervention may be beneficial. Surgery involves debriding, or surgically removing, tissue that is irritating the rotator cuff. This may be done with either open or arthroscopic techniques. Outcome is favorable in about 90% of the cases.

Section 27.2

Frozen Shoulder

Frozen shoulder, also called adhesive capsulitis, causes pain and stiffness in the shoulder. Over time, the shoulder becomes very hard to move.

Frozen shoulder occurs in about 2% of the general population. It most commonly affects people between the ages of 40 and 60, and occurs in women more often than men.

Anatomy

Your shoulder is a ball-and-socket joint made up of three bones: your upper arm bone (humerus), your shoulder blade (scapula), and your collarbone (clavicle).

The head of the upper arm bone fits into a shallow socket in your shoulder blade. Strong connective tissue, called the shoulder capsule, surrounds the joint.

To help your shoulder move more easily, synovial fluid lubricates the shoulder capsule and the joint.

Description

In frozen shoulder, the shoulder capsule thickens and becomes tight. Stiff bands of tissue—called adhesions—develop. In many cases, there is less synovial fluid in the joint.

The hallmark sign of this condition is being unable to move your shoulder—either on your own or with the help of someone else. It develops in three stages:

Freezing

In the "freezing" stage, you slowly have more and more pain. As the pain worsens, your shoulder loses range of motion. Freezing typically lasts from six weeks to nine months.

Frozen

Painful symptoms may actually improve during this stage, but the stiffness remains. During the four to six months of the "frozen" stage, daily activities may be very difficult.

Thawing

Shoulder motion slowly improves during the "thawing" stage. Complete return to normal or close to normal strength and motion typically takes from six months to two years.

Cause

The causes of frozen shoulder are not fully understood. There is no clear connection to arm dominance or occupation. A few factors may put you more at risk for developing frozen shoulder.

Diabetes: Frozen shoulder occurs much more often in people with diabetes, affecting 10% to 20% of these individuals. The reason for this is not known.

Other diseases: Some additional medical problems associated with frozen shoulder include hypothyroidism, hyperthyroidism, Parkinson's disease, and cardiac disease.

Immobilization: Frozen shoulder can develop after a shoulder has been immobilized for a period of time due to surgery, a fracture, or other injury. Having patients move their shoulders soon after injury or surgery is one measure prescribed to prevent frozen shoulder.

Symptoms

Pain from frozen shoulder is usually dull or aching. It is typically worse early in the course of the disease and when you move your arm. The pain is usually located over the outer shoulder area and sometimes the upper arm.

Doctor Examination

Physical Examination

After discussing your symptoms and medical history, your doctor will examine your shoulder. Your doctor will move your shoulder carefully in all directions to see if movement is limited and if pain occurs with the motion. The range of motion when someone else moves your shoulder is called "passive range of motion." Your doctor will compare this to the range of motion you display when you move your shoulder on your own ("active range of motion"). People with frozen shoulder have limited range of motion both actively and passively.

Imaging Tests

Other tests that may help your doctor rule out other causes of stiffness and pain include:

X-rays: Dense structures, such as bone, show up clearly on X-rays. X-rays may show other problems in your shoulder, such as arthritis.

Magnetic resonance imaging (MRI) and ultrasound: These studies can create better images of problems with soft tissues, such as a torn rotator cuff.

Treatment

Frozen shoulder generally gets better over time, although it may take up to three years.

The focus of treatment is to control pain and restore motion and strength through physical therapy.

Nonsurgical Treatment

More than 90% of patients improve with relatively simple treatments to control pain and restore motion.

Non-steroidal anti-inflammatory medicines: Drugs like aspirin and ibuprofen reduce pain and swelling.

Steroid injections: Cortisone is a powerful anti-inflammatory medicine that is injected directly into your shoulder joint.

Physical therapy: Specific exercises will help restore motion. These may be under the supervision of a physical therapist or via a home program. Therapy includes stretching or range of motion exercises for the shoulder. Sometimes heat is used to help loosen the shoulder up before the stretching exercises.

Surgical Treatment

If your symptoms are not relieved by therapy and anti-inflammatory medicines, you and your doctor may discuss surgery. It is important to talk with your doctor about your potential for recovery continuing with simple treatments, and the risks involved with surgery.

The goal of surgery for frozen shoulder is to stretch and release the stiffened joint capsule. The most common methods include manipulation under anesthesia and shoulder arthroscopy.

- **Manipulation under anesthesia:** During this procedure, you are put to sleep. Your doctor will force your shoulder to move which causes the capsule and scar tissue to stretch or tear. This releases the tightening and increases range of motion.

- **Shoulder arthroscopy:** In this procedure, your doctor will cut through tight portions of the joint capsule. This is done using pencil-sized instruments inserted through small incisions around your shoulder.

In many cases, manipulation and arthroscopy are used in combination to obtain maximum results. Most patients have very good outcomes with these procedures.

Recovery: After surgery, physical therapy is necessary to maintain the motion that was achieved with surgery. Recovery times vary, from six weeks to three months. Although it is a slow process, your commitment to therapy is the most important factor in returning to all the activities you enjoy.

Long-term outcomes after surgery are generally good, with most patients having reduced or no pain and greatly improved range of motion. In some cases, however, even after several years, the motion does not return completely and a small amount of stiffness remains.

Although uncommon, frozen shoulder can recur, especially if a contributing factor like diabetes is still present.

Chapter 28

Rotator Cuff Tendonitis

The rotator cuff is a group of muscles and tendons that attach to the bones of the shoulder joint, allowing the shoulder to move and keeping it stable.

- Rotator cuff tendinitis refers to irritation of these tendons and inflammation of the bursa (a normally smooth layer) lining these tendons.

- A rotator cuff tear occurs when one of the tendons is torn from overuse or injury.

Causes

The shoulder joint is a ball and socket type joint where the top part of the arm bone (humerus) forms a joint with the shoulder blade (scapula). The rotator cuff holds the head of the humerus into the scapula and controls movement of the shoulder joint.

The tendons of the rotator cuff pass underneath a bony area on their way to attaching the top part of the arm bone. When these tendons become inflamed, they can become more frayed over this area during shoulder movements. Sometimes, a bone spur may narrow the space even more.

This problem is called rotator cuff tendinitis, or impingement syndrome, and may be due to:

Excerpted from "Rotator Cuff Problems," © 2011 A.D.A.M., Inc. Reprinted with permission.

- keeping the arm in the same position for long periods of time, such as doing computer work or hairstyling;

- sleeping on the same arm each night;

- playing sports requiring the arm to be moved over the head repeatedly as in tennis, baseball (particularly pitching), swimming, and lifting weights over the head;

- working with the arm overhead for many hours or days (such as painters and carpenters);

- poor control or coordination of your shoulder and shoulder blade muscles.

Poor posture over many years and the usual fraying of the tendons that occurs with age may also lead to rotator cuff tendinitis.

Symptoms

Early on, pain occurs with overhead activities and lifting your arm to the side. Activities include brushing hair, reaching for objects on shelves, or playing an overhead sport.

- Pain is more likely in the front of the shoulder and may radiate to the side of the arm. However, this pain always stops before the elbow. If the pain travels beyond the arm to the elbow and hand, this may indicate a pinched nerve.

- There may also be pain with lowering the shoulder from a raised position.

At first, this pain may be mild and occur only with certain movements of the arm. Over time, pain may be present at rest or at night, especially when lying on the affected shoulder.

You may have weakness and loss of motion when raising the arm above your head. Your shoulder can feel stiff with lifting or movement. It may become more difficult to place the arm behind your back.

Exams and Tests

A physical examination may reveal tenderness over the shoulder. Pain may occur when the shoulder is raised overhead. There is usually weakness of the shoulder when it is placed in certain positions.

X-rays of the shoulder may show a bone spur. They can be done in your doctor's office.

If your doctor feels you may have a rotator cuff tear, you may have one or more of the following tests:

- An ultrasound test uses sound waves to create an image of the shoulder joint. It can often show a tear in the rotator cuff.

- MRI [magnetic resonance imaging] of the shoulder may show swelling or a tear in the rotator cuff.

Sometimes, a special imaging test called arthrography is needed to diagnose a rotator cuff tear. Your doctor will inject contrast material into your shoulder joint. Then either an X-ray, CT [computed tomography] scan, or MRI scan are used to take a picture of it. Contrast is usually used when your doctor suspects a small rotator cuff tear.

Treatment

Treatment involves resting the shoulder and avoiding activities that cause pain. It may involve:

- ice packs applied 20 minutes at a time, three to four times a day to the shoulder;

- taking drugs like ibuprofen and naproxen to help reduce swelling and pain;

- avoiding or reducing activities that cause or worsen your symptoms.

You should start physical therapy to learn exercises to stretch and strengthen the muscles of your rotator cuff.

If the pain persists or if therapy is not possible because of severe pain, a steroid injection may reduce pain and swelling in the injured tendons, to allow effective therapy.

With rest and exercise, symptoms often improve or go away. However, this may take weeks or months to occur.

Arthroscopic surgery can remove inflamed tissue and part of the bone that lies over the rotator cuff. Removing the bone may relieve the pressure on the tendons.

Outlook (Prognosis)

Many people recover full function after a combination of medications, physical therapy, and steroid injections after an episode of rotator cuff tendonitis. Some may need to change or reduce the amount of time they play certain sports to remain pain-free.

Prevention

Avoid repetitive overhead movements. Develop shoulder strength in opposing muscle groups.

Chapter 29

Problems with Shoulder Instability

Chapter Contents

Section 29.1

Shoulder Instability

"Multidirectional Shoulder Instability," reprinted with permission from Children's Memorial Hospital, Chicago, IL (www.childrens memorial.org). All rights reserved. Reviewed by David A. Cooke, MD, FACP, August 2011.

Your upper arm bone (humerus) rests in a shallow socket to form the main part of your shoulder joint. The capsule and ligaments are the structures that hold the bones of the shoulder together. If these structures don't hold the bones together as tightly as they should, the shoulder joint may feel too loose. This looseness allows the humerus to partially slide out of its socket, a condition called shoulder subluxation. The humerus may even come all the way out of its socket; this is called a shoulder dislocation.

With multidirectional shoulder instability, the shoulder is loose in a way that allows the humerus to have extra movement in several directions.

How It Occurs

Some individuals have naturally loose ligaments which can predispose them to instability. Shoulder instability can also occur in people who regularly perform shoulder motions that stretch out the joint capsule; gymnasts, pitchers, volleyball players, and swimmers are at higher risk for shoulder instability. Sometimes a sudden injury will cause increased symptoms. With multidirectional instability, the shoulder is loose with motions in several directions. This is different from patients who have instability following a shoulder dislocation that occurs as a result of a traumatic injury; these individuals generally have looseness in only one direction.

Signs and Symptoms

The main sign is pain in your shoulder. The pain can start suddenly or slowly. Certain motions or positions (for example winding up to throw a ball) may aggravate the pain. You may notice that your shoulder feels loose or that your arm feels weak.

Diagnosis

Your doctor will look at your shoulder, perform maneuvers to test for instability, and may take X-rays and/or send you for an MRI [magnetic resonance imaging] to examine the structure of the shoulder and rule out other conditions.

Treatment

- **Rest:** Avoid painful activities or activities that stress the joint

- **Ice:** Helps control pain, especially after exercise

- **Medication:** May be given to manage pain such as ibuprofen (Motrin, Advil) or naproxen (Aleve)

- **Rehabilitation:** You may need therapy treatments for six to eight weeks or more:
    - physical therapy to strengthen the muscles that control and stabilize the shoulder joint;
    - specific exercises for certain sports;
    - learn how to modify activities to prevent re-injury;
    - you will need to continue your physical therapy exercises at home to prevent further injury.

- **Surgery:** Most patients have significant improvement in their symptoms with physical therapy. Surgery is considered if other treatments fail. Many different procedures may be used to correct shoulder instability. The goal is to fix the cause. The doctor may use an arthroscope (a small surgical camera placed into small incisions) or make a larger incision for your surgery. After surgery, physical therapy is required to regain strength and range-of-motion.

Returning to Activity and Sports

The goal is to return to sports as quickly and safely as possible. If you return to sports or activities too soon, or play with pain, the injury may worsen. Everyone recovers from injury at a different rate. Your doctor will work with you to determine when you can resume athletic activities. Regaining full range of motion and strength is vitally important, as well as improving the overall stability of the joint.

Preventing Shoulder Instability

- Do regular exercise to strengthen the supporting muscles.

- Use proper athletic training methods.

- Do not increase exercise duration or intensity more than 10% per week.

- Modify activities to prevent excessive external rotation and overhead motions of the shoulder.

- *Do not play through pain. Pain is a sign of injury, stress, or overuse.* Rest is required to allow time for the injured area to heal. If pain does not resolve after a couple days of rest, consult your physician. The sooner an injury is identified, the sooner proper treatment can begin. The result is shorter healing time and faster return to sport.

Section 29.2

Shoulder Dislocation

"Shoulder Dislocation," © 2005 St. John's Hospital (www.st-johns.org). All rights reserved. Reprinted with permission. Reviewed by David A. Cooke, MD, FACP, August 2011.

Introduction

The shoulder is the most frequently dislocated major joint in the body. In some sports, shoulder joint dislocations are more common than all other joint dislocations combined. Anterior, or forward, dislocations account for between 80% and 95% of all shoulder girdle dislocations. Shoulder instability can range from a vague sense of shoulder dysfunction, resulting in non-traumatic instability, to traumatic dislocation.

Mechanism of Injury

If the arm is externally rotated and abducted (moved away and upward from the body) this force pushes the arm beyond the limits of the capsule and the ligaments surrounding the shoulder joint. The greater tuberosity of the humerus is levered against the acromial process and the coracoacromial ligament. This tears the inferior shoulder ligaments, the anterior capsule, and perhaps the labrum. The humeral head slips out, commonly in a downward and forward direction. When the arm is dropped to the side, the head usually comes to rest under the coracoid process.

Symptoms

The athlete usually knows that the shoulder has dislocated and is very alarmed and apprehensive. There is intense pain with initial dislocation (though recurrent dislocations may be much less painful). There may be tingling and numbness down into the hand.

Diagnosis

Immediate recognition of an anterior dislocation is often possible due to the characteristic position of the athlete's arm.

- There is a sharp contour of the affected limb in comparison to the opposite side.

- There is a prominent acromion process.

- The humeral head is below the coracoid process.

- The athlete is resistive to any attempt to lift the arm out to the side or internally rotate the arm (i.e., the arm can not be brought across the chest).

At the scene of the injury, it is important to examine the sensation of the arm, the strength (this may be difficult due to pain), the radial pulse, and peripheral circulation.

Complications

1. Damage to the nerves around the shoulder joint

2. Rotator cuff tears in conjunction with an anteroinferior dislocation, even in young athletes

3. Fractures of the humeral head and glenoid—relatively frequent in the older athlete (the greater tuberosity is the area most commonly fractured, due to its shearing against the acromion process and the coracoacromial ligament)

267

Management

The ideal time to reduce a shoulder dislocation is immediately after it occurs. If there is a delay before the shoulder is reduced, pain and involuntary muscle spasm can make reduction difficult.

Reduction should be done by a physician, and an evaluation of the neurological and vascular structures should be performed and recorded before reduction. If possible, X-rays should be taken before reduction is attempted; post-reduction X-rays should always be taken.

In the acute phase of an injury, if a physician is not present to reduce the injury, the athlete's shoulder should be splinted and supported with bandages. Ice should also be applied at this time to reduce swelling, inflammation, and muscle spasm. The athlete should then be transported to the emergency room.

For anterior dislocation, after closed reduction, the shoulder is immobilized with a sling. In the first two weeks after reduction, a program of strong isometric shoulder work is instituted to minimize muscle wasting. From two to six weeks after injury, the sling is removed for exercises several times a day. The emphasis is still on isometric activities, with shoulder medial and lateral rotator isometric exercises being added. Concentric exercise through a limited range is permitted, as long as the movement is controlled.

Treatment progression is aimed at further restoration of range of motion, continued strengthening of the appropriate muscle groups, increasing speed of movement activity to functional levels, improving control of shoulder mechanics, increasing endurance, and continuing to restore proprioceptive control. As shoulder function improves, the athlete may work up to heavier weights or begin using various exercise devices, such as Nautilus or isokinetic machines, elastic tubing, pulleys, a broomstick, or T-bar routine. Plyometrics and use of medicine balls are helpful in later stages of rehabilitation to teach functional stabilization and control.

If the problem is one of recurrent shoulder instability, the rehabilitation process follows a similar path, ensuring especially that exercises demonstrate activation of the appropriate muscle or muscle groups and that the proper functional control is achieved. Surgical repair may be necessary in cases of recurrent dislocation.

Conclusion

Shoulder dislocation is a common problem among athletes. In this section we have focused on the most common form of dislocation, anterior dislocation. Return to sports and activities is definitely the goal of rehabilitation. Complications can best be avoided by following the correct procedures at the onset of the injury. The rehabilitation process is tailored to each individual athlete and sport. If managed correctly, most can return to prior function.

Section 29.3

Shoulder Separation and Acromioclavicular (AC) Injuries

Introduction

Injuries to the acromioclavicular (AC) joint are common in athletes. However, these problems are often confused with other problems associated with the shoulder. This injury is approximately five times more common in men than in women.

Mechanisms of Injury

1. The athlete falls on the point of the shoulder, forcing the acromion and the coracoid process downward.

2. The athlete falls on the outstretched hand, transmitting the force up to the arm and through the acromioclavicular joint.

3. The athlete falls on the outstretched hand, which is at a right angle to the body. Contact is then made by the opposition against the shoulder, forcing the shoulder forward on a fixed arm.

AC joint injuries are classified as types I through VI, according to the severity of the injury and the ligaments involved. In this section we will focus on types I, II and III. Types IV–VI are rare modifications of type III injuries and require surgical repair.

Type I

Strain of the acromioclavicular ligament or capsule. Coracoclavicular ligament is intact. There is generally tenderness and swelling over the AC joint. There is minimal limitation of range of motion and the clavicle is stable.

Type II

Severe sprain of the AC ligament. Partial strain or stretching of the coracoclavicular ligament. There is increased swelling and tenderness over the joint and some tenderness over the ligaments. The shoulder motion is considerably limited due to pain. There is slight elevation of the clavicle relative to the acromion process.

Type III

Complete tearing of the AC and coracoclavicular ligaments. There is often damage to the shoulder muscles surrounding the area. The athlete supports the arm, as the symptoms are markedly increased when the arm hangs. There is significant tenderness and swelling and an obvious elevation of the clavicle relative to the acromion process.

The clinical differentiation of these injuries by type is based on physical examination. X-rays may be useful to exclude fractures of the clavicle, acromion, coracoid, or humerus. It is important to differentiate AC joint lesions from contusions to the end of the clavicle ("shoulder pointer"). A shoulder pointer implies a contusion only; there is no ligamentous involvement.

Management

Type I

Rest and application of ice usually result in cessation of discomfort within two weeks. Full return to activity should not be allowed until the patient has painless full range of motion. A sling should be initially applied. This is then followed by rehabilitation exercises to restore normal shoulder function quickly. A donut pad can be worn over the acromioclavicular joint if the athlete participates in contact sports.

Type II

At the onset of the injury, ice is again applied. The joint needs to be immobilized for two to four weeks, depending on the severity of the injury. Application of ice and rest are indicated as for type I injuries. The athlete will also require extensive rehabilitation and may not return to sports for up to eight weeks.

Type III

The management of type III injuries remains controversial. In the acute phase, ice application and rest are important. These injuries have been managed with surgical and non-surgical treatment. Support for non-operative treatment is well-documented in medical literature, and the current trend is reflective of this. In general, use of a sling is recommended for approximately four weeks, followed by gentle movement and strengthening. Guarded return to work and sports is allowed over the subsequent three months, dependent upon the return of full, painless range of motion and stability of the joint. Participation in contact sports is usually permitted three to five months after the injury, depending upon functional recovery. Operative management of acute injuries is generally reserved for high-level pitchers or patients with open injuries, nerve damage, or severe dislocations.

Complications

1. Pain, disability, and decrease in shoulder range of motion may occasionally be troublesome.

2. Degenerative changes may involve the acromion, resulting in spur formation which leads not only to pain in the AC joint, but impingement of the rotator cuff.

3. Calcification can develop over the end of the clavicle and render this area painful.

4. An unreduced separation may result in cosmetic deformity, consisting of a bulge over the end of the clavicle.

Rehabilitation

Rehabilitation exercises for the entire shoulder girdle muscle complex should continue until pre-injury power, strength, endurance, and flexibility are obtained. Attaining full shoulder range of motion is the first goal of rehabilitation. Static contraction exercises for all planes of motion can be started early and later progressed to resisted strengthening for all shoulder movements in straight planes and diagonals. Rotator cuff and scapula stabilizer muscle strengthening may

271

be necessary. Resistance for exercise may be in the form of elastic tubing, weights, isotonic exercises on a Universal gym or Nautilus, and isokinetic exercises with Cybex or BTE.

Conclusion

Our understanding of the acromioclavicular joint and its associated injuries has increased during the last three decades. Injuries to this joint are classified as acute or chronic and by severity of displacement. Most are treated non-operatively. In AC sprains, return to sporting activities is dependent upon the achievement of full range of motion and strength with stability comparable to the uninjured shoulder.

Chapter 30

Muscle Tears and Tendon Injuries

Chapter Contents

Section 30.1

Shoulder Joint and Labral Tears

"Shoulder Joint Tear (Glenoid Labrum Tear)," reproduced with permission from *Your Orthopaedic Connection.* © American Academy of Orthopaedic Surgeons (www.aaos.org), Rosemont, IL, 2001. Reviewed by David A. Cooke, MD, FACP, September 2011.

Advances in medical technology are enabling doctors to identify and treat injuries that went unnoticed 20 years ago. For example, physicians can now use miniaturized television cameras to see inside a joint. With this tool, they have been able to identify and treat a shoulder injury called a glenoid labrum tear.

Anatomy

The shoulder joint has three bones: the shoulder blade (scapula), the collarbone (clavicle), and the upper arm bone (humerus). The head of the upper arm bone (humeral head) rests in a shallow socket in the shoulder blade called the glenoid. The head of the upper arm bone is usually much larger than the socket, and a soft fibrous tissue rim called the labrum surrounds the socket to help stabilize the joint. The rim deepens the socket by up to 50% so that the head of the upper arm bone fits better. In addition, it serves as an attachment site for several ligaments.

Risk Factors/Prevention

Injuries to the tissue rim surrounding the shoulder socket can occur from acute trauma or repetitive shoulder motion. Examples of traumatic injury include:

- falling on an outstretched arm;
- a direct blow to the shoulder;
- a sudden pull, such as when trying to lift a heavy object;
- a violent overhead reach, such as when trying to stop a fall or slide.

Throwing athletes or weightlifters can experience glenoid labrum tears as a result of repetitive shoulder motion.

274

Symptoms

The symptoms of a tear in the shoulder socket rim are very similar to those of other shoulder injuries. Symptoms include:

- pain, usually with overhead activities;
- catching, locking, popping, or grinding;
- occasional night pain or pain with daily activities;
- a sense of instability in the shoulder;
- decreased range of motion;
- loss of strength.

Diagnosis

If you are experiencing shoulder pain, your doctor will take a history of your injury. You may be able to remember a specific incident or you may note that the pain gradually increased. The doctor will do several physical tests to check range of motion, stability, and pain. In addition, the doctor will request X-rays to see if there are any other reasons for your problems.

Because the rim of the shoulder socket is soft tissue, X-rays will not show damage to it. The doctor may order a computed tomography (CT) scan or magnetic resonance imaging (MRI) scan. In both instances, a contrast medium may be injected to help detect tears. Ultimately, however, the diagnosis will be made with arthroscopic surgery.

Tears can be located either above (superior) or below (inferior) the middle of the glenoid socket.

A SLAP lesion (superior labrum, anterior [front] to posterior [back]) is a tear of the rim above the middle of the socket that may also involve the biceps tendon.

A tear of the rim below the middle of the glenoid socket that also involves the inferior glenohumeral ligament is called a Bankart lesion.

Tears of the glenoid rim often occur with other shoulder injuries, such as a dislocated shoulder (full or partial dislocation).

Treatment

Until the final diagnosis is made, your physician may prescribe anti-inflammatory medication and rest to relieve symptoms. Rehabilitation exercises to strengthen the rotator cuff muscles may also be recommended. If these conservative measures are insufficient, your physician may recommend arthroscopic surgery.

During arthroscopic surgery, the doctor will examine the rim and the biceps tendon. If the injury is confined to the rim itself, without involving the tendon, the shoulder is still stable. The surgeon will remove the torn flap and correct any other associated problems. If the tear extends into the biceps tendon or if the tendon is detached, the shoulder is unstable. The surgeon will need to repair and reattach the tendon using absorbable tacks, wires, or sutures.

Tears below the middle of the socket are also associated with shoulder instability. The surgeon will reattach the ligament and tighten the shoulder socket by folding over and "pleating" the tissues.

Rehabilitation

After surgery, you will need to keep your shoulder in a sling for three to four weeks. Your physician will also prescribe gentle, passive, pain-free range-of-motion exercises. When the sling is removed, you will need to do motion and flexibility exercises and gradually start to strengthen your biceps. Athletes can usually begin doing sport-specific exercises six weeks after surgery, although it will be three to four months before the shoulder is fully healed.

Section 30.2

Rotator Cuff Tears

"Rotator Cuff Tears," reproduced with permission from
Your Orthopaedic Connection. © American Academy of Orthopaedic
Surgeons (www.aaos.org), Rosemont, IL, 2001.

A rotator cuff tear is a common cause of pain and disability among adults. In 2008, close to 2 million people in the United States went to their doctors because of a rotator cuff problem.

A torn rotator cuff will weaken your shoulder. This means that many daily activities, like combing your hair or getting dressed, may become painful and difficult to do.

Anatomy

Your shoulder is made up of three bones: your upper arm bone (humerus), your shoulder blade (scapula), and your collarbone (clavicle). The shoulder is a ball-and-socket joint: the ball, or head, of your upper arm bone fits into a shallow socket in your shoulder blade.

Your arm is kept in your shoulder socket by your rotator cuff. The rotator cuff is a network of four muscles that come together as tendons to form a covering around the head of the humerus. The rotator cuff attaches the humerus to the shoulder blade and helps to lift and rotate your arm.

There is a lubricating sac called a bursa between the rotator cuff and the bone on top of your shoulder (acromion). The bursa allows the rotator cuff tendons to glide freely when you move your arm. When the rotator cuff tendons are injured or damaged, this bursa can also become inflamed and painful.

Description

When one or more of the rotator cuff tendons is torn, the tendon no longer fully attaches to the head of the humerus. Most tears occur in the supraspinatus muscle and tendon, but other parts of the rotator cuff may also be involved.

In many cases, torn tendons begin by fraying. As the damage progresses, the tendon can completely tear, sometimes with lifting a heavy object.

There are different types of tears.

- **Partial tear:** This type of tear damages the soft tissue, but does not completely sever it.

- **Full-thickness tear:** This type of tear is also called a complete tear. It splits the soft tissue into two pieces. In many cases, tendons tear off where they attach to the head of the humerus. With a full-thickness tear, there is basically a hole in the tendon.

Cause

There are two main causes of rotator cuff tears: injury and degeneration.

Acute Tear

If you fall down on your outstretched arm or lift something too heavy with a jerking motion, you can tear your rotator cuff. This type of tear can occur with other shoulder injuries, such as a broken collarbone or dislocated shoulder.

Degenerative Tear

Most tears are the result of a wearing down of the tendon that occurs slowly over time. This degeneration naturally occurs as we age. Rotator cuff tears are more common in the dominant arm. If you have a degenerative tear in one shoulder, there is a greater risk for a rotator cuff tear in the opposite shoulder—even if you have no pain in that shoulder.

Several factors contribute to degenerative, or chronic, rotator cuff tears.

- **Repetitive stress:** Repeating the same shoulder motions again and again can stress your rotator cuff muscles and tendons. Baseball, tennis, rowing, and weightlifting are examples of sports activities that can put you at risk for overuse tears. Many jobs and routine chores can cause overuse tears, as well.

- **Lack of blood supply:** As we get older, the blood supply in our rotator cuff tendons lessens. Without a good blood supply, the body's natural ability to repair tendon damage is impaired. This can ultimately lead to a tendon tear.

- **Bone spurs:** As we age, bone spurs (bone overgrowth) often develop on the underside of the acromion bone. When we lift our arms, the spurs rub on the rotator cuff tendon. This condition is called shoulder impingement and over time will weaken the tendon and make it more likely to tear.

Risk Factors

Because most rotator cuff tears are largely caused by the normal wear and tear that goes along with aging, people over 40 are at greater risk.

People who do repetitive lifting or overhead activities are also at risk for rotator cuff tears. Athletes are especially vulnerable to overuse tears, particularly tennis players and baseball pitchers. Painters, carpenters, and others who do overhead work also have a greater chance for tears.

Although overuse tears caused by sports activity or overhead work also occur in younger people, most tears in young adults are caused by a traumatic injury, like a fall.

Symptoms

The most common symptoms of a rotator cuff tear include:

- pain at rest and at night, particularly if lying on the affected shoulder;

- pain when lifting and lowering your arm or with specific movements;

- weakness when lifting or rotating your arm;

- crepitus or crackling sensation when moving your shoulder in certain positions.

Tears that happen suddenly, such as from a fall, usually cause intense pain. There may be a snapping sensation and immediate weakness in your upper arm.

Tears that develop slowly due to overuse also cause pain and arm weakness. You may have pain in the shoulder when you lift your arm to the side, or pain that moves down your arm. At first, the pain may be mild and only present when lifting your arm over your head, such as reaching into a cupboard. Over-the-counter medication, such as aspirin or ibuprofen, may relieve the pain at first.

Over time, the pain may become more noticeable at rest, and no longer goes away with medications. You may have pain when you lie on the painful side at night. The pain and weakness in the shoulder may make routine activities such as combing your hair or reaching behind your back more difficult.

Doctor Examination

Medical History and Physical Examination

Your doctor will test your range of motion by having you move your arm in different directions.

After discussing your symptoms and medical history, your doctor will examine your shoulder. He or she will check to see whether it is tender in any area or whether there is a deformity. To measure the range of motion of your shoulder, your doctor will have you move your arm in several different directions. He or she will also test your arm strength.

Your doctor will check for other problems with your shoulder joint. He or she may also examine your neck to make sure that the pain is not coming from a "pinched nerve" and to rule out other conditions, such as arthritis.

Imaging Tests

Other tests which may help your doctor confirm your diagnosis include:

- **X-rays:** The first imaging tests performed are usually X-rays. Because X-rays do not show the soft tissues of your shoulder like the rotator cuff, plain X-rays of a shoulder with rotator cuff pain are usually normal or may show a small bone spur.

- **MRI or ultrasound:** These studies can better show soft tissues like the rotator cuff tendons. They can show the rotator cuff tear, as well as where the tear is located within the tendon and the size of the tear. An MRI can also give your doctor a better idea of how "old" or "new" a tear is because it can show the quality of the rotator cuff muscles.

Treatment

If you have a rotator cuff tear and you keep using it despite increasing pain, you may cause further damage. A rotator cuff tear can get larger over time.

Chronic shoulder and arm pain are good reasons to see your doctor. Early treatment can prevent your symptoms from getting worse. It will also get you back to your normal routine that much quicker.

The goal of any treatment is to reduce pain and restore function. There are several treatment options for a rotator cuff tear, and the best option is different for every person. In planning your treatment, your doctor will consider your age, activity level, general health, and the type of tear you have.

There is no evidence of better results from surgery performed near the time of injury versus later on. For this reason, many doctors first recommend nonsurgical management of rotator cuff tears.

Nonsurgical Treatment

In about 50% of patients, nonsurgical treatment relieves pain and improves function in the shoulder. Shoulder strength, however, does not usually improve without surgery.

Nonsurgical treatment options may include:

- **Rest:** Your doctor may suggest rest and limiting overhead activities. He or she may also prescribe a sling to help protect your shoulder and keep it still.

- **Activity modification:** Avoid activities that cause shoulder pain.

- **Non-steroidal anti-inflammatory medication:** Drugs like ibuprofen and naproxen reduce pain and swelling.

- **Strengthening exercises and physical therapy:** Specific exercises will restore movement and strengthen your shoulder. Your exercise program will include stretches to improve flexibility and range of motion. Strengthening the muscles that support your shoulder can relieve pain and prevent further injury.

- **Steroid injection:** If rest, medications, and physical therapy do not relieve your pain, an injection of a local anesthetic and a cortisone preparation may be helpful. Cortisone is a very effective anti-inflammatory medicine.

The chief advantage of nonsurgical treatment is that it avoids the major risks of surgery, such as:

- infection;

- permanent stiffness;

- anesthesia complications;

- sometimes lengthy recovery time.

The disadvantages of nonsurgical treatment are:

- no improvements in strength;
- size of tear may increase over time;
- activities may need to be limited.

Surgical Treatment

Your doctor may recommend surgery if your pain does not improve with nonsurgical methods. Continued pain is the main indication for surgery. If you are very active and use your arms for overhead work or sports, your doctor may also suggest surgery.

Other signs that surgery may be a good option for you include:

- your symptoms have lasted 6 to 12 months;
- you have a large tear (more than 3 cm);
- you have significant weakness and loss of function in your shoulder;
- your tear was caused by a recent, acute injury.

Surgery to repair a torn rotator cuff most often involves re-attaching the tendon to the head of humerus (upper arm bone). There are a few options for repairing rotator cuff tears. Your orthopaedic surgeon will discuss with you the best procedure to meet your individual health needs.

Read more about surgical treatment options at http://orthoinfo.aaos .org/topic.cfm?topic=A00406.

Section 30.3

Biceps Tendon Injuries

The biceps muscle is in the front of your upper arm. It helps you bend your elbow and rotate your arm. It also helps keep your shoulder stable.

Tendons attach muscles to bones. Your biceps tendons attach the biceps muscle to bones in the shoulder and in the elbow. If you tear the biceps tendon at the shoulder, you may lose some strength in your arm and be unable to forcefully turn your arm from palm down to palm up.

Many people can still function with a biceps tendon tear and only need simple treatments to relieve symptoms. Some people require surgery to repair the torn tendon.

Anatomy

There are two attachments of the biceps tendon at the shoulder joint.

Your shoulder is a ball-and-socket joint made up of three bones: your upper arm bone (humerus), your shoulder blade (scapula), and your collarbone (clavicle).

The head of your upper arm bone fits into a rounded socket in your shoulder blade. This socket is called the glenoid. A combination of muscles and tendons keeps your arm bone centered in your shoulder socket. These tissues are called the rotator cuff. They cover the head of your upper arm bone and attach it to your shoulder blade.

The upper end of the biceps muscle has two tendons that attach it to bones in the shoulder. The long head attaches to the top of the shoulder socket (glenoid). The short head attaches to a bump on the shoulder blade called the coracoid process.

Description

Biceps tendon tears can be either partial or complete.

- **Partial tears:** Many tears do not completely sever the tendon.
- **Complete tears:** A complete tear will split the tendon into two pieces.

In many cases, torn tendons begin by fraying. As the damage progresses, the tendon can completely tear, sometimes with lifting a heavy object.

The long head of the biceps tendon is more likely to be injured. This is because it is vulnerable as it travels through the shoulder joint to its attachment point in the socket. Fortunately, the biceps has two attachments at the shoulder. The short head of the biceps rarely tears. Because of this second attachment, many people can still use their biceps even after a complete tear of the long head.

When you tear your biceps tendon, you can also damage other parts of your shoulder, such as the rotator cuff tendons.

Cause

There are two main causes of biceps tendon tears: injury and overuse.

Injury

If you fall hard on an outstretched arm or lift something too heavy, you can tear your biceps tendon.

Overuse

Many tears are the result of a wearing down and fraying of the tendon that occurs slowly over time. This naturally occurs as we age. It can be worsened by overuse—repeating the same shoulder motions again and again.

Overuse can cause a range of shoulder problems, including tendonitis, shoulder impingement, and rotator cuff injuries. Having any of these conditions puts more stress on the biceps tendon, making it more likely to weaken or tear.

Risk Factors

Your risk for a tendon tear increases with:

Age: Older people have put more years of wear and tear on their tendons than younger people.

Heavy overhead activities: Too much load during weightlifting is a prime example of this risk, but many jobs require heavy overhead lifting and put excess wear and tear on the tendons.

Shoulder overuse: Repetitive overhead sports—such as swimming or tennis—can cause more tendon wear and tear.

Smoking: Nicotine use can affect nutrition in the tendon.

Corticosteroid medications: Using corticosteroids has been linked to increased muscle and tendon weakness.

Symptoms

- Sudden, sharp pain in the upper arm
- Sometimes an audible pop or snap
- Cramping of the biceps muscle with strenuous use of the arm
- Bruising from the middle of the upper arm down toward the elbow
- Pain or tenderness at the shoulder and the elbow
- Weakness in the shoulder and the elbow
- Difficulty turning the arm palm up or palm down
- Because a torn tendon can no longer keep the biceps muscle tight, a bulge in the upper arm above the elbow ("Popeye Muscle") may appear, with a dent closer to the shoulder

Doctor Examination

Medical History and Physical Examination

After discussing your symptoms and medical history, your doctor will examine your shoulder. The diagnosis is often obvious for complete ruptures because of the deformity of the arm muscle ("Popeye Muscle").

Partial ruptures are less obvious. To diagnose a partial tear, your doctor may ask you to bend your arm and tighten the biceps muscle. Pain when you use your biceps muscle may mean there is a partial tear.

It is also very important that your doctor identify any other shoulder problems when planning your treatment. The biceps can also tear near the elbow, although this is less common. A tear near the elbow will cause a "gap" in the front of the elbow. Your doctor will check your arm for damage to this area.

In addition, rotator cuff injuries, impingement, and tendonitis are some conditions that may accompany a biceps tendon tear. Your doctor may order additional tests to help identify other problems in your shoulder.

Imaging Tests

X-rays: Although X-rays cannot show soft tissues like the biceps tendon, they can be useful in ruling out other problems that can cause shoulder and elbow pain.

MRI: These scans create better images of soft tissues. They can show both partial and complete tears.

Treatment

Nonsurgical Treatment

For many people, pain from a long head of biceps tendon tear resolves over time. Mild arm weakness or arm deformity may not bother some patients, such as older and less active people.

In addition, if you have not damaged a more critical structure, such as the rotator cuff, nonsurgical treatment is a reasonable option. This can include:

Ice: Apply cold packs for 20 minutes at a time, several times a day to keep down swelling. Do not apply ice directly to the skin.

Nonsteroidal anti-inflammatory medications: Drugs like ibuprofen, aspirin, or naproxen reduce pain and swelling.

Rest: Avoid heavy lifting and overhead activities to relieve pain and limit swelling. Your doctor may recommend using a sling for a brief time.

Physical therapy: Flexibility and strengthening exercises will restore movement and strengthen your shoulder.

Surgical Treatment

Surgical treatment for a long head of the biceps tendon tear is rarely needed. However, some patients who require complete recovery of strength, such as athletes or manual laborers, may require surgery. Surgery may also be the right option for those with partial tears whose symptoms are not relieved with nonsurgical treatment.

Procedure: Several new procedures have been developed that repair the tendon with minimal incisions. The goal of the surgery is to re-anchor the torn tendon back to the bone. Your doctor will discuss with you the options that are best for your specific case.

Complications: Complications with this surgery are rare. Re-rupture of the repaired tendon is uncommon.

Rehabilitation: After surgery, your shoulder may be immobilized temporarily with a sling.

Your doctor will soon start you on therapeutic exercises. Flexibility exercises will improve range of motion in your shoulder. Exercises to strengthen your shoulder will gradually be added to your rehabilitation plan.

Be sure to follow your doctor's treatment plan. Although it is a slow process, your commitment to physical therapy is the most important factor in returning to all the activities you enjoy.

Surgical outcome: Successful surgery can correct muscle deformity and return your arm's strength and function to nearly normal.

Chapter 31

Collarbone Injuries

Chapter Contents

Section 31.1

Collarbone Fractures

"Clavicle Fracture," by David Edell, MEd, ATC, LAT, CSCS.
© 2010 David Edell. Reprinted with permission from
www.AthleticAdvisor.com.

The clavicle is an *S*-shaped bone that ties the appendicular skeleton to the axial skeleton. It serves as the only direct bony attachment of the arm to the trunk. Embryonically, the central clavicle ossifies first, providing most of the linear growth for the first five years of life. After five years of age, the medial and lateral physeal plates develop. The medial physeal plate is responsible for the majority of the remaining clavicle growth until adulthood. The medial physis eventually closes by 25 years of age.

Clavicle fractures are common injuries for active adults and children. Determination of a clavicle fracture is often not difficult when an appropriate history and examination is completed. X-rays often are used only as a validation of the initial, history-based diagnosis. Most clavicular fractures heal very well with appropriate bracing and do not require surgical intervention.

Clavicle fractures account for approximately 5% of all fracture types. The incidence of clavicle fractures seems to be increasing; this may be due to increasing participation in contact sports and/or increasing motor vehicle accidents.

The most common mechanism of injury for a clavicle fracture is falling on the tip of the shoulder or a direct blow to the front of the shoulder. Additionally, a fall on the outstretched arm may result in a clavicle fracture. Studies have also shown that the mechanism of injury does not correlate to the location of the fracture.

Clavicle fractures were first classified by Dr. F. L. Allman in 1967. The fractures are classified relative to where the injury has occurred. Group 1 fractures account for approximately 80% of all fractures. Group 2 fractures represent 12%–15%. And Group 3 fractures are the least common, accounting for approximately 5%–7% of clavicle fractures.

Examination

The athlete will present with a history of a fall or a blow to the shoulder. The athlete may have heard or felt a "pop," "snap," or "crack" during the injury. The athlete then describes the mechanism of injury followed by localized pain, swelling, crepitus with movement, and an increasing loss of shoulder motion.

The athlete will hold the arm hanging "pinned against the side" or will support the elbow and forearm with the opposite hand. Visually, there may be a deformity noticed along the clavicle. Palpation of the deformity will elicit focal pain, crepitus, and occasionally motion. The skin may be "tented" if the fracture is displaced. Rarely is an open clavicle fracture seen.

If the fracture is nondisplaced, a bump or deformity may not be present. However, palpation of the fracture site and active shoulder motion should still produce focal pain at the fracture site.

Neurological damage is rare with clavicle fractures. However, if the fracture is severely displaced, damage can occur to the medial cord of the brachial plexus. Due to this possibility, a neurological examination should be performed to rule out ulnar nerve dysesthesia.

Imaging

Plain film radiographs are used to confirm the history-based diagnosis, evaluate fracture position and alignment, classify the fracture, and follow healing on follow-up visits. Most physicians will order a standard shoulder series consisting of: an anteroposterior (AP) view with the humerus in internal rotation, an AP view with the humerus in external rotation, an axillary lateral view, and a scapulolateral view.

The AP view will best visualize the fractured clavicle. Clavicle fractures are easily visualized in X-rays.

Treatment

Treatment of most clavicle fractures is very straightforward. The athlete is placed in a sling and swath or a figure eight brace to immobilize the arm. If the fracture is not displaced significantly, a simple sling (with or without a swath) provides ample protection of the fracture to allow for healing.

The treating physician may use a figure eight brace with a displaced fracture. The figure eight brace holds the shoulders in a retracted position. This pulls the clavicle into a "normal" alignment to help reduce the displaced fracture. The figure eight brace should be tightened periodically during the day to maintain traction. Excessive tightening of the brace can lead to skin lesions, edema from venous obstruction, and brachial plexus palsy.

Rehabilitation begins immediately after the injury. Early rehab should focus on pain reduction, swelling reduction, range of motion exercises, and gentile strengthening. All of the rehabilitation exercises should follow the adage "use pain as your guide."

During the acute phase of the healing process, strength and ROM [range of motion] activities should be performed for the fingers, wrist, and elbow. Gripping exercises, wrist curls, and elbow flexion and extension will help to reduce swelling in the lower arm that results from the injury and use of a sling.

As pain in the shoulder declines and healing is demonstrated on X-ray (usually two to three weeks post injury), shoulder exercises for ROM may begin. As the healing progresses and pain decreases the rehabilitation advances to strength-building exercises.

Athletes who suffer clavicle fractures will return to full athletic participation with little morbidity. Full return in children is expected in 6 weeks. Full return for adolescents and adults is usually 6 to 12 weeks.

Section 31.2

Sternoclavicular Joint Separation

The sternoclavicular (SC) joint is the pivot on which the shoulder girdle moves on the trunk. It is located at the junction of the collar bone and the breast bone. Dislocation of this joint most often results from a fall onto the shoulder.

The type of treatment your physician prescribes will depend entirely on the type of injury to your joint.

Anterior or forward dislocations are the most common and can sometimes occur with minimal trauma in patients with generalized looseness in their joints. Posterior dislocation of the sternoclavicular joint is less common than the anterior type but is potentially much more serious. Damage to important structures located behind the sternoclavicular joint (arteries, veins, nerves, esophagus, trachea) can cause difficulty breathing and swallowing, poor circulation to the arm and hand, and nerve damage.

Treatment

Most severe dislocations are of the anterior type and can be treated by pulling, pushing, and moving the clavicle until it pops back into joint. This procedure can be very painful and most patients will be given general anesthesia and perhaps muscle relaxants before the procedure. After the closed reduction is performed, the SC joint will have to be held perfectly still. The physician will most likely recommend the patient continue with pain medication while wearing a figure-eight strap for at least six weeks. With anterior dislocations, redislocation is common but is often not very painful and can be tolerated without surgery.

Posterior sternoclavicular dislocations should always be reduced in the operating room and are usually stable after reduction. They are also more likely to require an open (requiring a surgical incision) reduction than the anterior type. Postoperatively they are treated like their anterior counterpart but are more often stable over the long term.

In patients with chronic instability of the sternoclavicular joint, surgery may be indicated. In chronic posterior instability, potential for damage to important neurovascular structures is a good reason for surgical reduction and stabilization. For individuals with chronic anterior instability engaged in strenuous activities such as sports, aching, swelling, as well as rapid fatigue may result. In addition, the onset of age and osteoarthritic changes may cause permanent stiffness and aching and restrict the full range of normal movement of the shoulder. These symptoms comprise the rare indications for surgical intervention.

Part Six

Injuries to the Elbows, Wrists, and Hands

Chapter 32

Arm and Wrist Injuries

Chapter Contents

Section 32.1

Arm Fractures

"Broken Arm," reproduced with permission from
Your Orthopaedic Connection. © American Academy of Orthopaedic
Surgeons (www.aaos.org), Rosemont, IL, 2007.

A broken arm is a common injury. About one in every 20 fractures involve the upper arm bone (humerus). Children are more likely to break the lower arm bones (radius and ulna).

Falling on an outstretched hand or being in a car crash or some other type of accident is usually the cause of a broken arm.

Symptoms

Most people know right away if their arm broke, because there may be a snap or a loud cracking sound. The broken arm may appear deformed and be swollen, bruised, and bleeding.

A person with a broken arm usually has:

- extreme pain at the site of the injury;

- pain increased by any movement;

- loss of normal use of the arm.

Diagnosis

The doctor will need to know exactly what happened. He or she will examine the broken arm and check for other injuries, such as nerve damage.

The doctor may want to see if the patient can flex and extend the wrist and fingers.

Sometimes, the doctor may use X-rays or other diagnostic imaging tools to see the bones of both the injured and uninjured arms.

If the patient is a child, the long bones of the arm are probably still growing. This makes the examination for any damage to growth plates very important.

Treatment

First Aid

First, make sure the injured person is out of the way of further harm.

- Emergency services should be called if there is serious bleeding or if there is reason to suspect multiple broken bones or other injuries.

- Do not try to move the broken arm. This can cause further damage to blood vessels, nerves, and soft tissues.

- If a broken bone sticks out from the skin (open fracture), do not try to push it back in.

Second, make sure the patient is stabilized.

- Check that the breathing is normal and the pulse is good.

- Bleeding can be slowed and swelling reduced by applying pressure and elevating the injured arm above the level of the person's heart.

- Avoid contaminating the area by lightly covering the site with a clean, dry cloth or bandage until medical help arrives.

Third, if medical help is not available, and the patient must be moved, immobilize the broken arm using a temporary splint and/or sling.

- **Temporary splints:** A temporary splint can be made using wood or rolled up magazines. The joint should be immobilized above and below the site of the injury. Each end of the splint should extend far beyond the injured region and be fastened using cloth, belts, or tape. Avoid any constriction of the arm with the supporting strap.

- **Slings:** A sling can stabilize the injury and support the splint. A broken arm sling can be as simple as a loop of cloth supported from the neck.

Fourth, take the injured person to a doctor or emergency room right away.

Nonsurgical Treatment

The doctor may need to move pieces of bone back into their correct positions (a process called reduction). Depending upon the severity of injury, the patient may or may not need anesthesia. Those with more serious fractures may require surgery.

With the broken bone back in place, the doctor immobilizes the arm (fracture bracing). Most patients are fitted with a cast or splint. The doctor tells the patient how long to wear the cast or splint and removes it at the right time.

Rehabilitation

It may take from several weeks to several months for the broken arm to heal completely. Rehabilitation involves gradually increasing activities to restore muscle strength, joint motion, and flexibility.

The patient's cooperation is essential to the rehabilitation process. The patient must complete range of motion, strengthening, and other exercises prescribed by the doctor. Rehabilitation continues until the muscles, ligaments, and other soft tissues perform their functions normally.

Once rehabilitation is completed, the doctor may want to examine the arm and its function to make sure healing is complete.

Section 32.2

Wrist Fractures

What is a wrist fracture?

The wrist is made up of eight small bones and the two forearm
bones, the radius and ulna. The bones come together to form multiple
large and small joints. At each joint, the ends of the bones are lined
with a very smooth covering (cartilage). The bones are held together
by ligaments. The shape and design of these joints allow the wrist to
bend and straighten, move side-to-side, and rotate, as in twisting the
palm up or down.

A fracture may occur in any of these bones when enough force is
applied to the wrist, such as when falling down onto an outstretched
hand. Severe injuries may occur from a more forceful injury, such as a
car accident or a fall off a roof or ladder. Osteoporosis, a common condition in which the bone becomes thinner and more brittle, may make
one more susceptible to getting a wrist fracture with a simple fall.

The most commonly broken bone of the wrist is the radius. Many
people think that a fracture is different from a break, but they are
the same. When the wrist bone is broken, there is pain, swelling, and
decreased use of the hand and wrist. Often the wrist appears crooked
and deformed. Fractures of the small wrist bones, such as the scaphoid,
are unlikely to appear deformed.

Fractures may be simple with one or two large bone pieces that are
well aligned and stable. Other fractures are unstable, which implies
that the bone fragments tend to displace or shift, which may cause the
wrist to appear crooked. Some fractures break the normally smooth,
ball bearing–like joint surface; others will be near the joint but leave
the joint surface intact. Sometimes the bone is shattered into many
pieces, which usually makes it unstable. An open (compound) fracture
occurs when a bone fragment breaks through the skin. There is a
higher risk of infection with compound (open) fractures. The alignment
of the bones once healed may affect the wrist's function. If the bones

heal in a significantly altered position, there may be permanent limitations in motion with an increased risk of arthritis and pain.

How are they evaluated?

Examination and X-rays are needed so that your doctor can tell if there is a fracture and assess the position of the bones, in order to help determine the treatment. Occasionally a CT [computed tomography] scan may be helpful to get better detail of the fracture fragments. In addition to the bone, ligaments (the structures that hold the bones together), tendons, muscles, and nerves may be injured as well when the wrist is broken. These injuries may need to be treated in addition to the fracture. Whenever the bone protrudes through the skin, it is important to receive immediate care to minimize the risk of bony infection. When numbness in the fingers is present, it implies that the nerves have been injured.

How are they treated?

Treatment is dependent on many factors. Patient factors such as age, activity level, hobbies, occupation, hand dominance, prior injuries or wrist arthritis, and other medical problems are very important when considering treatment. Remember, it might only be your wrist, but we all need our hands to perform daily activities. Local factors relate to the bone quality (density—osteoporosis), while others relate to the fracture itself. Certain fractures are simple and in good position with the bone and joints well aligned, whereas others are fragmented into multiple pieces and may be badly displaced. Some fractures are stable and will stay in place, whereas others are unstable and might shift during treatment. It is very important to see a physician with an in-depth understanding of these factors in order to get optimal treatment and outcome.

A splint or cast may be used to treat a fracture that is not displaced, or to protect a fracture that has been set. Usually a cast is worn for several weeks depending on each patient's fracture and ability to heal the broken bone.

Other fractures may need surgery to properly set the bone and/or to stabilize it. Fractures may be stabilized with pins, screws, plates, rods, or external fixation. Plates and screws that can be placed through an incision on the bottom or top of the wrist are often used to hold the bone fragments in place and may allow early use of the hand and wrist. These implants are buried inside the wrist and usually do not require removal. External fixation is a method in which a frame outside the body is attached to pins which have been placed in the bone above and below the fracture site, in effect keeping it in traction until the bone heals. Sometimes arthroscopy is used in the evaluation and treatment of wrist fractures. Your hand surgeon will determine which treatment is the most appropriate in your individual case.

On occasion, bone may be missing or may be so severely crushed that there is a gap in the bone once it has been re-aligned. In such cases, a bone graft may be necessary. In this procedure, bone is taken from another part of the body, or bone bank or bone graft substitutes are used, to help fill the defect.

While the wrist fracture is healing, it is very important to keep the fingers and shoulder flexible, provided that there are no other injuries that would require that they be immobilized. Once the wrist has enough stability, motion exercises may be started for the wrist itself. Your hand surgeon will determine the appropriate timing for these exercises. Hand therapy is often used to help recover flexibility, strength, and function.

What kind of results can I expect?

Recovery time varies considerably, depending on the severity of the injury, associated injuries, and other factors as noted previously. It is not unusual for maximal recovery from a wrist fracture to take several months. Some patients may have residual stiffness or aching. If the surface of the joint was badly injured, arthritis may develop. On occasion, additional treatment or reconstructive surgery may be needed.

Section 32.3

Scaphoid Fractures

What Are Scaphoid Fractures?

The scaphoid bone is one of the eight small bones that make up the "carpal bones" of the wrist. There are two rows of bones, one closer to the forearm (proximal row) and the other closer to the hand (distal row). The scaphoid bone is unique in that it links the two rows together. This puts it at extra risk for injury, which accounts for it being the most commonly fractured carpal bone.

How Do Scaphoid Fractures Occur?

Fractures of the scaphoid occur most commonly from a fall on the outstretched hand. Usually it hurts at first, but the pain may improve quickly, over the course of days or weeks. Bruising is rare, and there is usually no visible deformity and only minimal swelling. Since there is no deformity, many people with this injury mistakenly assume that they have just sprained their wrist, leading to a delay in seeking evaluation. It is common for people who have fractured this bone to not become aware of it until months or years after the event.

Diagnosis of Scaphoid Fractures

Scaphoid fractures are most commonly diagnosed by X-rays of the wrist. However, when the fracture is not displaced, X-rays taken early (first week) may appear negative. A non-displaced scaphoid fracture could thus be incorrectly diagnosed as a "sprain." Therefore a patient who has significant tenderness directly over the scaphoid bone (which is located in the hollow at the thumb side of the wrist, or "snuffbox") should be suspected of having a scaphoid fracture and be splinted. An X-ray a couple of weeks later may then more clearly reveal the fracture. In questionable cases, MRI [magnetic resonance imaging] scan, CT scan, or bone scan may be used to help diagnose an acute scaphoid fracture. CT scan and/or MRI are also used to assess fracture displacement and configuration. Until a definitive diagnosis is made, the patient should remain splinted to prevent movement of a possible fracture.

Treatment of Scaphoid Fractures

If the fracture is non-displaced, it can be treated by immobilization in a cast that usually covers the forearm, hand, and thumb, and sometimes includes the elbow for the first phase of immobilization. Healing time in a cast can range from 6 to 10 weeks and even longer. This is because the blood supply to the bone is variable and can be disrupted by the fracture, impairing bony healing. Part of the bone might even die after fracture due to loss of its blood supply, particularly in the proximal third of the bone, the part closest to the forearm. If the fracture is in this zone, or if it is at all displaced, surgery is more likely to be recommended. With surgery, a screw or pins are inserted to stabilize the fracture, sometimes with a bone graft to help heal the bone. Surgery to place a screw may also be recommended in non-displaced cases to avoid prolonged casting.

Complications of Scaphoid Fractures

Non-union: If a scaphoid fracture goes unrecognized, it often will not heal. Sometimes, even with treatment, it may not heal because of poor blood supply. Over time, the abnormal motion and collapse of the bone fragments may lead to malalignment within the wrist and subsequent arthritis. If caught before arthritis has developed, surgery may be performed to try to get the scaphoid to heal.

Avascular necrosis: A portion of the scaphoid may die because of lack of blood supply, leading to collapse of the bone and later arthritis. Fractures in the proximal one third of the bone, the part closest to the forearm, are more vulnerable to this complication. Again, if arthritis has not developed, surgery to try to stabilize the fracture and restore circulation to the bone may be attempted.

Post-traumatic arthritis: If arthritis has already developed, salvage-type procedures may be considered, such as removal of degenerated bone or partial or complete fusion of the wrist joint.

Section 32.4

Wrist Sprains

What Is a Sprain?

A sprain is an injury to a ligament. Ligaments are the connective tissues that connect and stabilize one bone to another bone; they could be
thought of as very strong tape that holds the bones together at a joint.
The degree of ligament injury may vary over a wide range of severity.
Sprains are generally classified into three types: Grade I—stable injury to
a ligament; Grade II—partial tearing/stretching; and Grade III—complete
tear of the ligament, either within the mid-portion of the ligament, or as
an avulsion ("pulling away") from its attachment into bone. A sprain may
upset the normal coordinated movements of the wrist bones resulting in
persistent stiffness, pain, swelling, and possible instability.

How Do Wrist Sprains Occur?

A sprain of one or multiple wrist ligaments occurs when there is excessive loading or force transmitted across the wrist. These frequently
occur as the result of a fall forwards or backwards onto an outstretched
hand. Force may be applied in other ways, such as with a violent twisting injury (torsion). Often, these injuries are associated with sports and
other outdoor activities such as biking, skiing, or snowboarding.

What Are the Most Common Types of Wrist Sprains?

There are many ligaments which stabilize the wrist joint. One of the
most common ligament injuries involves the scapho-lunate ligament,
the ligament which links the scaphoid and lunate bones.

How Are Wrist Sprains Diagnosed?

The diagnosis of a wrist sprain includes a careful patient history (how
the injury occurred), a clinical examination, and diagnostic testing. The

patient typically presents with complaints of wrist pain and stiffness, and loss of strength is also common. Examination of the wrist will allow your hand surgeon to pinpoint tenderness and thus localize the site of injury, and also assess wrist stability. Usually X-rays are obtained to evaluate for potential fractures and for signs of ligament insufficiency. While ligaments themselves are not seen on X-rays, the consequence of a ligament injury may be appreciated indirectly based on abnormal alignment of the wrist bones. Additional diagnostic testing may be required, such as an MRI or an MRI-arthrogram, which involves an injection of contrast into the wrist to enhance the sensitivity of the MRI. Wrist arthroscopy is a very precise, direct way to examine the wrist ligaments. It is a surgical procedure in which a small scope and specialized instruments are placed into various parts of the wrist joint via several small (approximately three millimeter) incisions. However, the risks and benefits of the surgery must be considered relative to the severity of the wrist injury.

How Are Wrist Sprains Treated?

The goals of treating a wrist ligament injury are to:

- provide pain relief;
- minimize potential stiffness or loss of motion;
- restore wrist joint stability;
- reduce the risk of long-term consequences of an untreated wrist ligament injury (arthritis, pain, instability).

The treatment of a wrist sprain is guided by the severity of the injury. Similar to a sprained ankle, milder ligament sprains of the wrist may be treated with protected activity, supportive splinting or casting, strategies to minimize inflammation and discomfort, and gradual return to activity. Evaluation by a hand surgeon will help grade the severity of the injury, identify associated injuries, and determine the need for more specific diagnostic testing.

For less severe wrist sprains, the ligaments usually heal well— occasionally, the injury and healing response may cause stiffness and your hand surgeon may recommend stretching and motion exercises to minimize the potential for longer term loss of wrist mobility.

In the case of a ligament tear, treatment may or may not involve surgery; treatment depends on the specific ligament injury and individual patient needs and considerations. For certain injuries, wrist arthroscopy may be recommended to evaluate the wrist and to possibly trim loose or inflamed flaps from the injured ligament. If the findings are more severe, your surgeon may need to proceed with an open ligament repair or reconstruction. The ligaments themselves are not always very substantial, and so repairs may need to be augmented with additional tissue such as the joint capsule or various tendon grafts, especially if the injury is not being treated acutely. There is much research underway searching for better methods to treat these serious injuries. They include stronger and more precise ligament reconstructions using either local tissues (tendons) or distant tissues (ligaments from the hand or foot). Pins or screws are often used to help stabilize the repairs as well. Your surgeon will discuss the various options based on the specifics of your injury.

Chronic Wrist Sprains

Unrecognized or untreated ligament injuries may result in wrist instability which leads to progressive cartilage degeneration (arthritis) in the wrist joint. This arthritic change may result in pain, stiffness, and swelling; these symptoms may be intermittent and vary in their severity. A common pattern is seen with scapho-lunate ligament tears that alter the normal wrist joint mechanics. The unlinked scaphoid rotates away from the lunate. As a result of the abnormal rotation of the scaphoid, its joint surface no longer makes contact with the radius bone properly. Instead of broad contact along the entire joint surface, there is "edge on edge" contact of the joint, wearing it down in a predictable progressive pattern of arthritis. This form of arthritis is known as scapho-lunate advanced collapse, or "SLAC" wrist, which progresses to involve a greater amount of the wrist over time, thereby limiting treatment options. A good analogy is that of placing two spoons into a drawer; normally they are placed flush with one another, with the greatest surface area of contact. However, if the spoons are rotated slightly, they match up "edge on edge" and no longer have a good, broad surface area where they touch each other.

In the presence of a chronic wrist ligament injury and associated arthritis, mild/intermittent symptoms may be treated with splinting, activity modifications, and analgesics, such as anti-inflammatory medications. Persistent symptoms or a symptom flare may be treated with a steroid injection.

Should these conservative measures fail, surgery may be considered in order to remove the offending, arthritic joint surfaces, such as with a proximal row carpectomy (remove the arthritic first row of wrist bones, which includes the scaphoid), or scaphoidectomy and partial wrist fusion (remove the arthritic scaphoid bone and fuse four small wrist bones together for stability). In the case of more widespread wrist arthritis, wrist arthroplasty (joint replacement) or total wrist fusion may be performed.

Chapter 33

Elbow Injuries

Chapter Contents

Section 33.1

Elbow Fractures

What is the elbow?

The elbow is a hinge joint comprised of three bones—humerus, radius, and ulna. Ligaments hold the bones together to provide stability to the joint. Muscles and tendons originate and insert onto the bones around the elbow to provide force to move the bones and perform activities.

How do elbow fractures happen?

Elbow fractures may result from falling onto an outstretched arm, a direct impact to the elbow, or a twisting injury. Sprains, strains, or dislocations may occur at the same time as a fracture.

What are the signs and symptoms?

Pain, swelling, bruising, and stiffness in and around the elbow suggest a possible fracture. A snap or pop at the time of injury may be felt or heard. Skin openings may reflect communication between the bone and the outside environment. Visible deformity would indicate displacement of the bones or a dislocation of the elbow joint. It is always important to check for possible nerve and/or artery damage.

How are elbow fractures diagnosed?

X-rays are used to confirm if a fracture is present and if the bones are displaced. Sometimes a CT [computed tomography] scan might be necessary to get further detail, especially of the joint surface.

How are they treated?

Stiffness is a major concern after any elbow fracture. Treatment is therefore focused on maximizing early motion. Conservative treatment (sling, cast) is usually used when the bones are at low risk of moving out of place, or when the position of the bones is acceptable. Age is also an important factor when treating elbow fractures. Casts are used frequently in children, as their risk of developing stiffness is small; however, in an adult, elbow stiffness is much more likely. Fractures that are displaced or unstable are more likely to need surgery to realign and stabilize the fragments, or sometimes to remove bone fragments, and ideally allow for early motion. Whenever a fracture is open (skin broken over the fracture), urgent surgery is needed to clean out the tract and bone so as to minimize the risk of a deep infection.

Therapy is often utilized to maximize motion. This might include exercises, scar massage, modalities such as ultrasound, heat, ice, etc., and splints that stretch the joint (static progressive or dynamic splints).

Specific types of elbow fractures:

Radial head and neck fractures: Pain is usually worse with forearm rotation. It is critical to detect the presence of a mechanical blockage of motion from displaced fracture fragments. The specific type of treatment depends on the number and size of the fragments. Non-displaced fractures are treated with early motion. Complex fractures often require surgery to repair and stabilize the fragments, or to remove the radial head if the fragmentation is too severe, or occasionally to replace the radial head.

Olecranon fractures: Stable fractures can be initially treated with splint immobilization, followed by gradual motion exercises. Severely displaced or unstable fractures require surgery. The bone fragments are re-aligned and held together with pins and wires, or plates and screws.

Fractures of the distal humerus: These fractures occur commonly in children and in the elderly. Nerve and/or artery injuries can be associated with these types of fractures and must be carefully checked for. These fractures usually need surgery, except for those that are minimally or non-displaced, stable, and have no associated nerve or artery injury.

Section 33.2

Tennis Elbow

What is tennis elbow?

Tennis elbow is a form of tendonitis that causes pain over the bony prominence called the lateral epicondyle on the outside of the elbow. It is often referred to as lateral epicondylitis.

What causes it?

Tennis elbow is caused by repetitive stress on the muscles and tendons that are connected to the lateral epicondyle. These muscles extend along the top, or dorsal, side of the forearm to the wrist and are responsible for extending or bending back the wrist and fingers. The tendons are fibrous bands that connect the muscles to the bone, in this case the lateral epicondyle.

If too much stress is placed on these muscles and tendons, micro tears can occur at the site where the tendons attach to the lateral epicondyle. These micro tears cause pain that is usually localized at the lateral epicondyle but the pain can occasionally radiate down the forearm. Aging appears to make these tendons more prone to breakdown. Therefore, lateral epicondylitis is more common once we get in our fourth decade of life and beyond.

The pain increases with activities that require contraction of the affected muscles and tendons: shaking hands, turning doorknobs, picking up objects with the palm down, or hitting a backhand in tennis.

How do I know if I have tennis elbow?

No special tests are needed to make the diagnosis. This diagnosis is made by history and physician examination of the patient. The patient may present symptoms consistent with tennis elbow and has pain when pressure is applied to the outside of the elbow. The patient frequently cannot remember an injury, but will have noticed the pain either at the beginning or end of an activity that requires wrist and elbow movement.

X-rays are not always required when evaluating a patient with tennis elbow symptoms, but a doctor may wish to order them just to make certain that the bone structures of the elbow are normal.

How is tennis elbow treated?

Like many overuse injuries of sport, there is no sure-fire treatment. Rest itself does not necessarily cure the problem, but it may decrease the pain and allow healing to progress. Decreased activity with the elbow and wrist is generally preferred over absolute rest and complete inactivity. The healing of tennis elbow can take weeks to months.

Some physicians believe that the key to healing this overuse injury lies in increasing the circulation to the area while decreasing the tightness of the muscles. Therefore, stretching and strengthening exercises are frequently helpful.

The following exercise may help: Support the forearm on a flat surface with the wrist and hand free. Hold a one- to two-pound weight in the hand. Keeping the palm down, slowly extend the wrist. Bring it backward, or up, and then bend it forward, or down. The muscles on the top of the forearm should contract when the wrist is moved upward and stretch when the hand is moved downward.

To balance the forearm muscles, these exercises should be repeated with the palm facing up. Each exercise should be repeated 10 times slowly.

A loop of rubber tubing, with one end attached to a table leg or held on the floor with a foot, can be used to provide resistance instead of the weight. This will also increase circulation to the area.

A snug, but not tight, strap worn around the top of the forearm often decreases the pull of the muscles on the lateral epicondyle and lessens pain. When symptoms are present during everyday activities, the band should be worn during all waking hours. Occasionally, an elbow sleeve with a pad specially designed to put gentle pressure over the forearm muscles can be used. This sleeve has the advantage of not only changing the pull of the muscles, but keeping them warm as well, which increases their flexibility and circulation.

A physician may also prescribe ultrasound or electrical stimulation to increase circulation to the area.

Nonsteroidal anti-inflammatory medications like aspirin, ibuprofen, and ketoprofen or various prescription drugs can treat the symptoms and may decrease the pain and irritation in and around the tendon. However, it appears unlikely that these medications can actually evoke more rapid healing of the condition.

Icing the joint after activity may also decrease the irritation and relieve the pain.

If treatment with decreased activity, exercises, and medication is not effective, your physician may recommend a corticosteroid injection in the affected area. This can further decrease the pain and irritation. In some cases this is not effective and surgery can be considered for these resistant and chronic cases.

Tips for Preventing Injury

- Warm up well before play. Muscles and tendons are like Silly Putty and stretch more when they are warm. Make sure to keep the muscles and tendons warm as you play.

- Choose appropriate equipment and maintain it properly. A racquet handle that is too big or too small, strung too tightly or loosely, or has a too big or too small head, may increase stress to the elbow and wrist during play.

- Condition for the activity by stretching and strengthening all the muscles used in the sport. Also evaluate play techniques to make sure that they are not irritating the condition.

Section 33.3

Golfer's Elbow

What is golfer's elbow?

Golfer's elbow, also known as medial epicondylitis, is pain or inflammation on the inside of the arm near the elbow, where the muscles and tendons in the forearm attach to the elbow's interior bony area. In some cases, a partial tear of the tendon, which attaches the muscles to the bone of the elbow, may occur. Pain can be felt in the elbow, forearm, wrist, or fingers.

What causes golfer's elbow?

Golfer's elbow is often caused by the overuse or repetitive use of the muscles in the wrist or fingers. Despite its name, the condition is not solely caused by playing golf, although it is a common injury among those that play golf due to the overuse of the muscles implicated in this injury. The injury can occur from a sudden and abrupt injury to the tendons and muscles in the forearm or a sudden and severe force to the wrist or elbow, or more typically can occur over time due to repeated overuse of the muscles in the wrist and fingers. The condition is more common in men than women and often affects people that are involved in repetitive use activities for work or leisure that may stress the wrists or fingers.

What are the symptoms of golfer's elbow?

The symptoms of golfer's elbow include pain that is apparent near the inside area of the elbow. The pain can also radiate along the inside of the forearm, and may be felt through the wrist and fingers. The pain typically develops over time, increasing in severity, although it can come on more suddenly if an abrupt injury occurs rather than a repetitive use injury. The pain is often felt in a person's dominant arm, since that is the arm that is most often used for most movements, although it can occur in both arms, and pain may be felt when twisting the wrist or arm, squeezing an object, picking something up, or even shaking hands. In addition to pain, individuals with golfer's elbow may experience stiffness in the elbow, numbness or tingling in the fingers, or weakness in the wrist or hand.

How is golfer's elbow diagnosed?

Golfer's elbow can be diagnosed by a medical professional based on the description and location of pain. A medical professional will apply pressure to the area to determine pain and tenderness and will ask you to move your arm, elbow, wrist, and fingers to see how the movement affects discomfort. There are no medical tests that can diagnose the condition with certainty, however, and X-rays are typically normal.

When should I seek care for golfer's elbow?

If you experience repeated or continuous pain in the interior of your elbow, forearm, wrist, or fingers, you should see a medical professional so that a proper diagnosis can be made. By treating the injury and resting the affected area, you can avoid continued pain and worsening of the injury. If you have already been diagnosed with golfer's elbow and basic treatment (such as ice, rest, and over-the-counter pain and anti-inflammatory medications) does not alleviate future pain, it is best to seek the advice of a medical professional. If the pain is severe or comes on suddenly, if your elbow is inflamed, or if you can't bend the elbow, you should seek immediate medical advice.

What will the treatment for golfer's elbow consist of?

Typical treatment for golfer's elbow may involve over-the-counter nonsteroidal anti-inflammatory medications to reduce pain or inflammation, cortisone injections, application of ice, and a recommendation to avoid activity that causes pain while the injury heals. Once the pain has subsided, physical therapy is typically recommended to strengthen and stretch the tendons and muscles around the elbow and in the forearm and wrist to avoid repeated injury. A change in how activities and movements are done may be recommended, the limiting of some activities may be suggested, and the use of a brace, forearm strap, or elastic bandage worn near the elbow may curtail future pain and injury. If the injury and pain does not respond to traditional treatments, surgery may be a last resort option, although this is not often necessary.

Which muscle groups/joints are commonly affected from golfer's elbow?

The interior portion of the elbow, as well as the tendons and muscles that connect to the elbow in the forearm, are affected in individuals with golfer's elbow. Pain may also be felt in the wrist and fingers.

What type of results should I expect from the treatment for golfer's elbow?

If treatment for golfer's elbow is sought on a timely basis and is completed according to doctor's recommendations, most individuals will notice a complete or at least substantial improvement in the pain associated with the initial condition. It may take a number of months for the pain to diminish and reintroducing activity may cause the pain to return. Rest is best to help the elbow heal when re-injury occurs. Ongoing changes to activity levels or the use of different techniques or equipment may need to be incorporated into routine activities in order to avoid re-injury. In a small percentage of cases, surgery may be required to repair the muscles and tendons near the elbow in order to clear up the underlying injury and pain associated with golfer's elbow. When surgery is indicated, it is often successful in diminishing or alleviating pain.

Section 33.4

Ulnar Collateral Ligament Injuries (Thrower's Elbow)

"Throwers Elbow," by David Edell, MEd, ATC, LAT, CSCS.
© 2010 David Edell. Reprinted with permission from
www.AthleticAdvisor.com.

Overhand throwing places multiple stresses on the elbow joint. These stresses place demands on vulnerable immature elbows that can cause numerous injuries. Persistent elbow soreness, stiffness, and discomfort can lead not only to poor performance but can be significant indicators of debilitating injuries.

Baseball is one of the most popular participation sports for children in the USA, but repeated throwing, in skeletally immature athletes, can produce elbow injuries that threaten proper growth. It is estimated that 40% of 9- to 12-year-old throwing athletes sustain elbow injuries requiring medical intervention. Athletic trainers, physicians, and parents should be aware that persistent elbow pain after throwing can be a sign of a significant injury.

The skeletally immature elbow has secondary growth centers at the distal humerus (lower arm) radial head (thumb side of the forearm) and olecranon (tip of the elbow). When these structures are subjected to the stress of overhand throwing, the growth plates (physes) are vulnerable to injuries more than the adjacent muscles and tendons. The act of throwing places compressive forces on the lateral elbow, specifically the radial head and capitellum of the humerus. It also places distractive forces on the ulnar collateral ligament (MCL). Both of these forces can result in debilitating injuries that have lifelong implications.

These stresses are felt during the acceleration and follow-through phases of pitching. These phases place a valgus stress on the elbow, resulting in distraction forces on the medial joint complex and compressive forces on the radiocapitellar joint. Repeated overuse, exacerbated by poor mechanics, will result in failure of the tissues on either side of the elbow.

Medial Compartment Injuries

The distractive forces on the medial elbow can result in damage to the growth plates in skeletally immature athletes and disruption of the MCL in the mature athlete. Both of these injuries are potential career-ending injuries.

The skeletally mature athlete will often times tear the ligament rather than avulsing it from the bone. These injuries result in a reconstructive surgery referred to as "Tommy John Surgery." This is named for the first athlete that successfully returned to professional baseball following an MCL reconstruction.

The skeletally immature athlete is at potential risk for an avulsion fracture of the MCL from the medial epicondyle of the humerus. This type of injury may not be due to a one-time injury, but rather the result of repetitive stress. Due to this coaches and parents must be aware of soreness after throwing that does not resolve within 24 hours. Post exercise soreness should resolve within one day of the activity; pain that lingers longer may be a sign of significant injury.

Signs and symptoms of a medial compartment injury are: medial joint tenderness, pain with a valgus stress test, diffuse medial pain while palpating the flexor muscle wad, and pain with resisted pronation. The medial musculature becomes symptomatic while acting as a secondary restraint for the injured MCL.

In the event of persistent medial elbow pain, a physician should be consulted to rule out ligamentous injury. Bilateral X-rays should be performed to compare the amount of medial apophyseal separation at the distal humerus. A separation of greater than three millimeters is an indication for a surgical repair.

Treatment for the non-surgical cases should include rest and rehabilitation exercises. The athlete should not throw a ball until the elbow is completely pain free and full strength has returned. Rehabilitation exercises should focus on wrist flexors and extensors, forearm pronators and supinators, as well as the shoulder musculature. After the athlete is pain free he/she should begin an interval throwing program, gradually returning to full throwing activities. Any pain during the interval throwing program should be evaluated and the throwing progression adjusted to compensate.

Lateral Compartment Injuries

The same valgus stress that can lead to medial compartment injuries also places compressive forces on the lateral compartment that can result in damage. These compressive forces cause the radial head to impinge on the capitellum of the humerus. The capitellum has a tenu-ous vascular supply that makes this area predisposed to bony necrosis or osteochondritis dissecans (OCD). Some researchers feel there may also be a genetic predisposition for the formation of an OCD.

The repetitive forces of throwing cause subchondral (below the joint surface cartilage) bone fatigue that results in microfractures. Repeated trauma, and the limited blood supply to the area, does not allow these fractures to heal. This results in bone resorption and separation of an osteochondral fragment from its underlying bed. Without the osseous structural support, this separated fragment becomes avascular result-ing in a partial or complete loose body.

The resulting loose body can then impinge on other areas in the joint causing further damage. X-rays may also show radial head hy-pertrophy. This is a result of the increased surface contact with the capitellum.

Signs and symptoms of this type of injury include: loss of full range of motion, most commonly in a loss of extension; pain with throwing that does not resolve after rest; swelling; grinding with elbow motion; and a decrease in performance.

This injury usually results in surgical intervention to correct the damage. If this injury is not treated appropriately the damage to the joint surfaces may result in permanent loss of normal joint function. Many athletes who have dealt with this injury have complications that include: lack of full extension, loss of normal pronation and supination, and incontractable pain.

Section 33.5

Elbow (Olecranon) Bursitis

The olecranon bursa is a sac between the tip of the elbow bone and the overlying skin; it allows skin to move well over the bone. Olecranon "bursitis" is inflammation of the bursa. This can result from a direct blow (trauma) to the tip of the elbow or from leaning on the tip of the elbow for long periods of time. Medical conditions like gout and rheumatoid arthritis can be associated with olecranon bursitis. An infection also can result if the skin is punctured in that area.

In general, the first symptom is swelling at the tip of the elbow. Considerable swelling can occur even without pain. Motion of the elbow usually is normal unless there is a significant amount of swelling. Redness or warmth of the skin, tenderness of the bursa, or drainage (especially of pus) are warning signs of infection; if any of these are present, evaluation by a doctor as soon as possible is recommended.

A doctor usually will examine the elbow. X-rays might be taken; often, a "bone spur" or a "foreign body" (an object like pieces of gravel that should not be there) are found in patients with olecranon bursitis.

Most olecranon bursitis can be treated without surgery. Unless there are signs of infection, it is reasonable to "observe" this while avoiding leaning on the elbow. Ice and elevation can be helpful, as can an elbow pad. Symptoms often resolve. In some cases, the doctor might recommend removing fluid and injecting steroid into the bursa.

Infected olecranon bursitis usually is drained both to help get rid of the infection and to see what bacteria is causing the infection in order to choose which antibiotic will be effective.

Surgery might be recommended if either an infected or non-infected bursitis doesn't resolve without it.

Section 33.6

Dislocated Elbow

"Elbow Dislocations and Fracture-Dislocations," reproduced with permission from *Your Orthopaedic Connection*. © American Academy of Orthopaedic Surgeons (www.aaos.org), Rosemont, IL, 2007.

When the joint surfaces of an elbow are separated, the elbow is dislocated. Elbow dislocations can be complete or partial. In a complete dislocation, the joint surfaces are completely separated. In a partial dislocation, the joint surfaces are only partly separated. A partial dislocation is also called a subluxation.

Anatomy

Three bones come together to make up the elbow joint. The humerus is the bone in the upper arm. Two bones from the forearm (the radius and the ulna) form the lower part of the elbow. Each of these bones has a very distinct shape. Ligaments connected to the bones keep all of these bones in proper alignment.

The elbow is both a hinge joint and a ball and socket joint. As muscles contract and relax, two unique motions occur at the elbow.

- Bending occurs through a hinge joint that allows the elbow to bend and straighten. This is called flexion and extension, respectively.

- Rotation occurs though a ball and socket joint that allows the hand to be rotated palm up and palm down. This is called pronation and supination, respectively.

Injuries and dislocations to the elbow can affect either of these motions.

Cause

Elbow dislocations are not common. Elbow dislocations typically occur when a person falls onto an outstretched hand. When the hand hits the ground, the force is sent to the elbow. Usually, there is a turning motion in this force. This can drive and rotate the elbow out of its socket. Elbow dislocations can also happen in car accidents when the passengers reach forward to cushion the impact. The force that is sent through the arm can dislocate the elbow, just as in a fall.

The elbow is stable because of the combined stabilizing effects of bone surfaces, ligaments, and muscles. When an elbow dislocates, any or all of these structures can be injured to different degrees.

A *simple dislocation* does not have any major bone injury.

A *complex dislocation* can have severe bone and ligament injuries.

In the most *severe dislocations*, the blood vessels and nerves that travel across the elbow may be injured. If this happens, there is a risk of losing the arm.

Some people are born with greater laxity or looseness in their ligaments. These people are at greater risk for dislocating their elbows. Some people are born with an ulna bone that has a shallow groove for the elbow hinge joint. They have a slightly higher risk for dislocation.

Symptoms

A complete elbow dislocation is extremely painful and very obvious. The arm will look deformed and may have an odd twist at the elbow.

A partial elbow dislocation or subluxation can be harder to detect. Typically, it happens after an accident. Because the elbow is only partially dislocated, the bones can spontaneously relocate and the joint may appear fairly normal. The elbow will usually move fairly well, but there may be pain. There may be bruising on the inside and outside of the elbow where ligaments may have been stretched or torn. Partial dislocations can continue to recur over time if the ligaments never heal.

Diagnosis

The doctor will examine the arm. He will check for tenderness, swelling, and deformity. He will evaluate the skin and circulation to the arm. Pulses at the wrist will be checked. If the artery is injured at the time of dislocation, the hand will be cool to touch and may have a white or purple hue. This is caused by the lack of warm blood reaching the hand.

It is also important to check the nerve supply to the hand. If nerves have been injured during the dislocation, some or all of the hand may be numb and not able to move.

An X-ray is necessary to determine if there is a bone injury. X-rays can also help show the direction of the dislocation.

X-rays are the best way to confirm that the elbow is dislocated. If bone detail is difficult to identify on an X-ray, a computed tomography (CT) scan may be done. If it is important to evaluate the ligaments, a magnetic resonance image (MRI) can be helpful.

First, however, the doctor will set the elbow, without waiting for the CT scan or MRI. These studies are usually taken after the dislocated elbow has been put back in place.

Treatment

An elbow dislocation should be considered an emergency injury. The goal of immediate treatment of a dislocated elbow is to return the elbow to its normal alignment. The long-term goal is to restore function to the arm.

Nonsurgical Treatment

The normal alignment of the elbow can usually be restored in an emergency department at the hospital. Before this is done, sedatives and pain medications usually will be given. The act of restoring alignment to the elbow is called a reduction maneuver. It is done gently and slowly. Two people are usually required to perform this maneuver.

Simple elbow dislocations are treated by keeping the elbow immobile in a splint or sling for two to three weeks, followed by early motion exercises. If the elbow is kept immobile for a long time, the ability to move the elbow fully (range of motion) may be affected. Physical therapy can be helpful during this period of recovery.

Some people will never be able to fully open (extend) the arm, even after physical therapy. Fortunately, the elbow can work very well even without full range of motion. Once the elbow's range of motion improves, the doctor or physical therapist may add a strengthening program. X-rays may be taken periodically while the elbow recovers to ensure that the bones of the elbow joint remain well aligned.

Surgical Treatment

In a complex elbow dislocation, surgery may be necessary to restore bone alignment and repair ligaments. It can be difficult to realign a complex elbow dislocation and to keep the joint in line.

After surgery, the elbow may be protected with an external hinge. This device protects the elbow from dislocating again. If blood vessel or nerve injuries are associated with the elbow dislocation, additional surgery may be needed to repair the blood vessels and nerves and repair bone and ligament injuries.

Late reconstructive surgery can successfully restore motion to some stiff elbows. This surgery removes scar tissue and extra bone growth. It also removes obstacles to movement.

Over time, there is an increased risk for arthritis in the elbow joint if the alignment of the bones is not good, the elbow does not move and rotate normally, or the elbow continues to dislocate.

Research on the Horizon

Treatment for simple dislocations is usually straightforward and the results are usually good. Some people with complex dislocations still have some type of permanent disability at the elbow. Treatment is evolving to improve results for these people.

One of the areas being researched is the best time to schedule surgery for the treatment of a complex dislocation. For some patients with complex dislocations, it seems that a slight delay for final surgery may improve results by allowing swelling to decrease. The dislocation still needs to be reduced right away, but then a brace, splint, or external fixation frame may rest the elbow for about a week before a specialist surgeon attempts major reconstructive surgery.

Moving the elbow early appears to be good for recovery for both kinds of dislocations. Early movement with complex dislocations can be difficult, however. Pain management techniques encourage early movement. Improved therapy and rehabilitation techniques, such as continuous motion machines, dynamic splinting (spring-loaded assist devices), and progressive static splinting, can improve results.

Section 33.7

Ulnar Nerve Entrapment (Cubital Tunnel Syndrome)

What Is Cubital Tunnel Syndrome?

Cubital tunnel syndrome is a condition brought on by increased pressure on the ulnar nerve at the elbow. There is a bump of bone on the inner portion of the elbow (medial epicondyle) under which the ulnar nerve passes. This site is commonly called the "funny bone." At this site, the ulnar nerve lies directly next to the bone and is susceptible to pressure. When the pressure on the nerve becomes great enough to disturb the way the nerve works, then numbness, tingling, and pain may be felt in the elbow, forearm, hand, and/or fingers.

What Causes Cubital Tunnel Syndrome?

Pressure on the ulnar nerve at the elbow can develop in several ways. The nerve is positioned right next to the bone and has very little padding over it, so pressure on this can put pressure on the nerve. For example, if you lean your arm against a table on the inner part of the elbow, your arm may fall asleep and be painful from sustained pressure on the ulnar nerve. If this occurs repetitively, the numbness and pain may be more persistent. In some patients, the ulnar nerve at the elbow clicks back and forth over the bony bump (medial epicondyle) as the elbow is bent and straightened. If this occurs repetitively, the nerve may be significantly irritated.

Additionally, pressure on the ulnar nerve can occur from holding the elbow in a bent position for a long time, which stretches the nerve across the medial epicondyle. Such sustained bending of the elbow may tend to occur during sleep. Sometimes the connective tissue over the nerve becomes thicker, or there may be variations of the muscle structure over the nerve at the elbow that cause pressure on the nerve. Cubital tunnel syndrome occurs when the pressure on the nerve is significant enough, and sustained enough, to disturb the way the ulnar nerve works.

Signs and Symptoms of Cubital Tunnel Syndrome

Cubital tunnel syndrome symptoms usually include pain, numbness, and/or tingling. The numbness or tingling most often occurs in the ring and little fingers. The symptoms are usually felt when there is pressure on the nerve, such as sitting with the elbow on an arm rest, or with repetitive elbow bending and straightening. Often symptoms will be felt when the elbow is held in a bent position for a period of time, such as when holding the phone, or while sleeping. Some patients may notice weakness while pinching, occasional clumsiness, and/or a tendency to drop things. In severe cases, sensation may be lost and the muscles in the hand may lose bulk and strength.

Diagnosis of Cubital Tunnel Syndrome

Your physician will assess the pattern and distribution of your symptoms, and examine for muscle weakness, irritability of the nerve to tapping and/or bending of the elbow, and changes in sensation. Other medical conditions may need to be evaluated such as thyroid disease or diabetes. A test called electromyography (EMG) and/or nerve conduction study (NCS) may be done to confirm the diagnosis of cubital tunnel syndrome and stage its severity. This test also checks for other possible nerve problems, such as a pinched nerve in the neck, which may cause similar symptoms.

Treatment of Cubital Tunnel Syndrome

Symptoms may sometimes be relieved without surgery, particularly if the EMG/NCS testing shows that the pressure on the nerve is minimal. Changing the patterns of elbow use may significantly reduce the pressure on the nerve. Avoiding putting your elbow on hard surfaces may help, or wearing an elbow pad over the ulnar nerve and "funny bone" may help. Keeping the elbow straight at night with a splint also may help. A session with a therapist to learn ways to avoid pressure on the nerve may be needed.

When symptoms are severe or do not improve, surgery may be needed to relieve the pressure on the nerve. Many surgeons will recommend shifting the nerve to the front of the elbow, which relieves pressure and tension on the nerve. The nerve may be placed under a layor of fat, under the muscle, or within the muscle. Some surgeons may recommend trimming the bony bump (medial epicondyle). Following surgery, the recovery will depend on the type of surgery that was performed. Restrictions on lifting and/or elbow movement may be recommended. Therapy may be necessary. The numbness and tingling may improve quickly or slowly, and it may take several months for the strength in the hand and wrist to improve. Cubital tunnel symptoms may not completely resolve after surgery, especially in severe cases.

Section 33.8

Osteochondritis Dissecans of the Elbow (Little League Elbow)

What is little league elbow?

Little league elbow is a growth plate injury on the medial, or inner aspect of the elbow. The growth plate, also called the medial epicondylar apophysis, is the attachment site for the group of muscles that flex the wrist and rotate the forearm palm down. Another name for this sports injury is medial epicondylar apophysitis. It occurs in children and teens involved in sports that require repetitive throwing motions.

What causes little league elbow?

Little league elbow is caused by repetitive throwing. More specifically, there are two phases of the throwing motion that stress the growth plate. The first is the early acceleration phase. During this phase of throwing there is a pulling, or traction force applied to the growth plate on the inner elbow. The second phase of the throwing motion that stresses the elbow is when the ball is released. During this phase, there is a powerful inward and downward snap of the wrist. The growth plate in the elbow is vulnerable to injury because it is made up growth cartilage, a relatively soft substance that is not as strong as bone, muscle, or tendons. With repetitive throwing, and not enough rest between throwing activities, the growth cartilage weakens, begins to develop very small cracks, and may actually pull apart from the arm bone, like a screw pulling out of a plaster wall.

What are the symptoms of little league elbow?

The most striking symptom of little league elbow is pain at the inner elbow. The pain may be severe and occur abruptly after one hard throw, or it may occur gradually over the course of a season. There may also be swelling, redness, and warmth over the inner elbow.

What should I do if I think I have little league elbow?

The first and most important thing to do if little league elbow is suspected is to stop throwing. Ice should be applied for 15 to 20 minutes, and the elbow can be wrapped with an elastic bandage or a compression sleeve. All young throwers with elbow pain should see a doctor since X-rays may be needed to determine the extent of the growth plate injury.

How is little league elbow treated?

Treatment for little league elbow depends on the extent of the growth plate injury. Usually, if caught early, there is minimal separation of the growth plate and it can be treated with rest, ice, and compression wraps. The period of non-throwing may take four to six weeks to allow proper healing. Sometimes, if this sports injury is minor and caught early, an athlete will be allowed to bat or play an infield position such as first base. If the injury to the growth plate is more severe, or there is significant separation of the growth plate from the bone, casting may be necessary. On rare occasions, the injury is severe enough that surgical pinning is necessary to re-attach the growth plate fragment.

Once healing is complete, there will be a gradual return to throwing, usually during a two- to three-week period. This consists of a functional progression starting with very light throws from short distances and progressing to 50 pitches from the mound. This is best directed by a sports medicine physician or sports physical therapist.

Does little league elbow cause permanent damage?

Usually not. If caught early and treated properly, little league elbow will heal completely, and there will be no long-term effects to the growth plate. On rare occasions, the cartilage will degenerate, become fragmented, and break off inside the elbow joint, causing loose pieces that need to be surgically removed. This is more common on the lateral, or outside, of the elbow.

Can little league elbow be prevented?

There is no way to 100% guarantee that a young thrower will not develop little league elbow, but here are some ways to minimize the risk:

- Always warm up before throwing.

- Have a coach or parent count pitches. This is a much better and more accurate way to monitor stress on the elbow than counting innings.

- Remember hard throws when not pitching (playing infield, throwing at home, pitching lessons, PE class, etc).

- No curve balls or other breaking pitches until age 14 (or when the pitcher is shaving). Young pitchers should master control of the fastball and change-up before attempting to throw curve balls. The proper curve ball requires a large enough hand for finger placement across the top of the ball, so ball release does not put any stress on the wrist or elbow. Young pitchers' hands are too small for proper finger placement, and they must twist or torque the wrist and elbow to get the ball to rotate. This increases stress on the inner elbow growth plate.

- At the first sign of elbow pain, stop throwing, and see your doctor for an evaluation.

Chapter 34

Hand Injuries

Chapter Contents

Section 34.1

Hand Fractures

What is a fracture?

The hand is made up of many bones that form its supporting framework. This frame acts as a point of attachment for the muscles that make the wrist and fingers move. A fracture occurs when enough force is applied to a bone to break it. When this happens, there is pain, swelling, and decreased use of the injured part. Many people think that a fracture is different from a break, but they are the same. Fractures may be simple with the bone pieces aligned and stable. Other fractures are unstable and the bone fragments tend to displace or shift. Some fractures occur in the shaft (main body) of the bone, others break the joint surface. Comminuted fractures (bone is shattered into many pieces) usually occur from a high-energy force and are often unstable. An open (compound) fracture occurs when a bone fragment breaks through the skin. There is some risk of infection with compound fractures.

How does a fracture affect the hand?

Fractures often take place in the hand. A fracture may cause pain, stiffness, and loss of movement. Some fractures will cause an obvious deformity, such as a crooked finger, but many fractures do not. Because of the close relationship of bones to ligaments and tendons, the hand may be stiff and weak after the fracture heals. Fractures that injure joint surfaces may lead to early arthritis in those joints.

How are hand fractures treated?

Medical evaluation and X-rays are usually needed so that your doctor can tell if there is a fracture and to help determine the treatment. Depending upon the type of fracture, your hand surgeon may recommend one of several treatment methods.

A splint or cast may be used to treat a fracture that is not displaced, or to protect a fracture that has been set. Some displaced fractures may need to be set and then held in place with wires or pins without making an incision. This is called closed reduction and internal fixation.

Other fractures may need surgery to set the bone (open reduction). Once the bone fragments are set, they are held together with pins, plates, or screws. Fractures that disrupt the joint surface (articular fractures) usually need to be set more precisely to restore the joint surface as smooth as possible. On occasion, bone may be missing or be so severely crushed that it cannot be repaired. In such cases, a bone graft may be necessary. In this procedure, bone is taken from another part of the body to help provide more stability. Sometimes bone graft substitutes may be used instead of taking bone from another part of the body.

Fractures that have been set may be held in place by an "external fixator," a set of metal bars outside the body attached to pins which are placed in the bone above and below the fracture site, in effect keeping it in traction until the bone heals.

Once the fracture has enough stability, motion exercises may be started to try to avoid stiffness. Your hand surgeon can determine when the fracture is sufficiently stable.

What types of results can I expect from surgery for hand fractures?

Perfect alignment of the bone on X-ray is not always necessary to get good function. A bony lump may appear at the fracture site as the bone heals and is known as a "fracture callus." This functions as a "spot weld." This is a normal healing process and the lump usually gets smaller over time. Problems with fracture healing include stiffness, shift in position, infection, slow healing, or complete failure to heal. Smoking has been shown to slow fracture healing. Fractures in children occasionally affect future growth of that bone (see the brochure/web page on Fractures in Children [at http://www.assh.org/Professionals/ProdsSvcs/Store/Pages/FracturesinChildren.aspx]). You can lessen the chances of complication by carefully following your hand surgeon's advice during the healing process and before returning to work or sports activities. A hand therapy program with splints and exercises may be recommended by your physician to speed and improve the recovery process.

Section 34.2

Finger Sprains, Fractures, and Dislocations

Finger Sprains

A finger sprain is stretching or tearing of the ligaments that support the small joints of the finger. Ligaments are strong bands of tissue that connect bones to each other.

Treatment

In consultation with your doctor, treatment may include:

- **Rest:** Avoid using the injured finger.

- **Ice:** Apply ice or a cold pack to your finger for 15–20 minutes, four times a day, for several days or until the pain and swelling goes away. Ice helps to reduce pain and swelling in the sprained finger. Wrap the ice or cold pack in a towel. Do not apply the ice directly to your skin.

- **Compression:** Wrap an elastic compression bandage around your finger. This will limit swelling and support your finger. Be careful not to wrap too tightly or it can cut off the circulation to your finger.

- **Elevation:** Try to hold the injured hand above the level of your heart as much as possible for the first several days or until the swelling goes down (for example, up on a pillow). This will help drain fluid and reduce swelling.

- **Medication:** In consultation with your doctor, consider taking one of the following over-the-counter (OTC) drugs to help reduce inflammation and pain:
  - Ibuprofen (Motrin, Advil)
  - Naproxen (Aleve, Naprosyn)
  - Acetaminophen (Tylenol)

- Aspirin

- **Splinting and taping:** You may need to wear a splint to immobilize your finger. If you play sports, you may need to tape your finger to the finger next to it when you return to play. Your doctor can show you how to splint or tape your finger.

- **Surgery:** Surgery may be needed to repair a finger sprain if:

  - a small piece of bone has been broken off by the injury to the ligament; or

  - a ligament is torn completely.

Finger Fractures

Although a fractured finger is usually considered a minor incident, without the right treatment it can cause serious problems. In the normal hand, the bones all line up precisely. This allows for manual dexterity and precise movement with the thumb and fingers. When a finger bone is fractured it can result in improper alignment of the entire hand. In addition, if left untreated, a fractured finger can remain painful and stiff for a long time.

Treatment

Before proper healing can begin, the broken finger must be put back into place. In most cases, a cast or splint will be sufficient to hold the finger straight while protecting it from any further injury during the healing process. The neighboring fingers can be used as a splint as well. After about three weeks in a splint, X-rays may be needed to assess the healing progress. As soon as possible and with your physician's approval, you should begin using your hand again. Your physician should be able to recommend some everyday exercises to help reduce the finger's swelling and stiffness.

In addition, occasionally surgery is needed to realign the bone and maintain the position until the bone heals. Wires or small screws and plates are often used for this purpose.

Finger Dislocations

A finger dislocation is a joint injury in which the finger bones move apart or sideways so the ends of the bones are no longer aligned normally. Finger dislocations usually happen when the finger is bent backward beyond its normal limit of motion.

Treatment

A dislocated finger can be corrected with or without injecting local anesthesia. To correct the dislocation, the doctor will press against the displaced bone to dislodge the bone if it is caught against the side of the joint. As the end of the bone is freed, the doctor can pull outward to restore the bone to its correct position. This is called closed reduction. Once your finger joint is back in its normal position, you will wear a splint or tape the finger to another finger for three to six weeks, depending on the specific type of your dislocation.

If your doctor cannot straighten your finger using closed reduction or if your injured joint is not stable after closed reduction, your dislocated finger may need to be repaired surgically. Surgery also is used to treat finger dislocations that are complicated by large fractures or fractures that involves the joint.

Section 34.3

Thumb Strains (Skier's Thumb)

Skier's thumb, also referred to as gamekeeper's thumb, is an injury to the ulnar collateral ligament (UCL) in the thumb. A ligament is a rope-like tissue that attaches one bone to another. The UCL links the metacarpal bone (at the base of the thumb) with the proximal phalanx (the middle thumb bone). The injury can be partial, where only a part of the ligament is torn, or it can be complete (also called a rupture), where the entire ligament is torn into two pieces.

At times, when the ligament tears, it pulls a small chip of bone away with it; this is called an avulsion fracture. In some cases, the end of the torn ligament is folded over and trapped over one of the thumb muscles created a small bump; this is known as a Stener lesion. Skier's thumb got its name because the injury commonly occurs when a skier falls and the thumb is bent over a ski pole.

How It Occurs

Any strong force that pulls the thumb away from the rest of the hand can cause skier's thumb.

Signs and Symptoms

Pain is present at the base of the thumb in the web space between the thumb and index finger; the pain worsens with any movement of the thumb. In addition, there may be swelling, bruising, and a weak pinch and grasp. Wrist pain may also be present.

Diagnosis

The doctor will perform a good physical exam looking for laxity (looseness) of the ligament by pushing your thumb into different positions. The looser and less steady the joint is, the worse the injury likely is.

The doctor will likely obtain an X-ray of your thumb to evaluate for the presence of an avulsion fracture. X-rays show injuries to the bones but do not show injuries to the ligaments. In some cases, additional tests are needed, such as magnetic resonance imaging (MRI).

Treatment

Generally, skier's thumb can be treated with immobilization with a splint or cast to keep the joint from moving and allow the ligament to heal. The length and type of immobilization depend on the severity of injury. Some skier's thumb injuries require surgery followed by immobilization. Surgery is required if a Stener lesion is present, if the joint is extremely loose, or if an avulsion fracture occurs and the piece of avulsed bone is displaced from its original position. Physical therapy to help in regaining strength and motion is often part of the treatment regimen.

Return to Activity and Sports

The timing of return to play depends on the severity of injury and the type of treatment required. Many athletes are able to train and condition while wearing a rigid splint or cast. Athletes with milder injuries generally have full use of their thumb as early as four to six weeks after injury. Individuals who require surgery have a longer recovery. The physician may recommend a soft splint or taping for the first few weeks of return to activities.

Section 34.4

Mallet Finger (Baseball Finger)

"Mallet Finger (Extensor Tendon Injury of the Distal Interphalangeal Joint)," reprinted with permission from Children's Memorial Hospital, Chicago, IL (www.childrensmemorial.org). © 2010. All rights reserved.

Mallet finger is an injury involving the distal interphalangeal joint (DIP) which is the joint nearest the tip of the finger. It is caused either by an injury to the extensor tendon or to the bone where it inserts. The extensor tendon straightens the last joint of the finger.

How It Occurs

The most common type of injury is one which causes forced flexion of the DIP joint. This could be caused, for example, by getting hit by a ball on the tip of the finger, causing the tip of the finger to be bent downward suddenly and forcefully.

Signs and Symptoms

Most people with a mallet finger experience pain at the time of injury. Swelling often occurs at the DIP joint. This injury results in a person being unable to actively fully extend (straighten) the finger at the DIP, causing the tip of the finger to droop or drop. However, it is usually possible to passively extend the DIP joint. The inability to straighten the affected finger might not occur until several hours or days after the injury.

Diagnosis

Mallet finger is diagnosed by a physical exam by a doctor. X-rays are performed in order to evaluate the bones of the finger and to see if any displacement or avulsion (breaking off of a piece of bone) has occurred.

Treatment

Usually mallet finger can be treated with splinting. The splint stabilizes the joint so that the tendon and/or bone can heal. Only the DIP joint needs to be immobilized in the splint. Many different types of splints can be used; they can be placed:

1. on the top (dorsal aspect) of the finger;

2. the bottom (volar aspect) of the finger;

3. on either side (lateral aspect) of the finger.

The finger is held in extension, so that the DIP joint is held in a straight position, or in mild hyperextension, so that the DIP joint is curled slightly upwards. The splint will need to be in place for six to eight weeks. It is very important that the DIP joint never be allowed to bend during this time, even if the splint is being changed. The tip of the finger must be held while the splint is off so that there is no flexion or bending of the DIP joint. If a fracture has occurred or the finger cannot be passively extended, surgery may be necessary for healing.

Returning to Activities and Sports

Your doctor will let you know when your child may return to play. It is best to avoid contact sports during the first six to eight weeks of splinting so that the joint is not re-injured. Depending on the sport that your child plays, it may be possible to return to play immediately. However, it will be necessary to continue to wear the splint at all times, including while playing.

Preventing Mallet Finger

Mallet finger can be prevented by avoiding injuries which cause forced flexion of the DIP joint. The riskiest activities are ball sports. There are no exercises, braces, or equipment that will prevent mallet finger.

Section 34.5

Flexor Tendon Injuries

Flexor Tendons in the Hand and Forearm

The muscles that bend (flex) the fingers are called flexor muscles. These flexor muscles move the fingers through cord-like extensions called tendons, which connect the muscles to bone. The flexor muscles start at the elbow and forearm regions, turn into tendons just past the middle of the forearm, and attach to the bones of the fingers. In the finger, the tendons pass through fibrous rings called pulleys, which guide the tendons and keep them close to the bones, enabling the tendons to move the joints much more effectively.

Deep cuts on the palm side of the wrist, hand, or fingers can injure the flexor tendons and nearby nerves and blood vessels. The injury may appear simple on the outside, but is actually much more complex on the inside. When a tendon is cut, it acts like a rubber band, and its cut ends pull away from each other. A tendon that has not been cut completely through may still allow the fingers to bend, but can cause pain or catching, and may eventually tear all the way through. When tendons are cut completely through, the finger joints cannot bend on their own.

How Are Flexor Tendon Injuries Treated?

Tendon Healing

Tendons are made of living cells. If the cut ends of the tendon can be brought back together, healing begins through the cells that are inside of the tendon as well as the tissue outside of the tendon. Because the cut ends of a tendon usually separate after an injury, a cut tendon cannot heal without surgery.

Your doctor will advise you on how soon surgery is needed after a flexor tendon is cut. There are many ways to repair a cut tendon, and certain types of cuts need a specific type of repair. In the finger, it is important to preserve certain pulleys, and there is very little space between the tendon and pulley in which to perform a repair. Nearby nerves and blood vessels may need to be repaired as well. After surgery, and depending on the type of cut, the injured area can either be protected from movement or started on a very specific limited-movement program for several weeks. Your doctor may prescribe hand therapy for you after surgery. If unprotected finger motion begins too soon, the tendon repair is likely to pull apart. After four to six weeks, the fingers are allowed to move slowly and without resistance. Healing takes place during the first three months after the repair.

In most cases, full and normal movement of the injured area does not return after surgery. If it is hard to bend the finger using its own muscle power, it could mean that the repaired tendon has pulled apart or is bogged down in scar tissue. Scarring of the tendon repair is a normal part of the healing process. But in some cases, the scarring can make bending and straightening of the finger very difficult. Depending on the injury, your doctor may prescribe therapy to loosen up the scar tissue and prevent it from interfering with the finger's movement. If therapy fails to improve motion, surgery to release scar tissue around the tendon may be required.

Hand Therapy after Surgery

If a program of controlled, limited motion is selected as therapy for the first several weeks after surgery, it is important to work closely with a hand therapist and your surgeon to understand the therapy and follow set guidelines. The tendon repair might pull apart if your hand is used too soon or if therapy guidelines are not followed. In addition to regaining motion of the finger after a tendon injury, therapy will be helpful in softening scars and building grip strength.

Section 34.6

Extensor Tendon Injuries

What is an extensor tendon?

Extensor tendons, located on the back of the hand and fingers, allow
you to straighten your fingers and thumb. These tendons are attached
to muscles in the forearm. As the tendons continue into the fingers,
they become flat and thin. In the fingers, smaller tendons from small
muscles in the hand join these tendons. It is these small-muscle tendons that allow delicate finger motions and coordination.

How are extensor tendons injured?

Extensor tendons are just under the skin, directly on the bone, on
the back of the hands and fingers. Because of their location, even a
minor cut can easily injure them. Jamming a finger may cause these
thin tendons to rip apart from their attachment to the bone. After this
type of injury, you may have a hard time straightening one or more
joints. Treatment is necessary to return use to the tendon and finger.

How are extensor tendon injuries treated?

Cuts that split the tendon may need stitches, but tears caused by
jamming injuries are usually treated with splints. Splints stop the
healing ends of the tendons from pulling apart and should be worn at
all times until the tendon is fully healed. Your doctor will apply the
splint in the correct place and give you directions on how long to wear
it. Sometimes a pin is placed through the bone across the joint as an
internal splint in addition to the external splint.

What are the common extensor tendon injuries?

Mallet finger refers to the droop of the end joint where an extensor
tendon has been cut or separated from the bone. Sometimes a piece of

bone is pulled off with the tendon, but the result is the same: a fingertip that cannot actively straighten. Whether the tendon injury is caused by a cut or jammed finger, splinting is necessary. Often the cut tendon requires stitches. A splint is used to keep the fingertip straight until the tendon is healed. The size of the splint and length of time you will have to wear it is determined by the type and location of your injury. The splint should remain in place constantly during this time. The tendon may take four to eight weeks, or longer in some patients, to heal completely. Removing the splint early may result in drooping of the fingertip, which may then require additional splinting. Your physician will instruct you to remove the splint at the proper time. Sometimes there is a mild permanent droop, despite proper splint wear.

Boutonniere deformity describes the bent-down (flexed) position of the middle joint of the finger from a cut or tear of the extensor tendon at the middle joint. Treatment involves splinting the middle joint in a straight position until the injured tendon is fully healed. Sometimes, stitches are necessary when the tendon has been cut and even if the tendon is torn. If the injury is not treated, or if the splint is not worn properly, the finger can quickly become even more bent and finally stiffen in this position. Be sure to follow your doctor's instructions and wear your splint for a minimum of four to eight weeks. Your doctor will tell you when you may stop wearing the splint.

Lacerations or cuts on the back of the hand that go through the extensor tendons cause difficulty in straightening the finger at the large joint where the fingers join the hand. Stitching the tendon ends together is the usual way of treating these injuries, followed by splinting to protect the repair. The splint for a tendon injury in this area may include the wrist and part of the finger. Dynamic splinting, which is a splint with slings that allows some finger motion, may be used for injuries of this kind. The dynamic splint allows early movement and protects the healing tendon.

What can I expect as a result of my extensor tendon injury?

Extensor tendon injuries may form scar that causes the tendon to adhere to nearby bone and scar tissue, limiting the movement of the tendon. The scar tissue that forms may prevent full finger bending and straightening even with the best of treatment. Many factors can affect the seriousness of the injury, including fracture, infection, medical illnesses, and individual differences. To improve motion, hand therapy may be necessary. Surgery to free scar tissue may sometimes by helpful in serious cases of motion loss. Your physician will explain the risks and benefits of the various treatments of extensor tendon injuries.

Part Seven

Injuries to the Trunk, Groin, Upper Legs, and Knees

Chapter 35

Trunk and Groin Injuries

Chapter Contents

Section 35.1

Rib Stress Fractures

Overview

What is a rib stress fracture?

A stress fracture is an area in the bone where it has become weakened and microscopic cracks have gradually formed because the bone is repeatedly loaded and stressed. This is different from a regular "traumatic" bone fracture or break in which one event causes the bone to crack all at once. The cracks in stress fractures are often so small that they can't be seen on regular X-rays, but the area where the bone has built up some new bone ("callus") as it tries to heal is sometimes visible. A stress fracture can progress to become a complete fracture if it is not allowed to heal with a period of rest. Stress fractures can occur in almost any bone. A stress fracture of the rib is rare but can be seen in high-level athletes with significant demands of repetitive upper extremity activities, such as rowers or track and field athletes. Stress fractures in the legs and feet of runners are much more common due to the constant, repetitive impact forces with each stride.

What is the anatomy involved in a rib stress fracture?

Most commonly the first rib is the one involved in a rib stress fracture. There are 12 ribs on the right and 12 ribs on the left. The first rib is the top one and it can barely be felt deep in the space behind and above the collarbone (clavicle). The first rib connects the spine in the back to the breastbone (sternum) in the front. Large blood vessels (subclavian artery and vein) travel right over the first rib as they go to the arm. These vessels have corresponding grooves in the first rib where the vessels travel over the rib. These grooves make the rib thinner and weaker in those regions. Normally, the bone can withstand these forces, but when a stress fracture has formed, the repeated stress on the bone exceeds the rate at which the bone can repair itself.

Symptoms

How is a rib stress fracture diagnosed?

The athlete will usually notice gradual onset of pain in the side of the neck and upper back and/or pain in the back of the shoulder. This may gradually increase or come and go for weeks to months. The pain gets worse with activity and gets better with rest. The pain may be worsened by deep breaths, using the arm overhead, or by coughing. Rarely, the athlete may feel a pop or snap if the stress fracture all of a sudden becomes a complete fracture.

When the physician examines the athlete, a complete exam of the shoulder, neck, and arm will rule out other causes of the pain. The athlete will have tenderness directly over the first rib (behind the collarbone at the base of the neck). Squeezing the trapezius muscle at the base of the neck may be painful.

What imaging is used to diagnose a rib stress fracture?

If a stress fracture is suspected, X-rays of the rib will be taken. If the diagnosis is not clear, X-rays might also be taken of the neck and/or shoulder. On X-rays, a stress fracture may show up as a small crack, or the bone might be thickened in that area from trying to heal. If the stress fracture has gone on to become a complete fracture, there may be a very obvious crack visible. Often times, however, the stress fracture doesn't show up in the X-ray. In this case a bone scan, MRI [magnetic resonance imaging], or a CT [computed tomography] may be ordered.

A bone scan is a special test with a tracer that is injected into an IV. The tracer is taken up more strongly by areas of the bone that are trying to heal, so the stress fracture shows up as a bright spot. A CT scan is a special scan that shows the details of bone very well and can show small cracks and changes in bones. It can also show if there is an underlying cause of the fracture such a bone cyst, but this is very rare. An MRI may also reveal areas of increased inflammation and swelling in response to the stress reaction in the bone.

Causes

What may predispose me to getting a rib stress fracture as an athlete?

A rib stress fracture is not common, but they have been reported in many sports that have repetitive vigorous shoulder motions. These sports include baseball (especially pitching), dancing, tennis, golf, rowing, backpacking, wind surfing, and other sports. They have also been seen in people that do a lot of shoveling.

Often, there is no clear cause for the stress fracture, but there are some factors that sometimes contribute. A sudden increase in weightlifting or training could predispose to stress fractures. Poor mechanics when participating in the sport may also increase the risk of stress fracture. A poor diet, eating disorders such as anorexia, lack of vitamin D, lack of calcium, and insufficient rest may contribute. In some female athletes who train extensively, amenorrhea (infrequent menstrual periods) may lead to weaker bones and a predisposition to getting stress fractures. Rarely, a disease or a biochemical imbalance may contribute to weaker bones.

Prevention

How can I prevent them as an athlete?

Many stress fractures could be avoided by watching for and correcting the aforementioned factors. Work with a coach to be sure you are using the proper form and mechanics in your sport. Gradually increase training and weightlifting to give your body a chance to adjust. Get plenty of rest and be sure to eat a balanced nutritious diet with plenty of calcium and vitamin D. If a stress fracture is developing, it is important to recognize it and rest early to avoid further injury and the risk for secondary traumatic fracture.

Treatment

When is treatment without surgery appropriate and what does it entail?

Treatment without surgery is always the most appropriate first-line of treatment for a typical rib stress fracture. The key is "relative rest" which means don't do anything that causes significant pain or discomfort. The goal is to let the rib rest so it can heal itself. If stress is continually placed on it, it never gets a chance to heal. This usually means a period of four to six weeks without throwing or weightlifting with the affected shoulder, but lower body workouts can usually be continued without interruption or they can be modified so they do not cause rib pain. Once there is no pain during regular activities, then light lifting and throwing, or other sport specific activities, can be gradually added. If pain recurs, then the athlete must back off again and give it more time.

Other important elements of treatment include analyzing the training program, rest, and body mechanics of the athlete to identify and correct any contributing factors. Also, the diet should be examined to make sure nutrition is appropriate.

If the athlete has a history of multiple stress fractures or if the fracture is not healing, it may be appropriate to do some blood tests or special imaging to make sure there are not other, systemic factors involved.

The time for healing may vary significantly between athletes and must be individualized and discussed with the athlete's physician. If the stress fracture is not visible on X-rays, the athlete might return to full sports participation in 8–12 weeks. If the stress fracture has become a complete fracture, it may take 6–12 months.

Is surgery needed for rib stress fractures?

In the vast majority of cases, surgery is not needed. Even if the bone doesn't heal, the athlete can usually get back to their sport without surgery and without pain. However, there are some unusual reported cases of the bone healing with such a large mass of bone ("callus") that it impinges the underlying nerves and vessels and requires a "decompressive" surgery.

If you suspect that you have a rib stress fracture, it is critical to seek the urgent consultation of a local sports injuries doctor for appropriate care.

References

Coris EE, Higgins HW. First rib stress fractures in throwing athletes. *Am J Sports Med*. 2005;33:1400–1403.

Prisk VR, Hamilton WG. Stress fracture of the first rib in weight-trained dancers. *Am J Sports Med*. 2008;36:2444–2447.

Section 35.2

Exercise-Induced Hematuria

"Hematuria (Blood in the Urine)," National Kidney and Urologic
Diseases Information Clearinghouse (NKUDIC), National Institutes of
Health, September 2, 2010.

What is hematuria?

Hematuria is the presence of red blood cells (RBCs) in the urine.
In microscopic hematuria, the urine appears normal to the naked eye,
but examination with a microscope shows a high number of RBCs.
Gross hematuria can be seen with the naked eye—the urine is red or
the color of cola.

What causes hematuria?

Several conditions can cause hematuria, most of them not serious.
For example, exercise may cause hematuria that goes away in 24 hours.
Many people have hematuria without any other related problems.
Often no specific cause can be found. But because hematuria may
be the result of a tumor or other serious problem, a doctor should be
consulted.

How is hematuria diagnosed?

To find the cause of hematuria, or to rule out certain causes, the
doctor may order a series of tests, including urinalysis, blood tests,
kidney imaging studies, and cystoscopic examination.

- Urinalysis is the examination of urine for various cells and
  chemicals. In addition to finding RBCs, the doctor may find
  white blood cells that signal a urinary tract infection or casts,
  which are groups of cells molded together in the shape of the
  kidneys' tiny filtering tubes, that signal kidney disease.
  Excessive protein in the urine also signals kidney disease.

- Blood tests may reveal kidney disease if the blood contains high
  levels of wastes that the kidneys are supposed to remove.

- Kidney imaging studies include ultrasound, CT scan, or intravenous pyelogram (IVP). An IVP is an X-ray of the urinary tract. Imaging studies may reveal a tumor, a kidney or bladder stone, an enlarged prostate, or other blockage to the normal flow of urine.

- A cystoscope can be used to take pictures of the inside of the bladder. It has a tiny camera at the end of a thin tube, which is inserted through the urethra. A cystoscope may provide a better view of a tumor or bladder stone than can be seen in an IVP.

How is hematuria treated?

- Treatment for hematuria depends on the cause. If no serious condition is causing the hematuria, no treatment is necessary.

Section 35.3

Testicular Injuries

It hurts to even think about it. A baseball takes an unexpected bounce when you're crouched and waiting to field a grounder, an opponent misses a kick on the soccer field and his foot has only one place to go, or you're speeding along on your bike and you hit a big bump. All result in one really painful thing—a shot to the testicles, one of the most tender areas on a guy's body.

Testicular injuries are relatively uncommon, but guys should be aware that they can happen. So how can you avoid injury?

Why Do Testicular Injuries Happen and What Can You Do?

If you're a guy who plays sports, likes to lift weights and exercise a lot, or leads an all-around active life, you've probably come to find out that the testicles are kind of vulnerable and can be injured in a variety of ways.

Because they hang in a sac outside the body (the scrotum), the testicles are not protected by bones and muscles like other parts of your reproductive system and most of your other organs. Also, the location of the testicles makes them prime targets to be accidentally struck on the playing field or injured during strenuous exercise and activity.

The good news is that because the testicles are loosely attached to the body and are made of a spongy material, they're able to absorb most collisions without permanent damage. Testicles, although sensitive, can bounce back pretty quickly and minor injuries rarely have long-term effects. Also, sexual function or sperm production will most likely not be affected if you have a testicular injury.

You'll definitely feel pain if your testicles are struck or kicked, and you might also feel nauseated for a short time. If it's a minor testicular injury, the pain should gradually subside in less than an hour and any other symptoms should go away.

In the meantime, you can do a few things to help yourself feel better such as take pain relievers, lie down, gently support the testicles with supportive underwear, and apply ice packs to the area. At any rate, it's a good idea to avoid strenuous activity for a while and take it easy for a few days.

However, if the pain doesn't subside or you experience extreme pain that lasts longer than an hour; if you have swelling or bruising of the scrotum or a puncture of the scrotum or testicle; if you continue to have nausea and vomiting; or if you develop a fever, get to a doctor immediately. These are symptoms of a much more serious injury that needs to be addressed as soon as possible.

Serious Testicular Injuries

Examples of serious testicular injury are testicular torsion and testicular rupture. In the case of testicular torsion, the testicle twists around, cutting off its blood supply. This can happen due to a serious trauma to the testicles, strenuous activity, or even for no apparent reason.

Testicular torsion isn't common, but when it does happen, it most often occurs in guys ages 12 to 18. If it occurs, it is crucial to see a doctor as soon as possible—within six hours of the time the pain starts. Unfortunately, after six hours, there is a much greater possibility that complications could result, including reduced sperm production or the loss of the testicle. The problem may be fixed by a doctor manually untwisting the testicle. If that doesn't work, surgery will be necessary.

Testicular rupture can also happen, but it is a rare type of testicular trauma. This can happen when the testicle receives a forceful direct blow or when the testicle is crushed against the pubic bone (the bone that forms the front of the pelvis), causing blood to leak into the scrotum. Testicular rupture, like testicular torsion and other serious injuries to the testicles, causes extreme pain, swelling in the scrotum, nausea, and vomiting. To fix the problem, surgery is necessary to repair the ruptured testicle.

Seeing a Doctor

If you have to see a doctor, he or she will first need to know how long you have been experiencing pain and how severe your discomfort is. To rule out a hernia or other problem as the cause of the pain, the doctor will examine your abdomen and groin.

In addition, the doctor will look at your scrotum for swelling, color, and damage to the skin and examine the testicle itself. Because infections of the reproductive system or urinary tract can sometimes cause similar pain, your doctor may do a urine test to rule out a urinary tract infection or infection of the reproductive organs.

Preventing Testicular Injuries

It's wise to take precautions to avoid testicular injuries, especially if you play sports, exercise a lot, or just live an all-around active life. Here are some tips to keep your testicles safe and sound:

- **Protect your testicles.** Always wear an athletic cup or athletic supporter when playing sports or participating in strenuous activity. Athletic cups are usually made of hard plastic, are worn over the groin area, and provide a good degree of shielding and safety for the testicles. Cups are best used when participating in sports where your testicles might get hit or kicked, like football, hockey, soccer, or karate.

  An athletic supporter, or jock strap, is basically a cloth pouch that you wear to keep your testicles close to your body. Athletic supporters are best used when participating in strenuous exercise, cycling, or doing any heavy lifting.

- **Check your fit.** Make sure the athletic cup and/or athletic supporter is the right size. Safety equipment that's too small or too big won't protect you as effectively.

- **Keep your doctor informed.** If you play sports, you probably have regular physical exams by a doctor. If you experience testicular pain even occasionally, talk to your doctor about it.

- **Be aware of the risks of your sport or activity.** If you play a sport or participate in an activity with a high risk of injury, talk to your coach or doctor about any additional protective gear you should use.

Participating in sports and living an active life are great ways to stay fit and relieve stress. But it's important to make sure your testicles are protected. When you're exercising or playing sports, make sure that using protective gear is part of your routine and you'll be able to play hard without fear of testicular injury!

Chapter 36

Hip Injuries

Chapter Contents

Section 36.1

Hip Bursitis

What is bursitis?

Bursitis of the hip is a very common cause of hip pain. A bursa is a closed fluid-filled sac that functions as a gliding surface to reduce friction between tissues of the body. The major bursae (plural) are located adjacent to the tendons near the large joints, such as the shoulders, elbows, hips, and knees. When a bursa becomes inflamed, the condition is known as "bursitis." Most commonly, this is a non-infectious condition (aseptic bursitis) caused by inflammation resulting from a local soft tissue trauma or strain. On rare occasions, bursae can become infected (usually a bacterial infection). This condition is called septic bursitis.

What is hip bursitis?

There are several bursae around the hip, which can give rise to stiffness and pain around the hip joint, groin, and gluteal region. The trochanteric bursa is located on the side of the hip and is by far the most common hip bursa to become inflamed. Anatomically, it is separated significantly from the actual hip joint by tissue and bone. When inflamed it can cause considerable tenderness around the bony prominence on the side of the hip. As well as local pain in this region, trochanteric bursitis may give rise to pain radiating down the outer thigh, bottom, or even the groin.

The ischial bursa is located in the buttock area. It can cause dull pain in this area that is most noticeable climbing uphill. The pain sometimes occurs after prolonged sitting on hard surfaces, hence the names "weaver's bottom" and "tailor's bottom." The treatment of ischial bursitis differs considerably from that of trochanteric bursitis and will not be covered here.

A third bursa of the hip, the iliopsoas bursa, may also give rise to pain in the groin and the upper thigh. Although numerous other pathologies can mimic iliopsoas bursitis (arthritis, tendonitis, osteitis pubis, etc.), once a firm diagnosis is made, the physiotherapy treatment is usually quite straightforward. Manual treatment involves releasing and stretching muscles in the thigh and groin as well as restrengthening some of the posterior pelvic musculature.

What are the symptoms of trochanteric bursitis?

Trochanteric bursitis frequently causes tenderness on the outer hip, making it difficult for patients to lie on the involved side. It also causes a dull, burning pain on the outer hip that can radiate down the outer part of the thigh and even into the groin. It is often made worse with excessive walking or stair climbing.

How is trochanteric bursitis treated?

The treatment of any bursitis depends on whether or not it involves infection. Aseptic hip bursitis can be treated extremely successfully by physiotherapy. Treatment involves deep tissue release of the bottom muscles and iliotibial band and a series of muscle stretches that aim to minimize the pressure and friction over the bursa. Releasing the appropriate muscles may involve deep tissue massage techniques, injections of local anesthetic, or dry needling techniques. You will also be required to follow a regimented home program of stretches for these muscles. This may be followed by strengthening for the gluteus medius muscle (a large muscle deep within the pelvis). In some instances, orthotics (inserts to be worn in the shoe) may be suggested. This is generally a treatment of last resort, however, even in situations where considerable biomechanical deformity of the foot exists. Ensure you have exhausted other medical and physiotherapy treatment options before you incur the expense of an orthotic.

Stubborn (usually long-term) cases may require anti-inflammatory medication, aspiration of the bursal fluid, or corticosteroid injections to the region. Although the relief that follows a corticosteroid injection is usually very good, it remains important to continue with the stretching and strengthening regime for several weeks after the injection as this will significantly reduce the likelihood of reoccurrence. Iontophoresis with corticosteroids is another option for those patients wishing to avoid an injection though it is considerably more expensive and less successful than having the bursa injected with a corticosteroid.

Patients can often also benefit by weight reduction and proper footwear for exercise activities. Patients should avoid those activities that aggravated their symptoms whilst the problem is being treated.

Section 36.2

Hip Flexor Strains

"Hip Flexor Strain," by Jon Heck, MS, ATC. © 2004 Richard Stockton College Athletic Training. Reprinted with permission. Reviewed by David A. Cooke, MD, FACP, October 2011.

What Is It?

The hip flexors are a group of muscles that move the hip forward when running and walking. A great deal of stress is applied to this muscle group when sprinting and kicking. Over the last three to four years this injury has become fairly common in the media, as professional athletes often sustain it. You will hear announcers mention it as "...he's going to be unable to play today due to a hip flexor." Well actually, we all have "hip flexors," it's those with a hip flexor strain that have a problem. A strain can vary anywhere from stretching to a complete tear of the muscle tissue.

It Hurts Where?

All of the hip flexors are primarily located on the anterior upper thigh or hip. There are six main muscles involved with hip flexion and it can be very difficult to distinguish which of them is actually injured. Considering their location it makes sense that pain will always occur on the anterior upper thigh/hip. Symptoms will be associated with actions that move the leg forward or upward.

How Does It Happen?

Frequently a hip flexor strain is the result of an overly forceful contraction. This can occur during a sprint or a series of sprints. Soccer players are at high risk for this injury due to the powerful kicks associated with crossing passes, corner kicks, and shots on goal. The strain can also be the result of overuse (kicking/sprinting) and associated "micro traumas." A micro trauma can be considered a tiny imperceptible tear. These tiny tears accumulate over time and eventually result in a strain and pain.

Injury Progression

Generally, a first-degree strain involves stretching (or very minor tearing) damage to the muscle or tendon. A second-degree strain is associated with partial tearing of the muscle or tendon. And, worst-case scenario, a third-degree strain is a complete tear. Regarding injury progression, playing with any strain can easily lead to further damage and function loss. This is particularly true when the injury is related to overuse and has a gradual onset. Athletes often try to play through this, with no rehabilitation, and it results in a grade 1 strain becoming a grade 2.

Similar Injuries

Most often, a hip flexor strain can be confused with a groin strain (adductor strain). This is because the athlete will have pain on the anterior-medial hip. One differentiating factor is adductor strains cause pain with lateral movements (cutting), and hip flexor strains do not. It is possible to involve both muscle groups in an injury though. A quad strain will also present with symptoms similar to a hip flexor strain.

Treatment

As always, ice bags over the painful area for 20–25 minutes after training is a good place to start. It is essential to focus on the following: a gradual strengthening of all the hip musculature, working on proprioception (various balancing skills), and increasing flexibility (including hamstring and adductors). Time off from aggravating activities may also be necessary, but this depends on the severity of the injury and when rehabilitation has begun.

Participation Status

Athletes with a grade 1 strain can usually continue to participate as tolerated, implementing ice and rehabilitation. Athletes with a grade 2 injury will require some time off and rehabilitation. Time missed can vary from a few days to a few weeks here. Grade 3 hip flexor injuries are rare and will probably be season ending.

Section 36.3

Quadriceps Contusions and Hip Pointers

"Rehabilitation of Quadriceps Contusions and Hip Pointers in Sports," by Scott Brackett, Bruce Getz, ATC, and Teri Mingee, M.S., P.T., *Hughston Health Alert*, Summer 1998. © 1998 Hughston Sports Medicine Foundation, Inc. All rights reserved. Reprinted with permission. Reviewed by David A. Cooke, MD, FACP, August 2011.

Quadriceps contusions and hip pointers are common injuries in sports. Immediate and appropriate action is vital in preventing complications that can keep you from your normal activities for a prolonged time.

Treating Quadriceps Contusions

Immediately after a direct blow to the front part of the thigh, ice should be placed over the injury site, with the knee bent all the way. This position should be maintained for 20 minutes. Thereafter, ice should be continued for 20 minutes, every hour for the first 24 hours, with the knee straight. With the doctor's consent, a physical therapist or athletic trainer may use electrical stimulation with the ice to ease pain and swelling. After the ice is removed, a thick felt or foam compression pad over the injury site and an elastic wrap around the thigh can help provide support and reduce swelling. The compression pad must be in place when the athlete is not using ice. The athlete can start gentle, pain-free quad sets (tightening the quadriceps muscle and holding for five seconds). Crutches are used; however, the athlete is encouraged to walk as normally as possible, while placing minimal weight on the injured leg.

The Day After

For 20 minutes, every hour when possible (three times per day minimum), ice is applied with the knee straight. Quad sets should be continued, and the athlete can begin to try to bend the knee as far as possible without assistance and without pain. The athlete continues to walk with crutches until walking can be done without pain, limping, or swelling.

Recommendations

The athlete must work to regain full knee bending motion and gradually progress to pain-free strengthening and conditioning exercises, such as leg raises, stationary biking, and straight-ahead jogging. Certain activities, such as squatting, running downhill, and quick stopping and cutting, place a great deal of stress on the quadriceps. These activities should not be started until the athlete has full, pain-free motion and is jogging straight ahead without pain, limping, or swelling.

Preventing Reinjury

When the athlete is ready to return to action, a large pad that covers the front and sides of the thigh is used. An impact or pressure relief pad (a foam donut covered by a hard plastic shell, such as Orthoplast) is highly recommended. Prevention of quadriceps contusions may be possible with the use of large thigh pads that surround the front and sides of the thigh. In football, many position players (such as running backs) have large quadriceps muscles, but wear small pads when larger pads might instead offer better protection. In addition, the correct pants size is important to hold the thigh pad in place. Specialty girdles with built-in pockets for thigh pads can be used by any athlete in almost any sport.

Treating Hip Pointers

Hip pointers can be very painful and debilitating. Ice and crutches are the recommended immediate treatment. Electrical stimulation to relieve pain can also be used with the ice. Ice is continued for 20 minutes, every hour, until the pain resolves. The athlete can gradually return to jogging and sport-specific drills as the pain allows. When the athlete returns to participation, extreme care should be taken to protect the injured hip with proper padding. A good way to prevent a hip pointer is to make sure hip pads are large enough to come up over the crest of the hip bone. Football hip pads can be used by athletes for most sports to protect and prevent hip injuries.

Prevention of quadriceps contusions and hip pointers through appropriate padding should be taken seriously by the athletes, parents, coaches, and athletic trainers. Unfortunately, despite the best precautions, these injuries still can occur and appropriate treatment is important for a quick, safe return to play.

Chapter 37

Upper Leg Injuries

Chapter Contents

Section 37.1

Exertional Compartment Syndrome

"Compartment Syndrome," by David Edell, MEd, ATC, LAT, CSCS. © 2010
David Edell. Reprinted with permission from www.AthleticAdvisor.com.

Compartment syndromes are potentially serious athletic injuries.
A compartment syndrome is the result of unusually high pressure in
one of the four compartments in the lower leg. The compartments do
not tolerate vast changes in pressure. If the pressure increases too
much, pain and disability can result.

Anatomy

The four osseofascial compartments of the lower leg are: the anterior, the lateral, the superficial posterior, and the deep posterior. Each
of these compartments is bordered by bone and/or a very non-elastic
fascial covering.

Each of the compartments are "sealed" spaces containing muscles,
arteries, and nerves. Each compartment contains the following major
nerves, arteries, and veins: the deep peroneal nerve, and anterior tibial
artery and vein in the anterior; the superficial peroneal nerve in the
lateral; the saphenous nerve in the superficial posterior; and the tibial
nerve, posterior tibial artery and vein, and the peroneal artery and
vein in the deep posterior.

The muscles located in the compartments are as follows:

- **Anterior:** Tibialis anterior, extensor hallucis longus, extensor
  digitorum longus

- **Lateral:** Peroneus longus and brevis

- **Superficial posterior:** Gastrocnemius and soleus

- **Deep posterior:** Flexor hallucis longus, tibialis posterior, and
  flexor digitorum longus

The superficial and deep compartments' anatomical boundaries
can vary. Both compartments are commonly involved in exertional

compartment syndromes (ECS). The "soleus bridge" is a combination of fascia layers in the deep posterior compartment that are closely related to ECS. The bridge is formed by the transverse intermuscular septum and its intersection with the anterior and posterior fascial layers of the soleus. The bridge ultimately inserts on the posteromedial tibia. Due to its insertion point irritation of the bridge is often misdiagnosed as medial tibial stress syndrome. Also, increased compression of the bridge is seen in athletes with excessive rear foot pronation.

Evaluation

Acute compartment syndromes are medical emergencies that may require immediate surgical treatment. Acute compartment syndromes are usually the result of a traumatic incident such as a car accident. The shin is struck with an object that causes a deep contusion. The swelling from the contusion causes the increased pressure in the compartment. These injuries are most often seen in the emergency room and are not athletic injuries.

ECS is seen more often in the athletic community. Diagnosing this injury is one of exclusion. A complete examination should rule out medial tibial stress syndrome, stress fractures, and Achilles tendon injuries.

The athlete will present with pain that is present during weight bearing training. Activities such as running, stair climbing, and jumping are the most common offenders. Radiographs should be obtained to rule out occult stress fractures.

The physical examination may not yield any significant findings. With a true ECS, a physical examination must be conducted immediately after cessation of the offending physical activity. An exam at this time should reveal a tense compartment or swollen lower leg, paresthesia, and non-focal pain on palpation. The ECS sufferer will not have point tenderness over the medial tibial border as seen with medial tibial stress syndrome.

Definitive diagnosis of an ECS can be made with an intracompartmental pressure test. A catheter is inserted into the offending compartment to measure its pressure. Most often three pressure readings will be taken; resting, and one minute and five minutes post exercise. Most physicians rely solely on the post-exercise pressures to render a diagnosis. The pressures alone are not relative; they must show an elevation from the resting pressure along with a recurrence in symptoms.

Appropriate pressure reading are a subject of debate. Most physicians will follow these readings:

- **Normal resting pressure:** 10 mmHg [millimeters of mercury]
- **Abnormal resting pressure:** >20 mmHg
- **Abnormal exertional pressure:** >30 mmHg
- **Abnormal post-exercise pressure:** >25 mmHg

Once the diagnosis is confirmed with a positive compartment measurement, a treatment course is to be chosen. Conservative treatment is the first option. Rehabilitation should include: low-impact cross training, flexibility training, appropriate strength training for weakened muscles, and/or the use of orthotics to correct biomechanical abnormalities.

If conservative treatment fails, surgical intervention in the next step. A fasciotomy is the procedure of choice. A fasciotomy can be performed with one long incision over the affected compartment or with a newer method that involves two small incisions.

The fascia over the affected compartment one centimeter posterior to the intermuscular septum will allow the compartment to increase in size due to the accommodate the higher pressures that occur during exercise. If the anterior or lateral compartments are affected, the surgeon will often release both.

Anterior and lateral compartment releases have a high success rate. Release of the posterior and deep posterior compartments have a lower success rate. Researchers do not know the reason for this disparity.

Full activities may begin as soon as tolerated, usually three to four weeks after surgery.

Section 37.2

Femur Fracture

"Femur Shaft Fractures (Broken Thighbone)," reproduced with
permission from *Your Orthopaedic Connection*. © American Academy of
Orthopaedic Surgeons (www.aaos.org), Rosemont, IL, 2011.

Your thighbone (femur) is the longest and strongest bone in your
body. Because the femur is so strong, it usually takes a lot of force to
break it. Car crashes, for example, are the number one cause of femur
fractures.

The long, straight part of the femur is called the femoral shaft.
When there is a break anywhere along this length of bone, it is called
a femoral shaft fracture.

Types of Femoral Shaft Fractures

Femur fractures vary greatly, depending on the force that causes
the break. The pieces of bone may line up correctly or be out of alignment (displaced), and the fracture may be closed (skin intact) or open
(the bone has punctured the skin).

Doctors describe fractures to each other using classification systems.
Femur fractures are classified depending on:

- the location of the fracture (the femoral shaft is divided into
  thirds: distal, middle, proximal);

- the pattern of the fracture (for example, the bone can break in
  different directions, such as cross-wise, length-wise, or in the
  middle);

- whether the skin and muscle above the bone is torn by the injury.

The most common types of femoral shaft fractures include:

Transverse fracture: In this type of fracture, the break is a
straight horizontal line going across the femoral shaft.

Oblique fracture: This type of fracture has an angled line across
the shaft.

369

Spiral fracture: The fracture line encircles the shaft like the stripes on a candy cane. A twisting force to the thigh causes this type of fracture.

Comminuted fracture: In this type of fracture, the bone has broken into three or more pieces. In most cases, the number of bone fragments corresponds with the amount of force required to break the bone.

Open fracture: If a bone breaks in such a way that bone fragments stick out through the skin or a wound penetrates down to the broken bone, the fracture is called an open or compound fracture. Open fractures often involve much more damage to the surrounding muscles, tendons, and ligaments. They have a higher risk for complications—especially infections—and take a longer time to heal.

Cause

Femoral shaft fractures in young people are frequently due to some type of high-energy collision. The most common cause of femoral shaft fracture is a motor vehicle or motorcycle crash. Being hit by a car as a pedestrian is another common cause, as are falls from heights and gunshot wounds.

A lower-force incident, such as a fall from standing, may cause a femoral shaft fracture in an older person who has weaker bones.

Symptoms

A femoral shaft fracture usually causes immediate, severe pain. You will not be able to put weight on the injured leg, and it may look deformed—shorter than the other leg and no longer straight.

Doctor Examination

Medical History and Physical Examination

It is important that your doctor know the specifics of how you hurt your leg. For example, if you were in a car accident, it would help your doctor to know how fast you were going, whether you were the driver or a passenger, whether you were wearing your seat belt, and if the airbags went off. This information will help your doctor determine how you were hurt and whether you may be hurt somewhere else.

It is also important for your doctor to know whether you have other health conditions like high blood pressure, diabetes, asthma, or allergies. Your doctor will also ask you about any medications you take.

After discussing your injury and medical history, your doctor will do a careful examination. He or she will assess your overall condition, and then focus on your leg. Your doctor will look for:

- an obvious deformity of the thigh/leg (an unusual angle, twisting, or shortening of the leg);

- breaks in the skin;

- bruises;

- bony pieces that may be pushing on the skin.

After the visual inspection, your doctor will then feel along your thigh, leg, and foot looking for abnormalities and checking the tightness of the skin and muscles around your thigh. He or she will also feel for pulses. If you are awake, your doctor will test for sensation and movement in your leg and foot.

Imaging Tests

Other tests that will provide your doctor with more information about your injury include:

- **X-rays:** The most common way to evaluate a fracture is with X-rays, which provide clear images of bone. X-rays can show whether a bone is intact or broken. They can also show the type of fracture and where it is located within the femur.

- **Computed tomography (CT) scan:** If your doctor still needs more information after reviewing your X-rays, he or she may order a CT scan. A CT scan shows a cross-sectional image of your limb. It can provide your doctor with valuable information about the severity of the fracture. For example, sometimes the fracture lines can be very thin and hard to see on an X-ray. A CT scan can help your doctor see the lines more clearly.

Treatment

Nonsurgical Treatment

Most femoral shaft fractures require surgery to heal. It is unusual for femoral shaft fractures to be treated without surgery. Very young children are sometimes treated with a cast. For more information on that, see "Pediatric Thighbone (Femur) Fracture" [at http://orthoinfo .aaos.org/topic.cfm?topic=A00424].

371

Surgical Treatment

Timing of surgery: If the skin around your fracture has not been broken, your doctor will wait until you are stable before doing surgery. Open fractures, however, expose the fracture site to the environment. They urgently need to be cleansed and require immediate surgery to prevent infection.

For the time between initial emergency care and your surgery, your doctor will place your leg either in a long-leg splint or in skeletal traction. This is to keep your broken bones as aligned as possible and to maintain the length of your leg.

Skeletal traction is a pulley system of weights and counterweights that holds the broken pieces of bone together. It keeps your leg straight and often helps to relieve pain.

External fixation: In this type of operation, metal pins or screws are placed into the bone above and below the fracture site. The pins and screws are attached to a bar outside the skin. This device is a stabilizing frame that holds the bones in the proper position so they can heal.

External fixation is usually a temporary treatment for femur fractures. Because they are easily applied, external fixators are often put on when a patient has multiple injuries and is not yet ready for a longer surgery to fix the fracture. An external fixator provides good, temporary stability until the patient is healthy enough for the final surgery. In some cases, an external fixator is left on until the femur is fully healed, but this is not common.

Intramedullary nailing: Currently, the method most surgeons use for treating femoral shaft fractures is intramedullary nailing. During this procedure, a specially designed metal rod is inserted into the marrow canal of the femur. The rod passes across the fracture to keep it in position.

An intramedullary nail can be inserted into the canal either at the hip or the knee through a small incision. It is screwed to the bone at both ends. This keeps the nail and the bone in proper position during healing.

Intramedullary nails are usually made of titanium. They come in various lengths and diameters to fit most femur bones.

Plates and screws: During this operation, the bone fragments are first repositioned (reduced) into their normal alignment. They are held together with special screws and metal plates attached to the outer surface of the bone.

Plates and screws are often used when intramedullary nailing may not be possible, such as for fractures that extend into either the hip or knee joints.

Recovery

Most femoral shaft fractures take four to six months to completely heal. Some take even longer, especially if the fracture was open or broken into several pieces.

Weightbearing

Many doctors encourage leg motion early in the recovery period. It is very important to follow your doctor's instructions for putting weight on your injured leg to avoid problems.

In some cases, doctors will allow patients to put as much weight as possible on the leg right after surgery. However, you may not be able to put full weight on your leg until the fracture has started to heal. It is very important to follow your doctor's instructions carefully.

When you begin walking, you will most likely need to use crutches or a walker for support.

Physical Therapy

Because you will most likely lose muscle strength in the injured area, exercises during the healing process are important. Physical therapy will help to restore normal muscle strength, joint motion, and flexibility.

A physical therapist will most likely begin teaching you specific exercises while you are still in the hospital. The therapist will also help you learn how to use crutches or a walker.

Complications

Complications from Femoral Shaft Fractures

Femoral shaft fractures can cause further injury and complications.

- The ends of broken bones are often sharp and can cut or tear surrounding blood vessels or nerves.

- Acute compartment syndrome may develop. This is a painful condition that occurs when pressure within the muscles builds to dangerous levels. This pressure can decrease blood flow, which prevents nourishment and oxygen from reaching nerve and muscle cells. Unless the pressure is relieved quickly, permanent disability may result. This is a surgical emergency. During the procedure, your surgeon makes incisions in your skin and the muscle coverings to relieve the pressure.

- Open fractures expose the bone to the outside environment. Even with good surgical cleaning of the bone and muscle, the bone can become infected. Bone infection is difficult to treat and often requires multiple surgeries and long-term antibiotics.

Complications from Surgery

In addition to the risks of surgery in general, such as blood loss or problems related to anesthesia, complications of surgery may include:

- infection;

- injury to nerves and blood vessels;

- blood clots;

- fat embolism (bone marrow enters the blood stream and can travel to the lungs; this can also happen from the fracture itself without surgery);

- malalignment or the inability to correctly position the broken bone fragments;

- delayed union or nonunion (when the fracture heals slower than usual or not at all);

- hardware irritation (sometimes the end of the nail or the screw can irritate the overlying muscles and tendons).

Section 37.3

Quadriceps Tendon Rupture

A quadriceps tendon rupture occurs relatively infrequently and usually occurs in athletes older than 40 years. Injuries to the quadriceps tendon can be very disabling. They can cause significant loss of time from sport and work.

If not treated appropriately, these injuries can have many negative long-term sequelae; however, if diagnosed quickly and treated appropriately, one can expect a full recovery from a quadriceps tendon rupture.

What is the quadriceps tendon and why is it important?

The quadriceps tendon is the strong tendon that inserts on the top of the patella (knee cap). The quadriceps tendon is a confluence (coming together) of the four muscles that make up the muscles that extend the knee. These four muscles are: vastus medialis, vastus intermedius, vastus lateralis, and rectus femoris. These muscles are the strong muscle on the anterior (front) side of the femur (thigh bone). Their main action is to extend the knee and leg. All four of these muscles come together just above the patella and form a strong, thick tendon.

The quadriceps tendon is important because it allows the knee to be extended. If the quadriceps tendon is injured then the patient will not be able to extend their knee.

How does one suffer quadriceps tendon rupture?

The quadriceps tendon is injured most commonly from a forced eccentric contraction (contracting while lengthening) against an outside force. This can happen during high-energy accidents such as motor vehicle crashes and during sporting activities, or during low-energy injuries such as falls from a standing position.

What are some risk factors for a quadriceps tendon rupture?

Really there are very few risk factors. Most quadriceps tendon ruptures are the result of either direct or indirect trauma. There are some medical problems that can increase a person's chance of having a quadriceps tendon rupture including renal (kidney) disease, rheumatoid arthritis, chronic steroid use, and diabetes mellitus. However, even in patients with these disorders, the incidence of quadriceps tendon ruptures is still very low.

What are the signs and symptoms of a quadriceps tendon rupture?

Most people with a quadriceps tendon rupture will note the acute onset of pain and disability in the affected leg. Usually this is precipitated by a fall or other traumatic event. The pain will be located at the level of the knee or just above the knee joint. The patient with a complete rupture is unable to do a straight leg raise or extend their knee. These patients will have a difficult time walking on the affected leg.

On physical examination the patient will be acutely tender to palpation directly above the patella. There is oftentimes a palpable defect in this area when compared to the contralateral side (uninjured knee). The knee will have a large effusion (swelling in the knee). The patient will be unable to extend their knee. Some patients with a partial tear may still be able to extend their knee, but will have significant weakness when compared to the other leg.

What imaging studies are needed for a quadriceps tendon rupture?

Initially a patient who presents with pain and swelling in the knee should undergo plain radiographs (X-rays) of the affected knee. This will help to rule out a fracture as the cause of the problem. If these are negative, then a MRI [magnetic resonance imaging] scan can be obtained to evaluate the integrity of the quadriceps tendon.

The X-rays of a patient with a quadriceps tendon rupture may show patellar baja (a knee cap that is lower than normal). There may also be a small piece of bone that is torn off of the patella with the tendon that can be visualized on X-ray. The gold standard for diagnosis would be a MRI scan of the knee, which would evaluate all of the soft tissue structures in the knee including all of the cartilage and ligaments. This would also help to distinguish between a complete and partial tear.

What are some other injuries that can mimic a quadriceps tendon rupture?

There are many injuries to consider when a patient may have a quadriceps tendon rupture. These include: patellar (knee cap) fracture, patellar tendon rupture, fracture of the end of the femur (thigh bone) or top of the tibia (shin bone), ACL tear, and patellar dislocation. The diagnosis is confirmed by doing an appropriate physical examination and also through imaging studies.

What are the different types of quadriceps tendon ruptures and how are they treated?

Quadriceps tendon ruptures come in two main types: partial and complete tears. Distinguishing between the two is very important, as the treatment is vastly different.

Partial tears can sometimes be treated non-operatively. In order for a partial tear to be treated without surgery, the patient must be able to do a straight-leg raise and have good strength with this physical exam finding. If this is the case, treatment should commence immediately with immobilization of the leg in full extension (out straight) for a short period of time. Then range of motion exercises are started at between 3 to 6 weeks from the injury. After 6 weeks, quadriceps strengthening is begun. Typically, after 10 to 12 weeks the injury has healed. The patient may resume normal activities after they have full range of motion and quadriceps strength. This can be anywhere from 3 to 6 months after the injury. Return to sport is governed by the ability to pass functional tests specific to the sport (example: jumping for a basketball player).

Complete tears, as well as partial tears when the patient is unable to perform a straight-leg raise, are always treated with surgery. Without surgery, the patient will be unable to extend their knee and have significant long-term disability. Surgery is typically recommended within a few days to a week after the injury. If the patient's other medical problems prohibit the opportunity to perform the surgery safely in the first week, it can be delayed until the patient is medically fit for surgery.

What does the surgery involve for repair of a quadriceps tendon rupture?

Typically surgery involves making an incision on the front of the knee. Then strong sutures are placed into the tendon and tied back down to the top of the patella. Surgery generally takes between one and two hours. The patient is then placed into a knee immobilizer keeping the knee straight after surgery.

What type of rehabilitation is needed after surgery?

After surgery, the patient will start with gentle passive range of motion with their physical therapist. The patient will be able to weight bear with all of their weight on their leg after a week or two but will have to wear the brace they received after surgery locked straight for the first six weeks, except when doing their therapy. By six weeks post-op, the patient should have 90 degrees of flexion (bending) of the knee. After six weeks, progressive strengthening is started as well as increasing range of motion. Typically, the brace is discontinued at eight weeks from surgery. Light running is generally started at four months from surgery. Return to sport is governed by the ability to perform sport specific exercises and having adequate range of motion and strength. This is generally between six to eight months from the day of surgery. It should be noted that rehabilitation protocols are often very specific to the type of injury and the type of repair that was achieved at the time of surgery. This protocol is just an outline of "typical" rehabilitation.

What if I do not seek treatment for my quadriceps tendon rupture right away?

When quadriceps tendon ruptures are not identified early, it can be more difficult to fix with surgical repair. The quadriceps muscle is very powerful, therefore the tendon retracts proximally (up the thigh) and becomes harder to fix back to the patella with surgery. Surgical repair is still possible but may require special techniques to do so and an extended rehabilitation protocol.

What is the long-term prognosis for a quadriceps tendon rupture?

Most people who undergo treatment of a quadriceps tendon rupture will do well long-term. They will be able to return to work and sport after the appropriate rehabilitation. It is important to be very diligent with the appropriate prescribed physical therapy to ensure a good outcome. Re-tear of the tendon after surgical repair is rare unless something unexpected happens (ex: a fall during the early postoperative phase). The most common complication is loss of motion in the knee after surgical repair.

If you suspect that you have a quadriceps tendon rupture, it is critical to seek the urgent consultation of a local sports injuries doctor for appropriate care.

References

Ilan D, Tejwani N, Keschner M and Liebman, M. Quadriceps Tendon Rupture. *Journal of the American Academy of Orthopaedic Surgeons.* 2003;11:192–200.

Rauh, M and Parker, R. Patellar and Quadriceps Tendinopathies and Ruptures. DeLee and Drez *Orthopaedic Sports Medicine: Principles and Practice.* 2010. Chapter 22 1513–1525.

Section 37.4

Hamstring Injuries

This section begins with "Hamstring Injuries" and continues with "Hamstring Injury Treatment," both reprinted with permission from St. Elizabeth Community Hospital (http://redbluff.mercy.org). © 2011 Catholic Healthcare West. All rights reserved.

What Is the Hamstring Muscle and How Does It Strain or Tear?

The hamstrings are a group of muscles at the back of your thigh. The function of the hamstrings is to allow the leg to extend or straighten at the hip and flex or bend at the knee. The hamstring muscles are paired with the quadriceps muscle in the front of the thigh to allow us to bend and straighten our leg. When you bend your leg, the hamstring muscle contracts and the quadriceps muscle relaxes. When you straighten your leg, the quadriceps muscle contracts and the hamstring muscle relaxes. It is extremely important that there is a balance between the muscle strength of the hamstring and quadriceps muscles.

The quadriceps muscle is generally more powerful than the hamstring muscle, which means that the hamstring muscle fatigues more quickly than the quadriceps muscle. This fatigue does not allow for a balance in the relaxation and contraction of the hamstring and quadriceps, which can lead to hamstring strains or tears. Hamstring strains in young adolescents often occur because of the different rate at which bones and muscles grow at this stage. During a growth spurt, the bones can grow faster than muscles. As the bone grows, it can create a tight pull on the muscle and during an activity that creates stress on the muscle, the hamstring can stretch or tear away from its connection to the bone. Muscle strains can also result from inadequate stretching. This can be a contributing factor of hamstring strains in anyone who does not take the time to warm up prior to activity or training.

Individuals who are susceptible to hamstring strains and tears are:

- dancers, cheerleaders, etc.;
- runners, sprinters;
- adolescent athletes who are going through a growth spurt;
- athletes: football, soccer, skating, running;
- anyone who engages in activity without adequate warm-up/ stretching.

Symptoms

- Sudden sharp pain at the back of the thigh during exercise, usually occurs during a high velocity movement
- Tightness in the back of the thigh
- Pain when flexing the knee against resistance
- Spasm of the hamstring
- Swelling, depending on severity
- Limp or impaired mobility, depending on severity
- Possible gap in the muscle, if there is a complete tear
- Bruising

Diagnosis

Your physician will take a detailed history and thorough clinical exam. In general, hamstring injuries are readily apparent.

Treatment

Hamstring strains are classified as Grade 1, 2, or 3.

Grade 1 Hamstring Strain

- Minor tear within the muscle
- Tightness in the back of the thigh
- Minimal discomfort while walking
- Possible swelling

Grade 2 Hamstring Strain

- Partial tear in the muscle
- Possible limp when walking
- Pressure increases pain
- Flexing knee against resistance causes pain
- Sudden twinges of pain during activity
- Range of motion may be impaired

Grade 3 Hamstring Strain or Tear

- Complete rupture of the hamstring muscle
- Impaired mobility; may need crutches initially
- Severe pain; particularly when trying to flex knee
- Swelling

Initial Treatment of All Hamstring Strains

- Rest your hamstring; avoid any stress on it through sports or activity. Use crutches if necessary for a severe strain.
- Apply ice to the hamstring over a thin layer of cloth for 20 minutes, two to three times a day for the first 48 hours following injury.
- Use a wrap such as an ACE bandage or compression type device to decrease swelling and provide support as the muscle heals.
- Elevate the affected extremity above the level of the heart with pillows for the first 48 hours when at rest.

Other Effective Methods of Treatment

- Non-steroidal, anti-inflammatory medications such as Advil or Aleve can decrease pain and swelling.

- Begin a stretching program as soon as the pain/swelling decrease.

- Start a strengthening program to rebuild the strength of the injured hamstring and prevent further recurrence.

- Possible referral to physical therapy.

Your physician will monitor your progress and evaluate when it is appropriate for you to return to full activity. Prevention of hamstring injuries: It is easier to prevent hamstring injuries than to recover from them. Stretching before and after an activity is the greatest way to prevent a hamstring strain or tear.

Chapter 38

Knee Injury Basics

What do the knees do? How do they work?

The knee is the joint where the bones of the upper leg meet the bones of the lower leg, allowing hinge-like movement while providing stability and strength to support the weight of the body. Flexibility, strength, and stability are needed for standing and for motions like walking, running, crouching, jumping, and turning.

Several kinds of supporting and moving parts, including bones, cartilage, muscles, ligaments, and tendons, help the knees do their job. Each of these structures is subject to disease and injury. Knee problems can interfere with many things, from participation in sports to simply getting up from a chair and walking.

What causes knee problems?

Disease: A number of diseases can affect the knee. The most common is arthritis. Although arthritis technically means "joint inflammation," the term is used loosely to describe many different diseases that can affect the joints.

Injury: Knee injuries can occur as the result of a direct blow or sudden movements that strain the knee beyond its normal range of motion. Sometimes knees are injured slowly over time. Problems with

This chapter excerpted from "Questions and Answers about Knee Problems," National Institute of Arthritis and Musculoskeletal and Skin Diseases (www.niams .nih.gov), May 2010.

the hips or feet, for example, can cause you to walk awkwardly, which throw off the alignment of the knees and lead to damage. Knee problems can also be the result of a lifetime of normal wear and tear.

What are the parts of the knee?

Bones and cartilage: The knee joint is the junction of three bones: the femur (thigh bone or upper leg bone), the tibia (shin bone or larger bone of the lower leg), and the patella (kneecap). The patella sits over the other bones at the front of the knee joint and slides when the knee moves. It protects the knee and gives leverage to muscles.

The ends of the three bones in the knee joint are covered with articular cartilage, a tough, elastic material that helps absorb shock and allows the knee joint to move smoothly. Separating the bones of the knee are pads of connective tissue called menisci. The two menisci in each knee act as shock absorbers, cushioning the lower part of the leg from the weight of the rest of the body as well as enhancing stability.

Muscles: There are two groups of muscles at the knee. The four quadriceps muscles on the front of the thigh work to straighten the knee from a bent position. The hamstring muscles, which run along the back of the thigh from the hip to just below the knee, help to bend the knee.

Tendons and ligaments: The quadriceps tendon connects the quadriceps muscle to the patella and provides the power to straighten the knee. The following four ligaments connect the femur and tibia and give the joint strength and stability:

- The medial collateral ligament, which runs along the inside of the knee joint, provides stability to the inner (medial) part of the knee.

- The lateral collateral ligament, which runs along the outside of the knee joint, provides stability to the outer (lateral) part of the knee.

- The anterior cruciate ligament, in the center of the knee, limits rotation and the forward movement of the tibia.

- The posterior cruciate ligament, also in the center of the knee, limits backward movement of the tibia.

How are knee problems diagnosed?

Medical history: During the medical history, the doctor asks how long symptoms have been present and what problems you are having using your knee. In addition, the doctor will ask about any injury, condition, or health problem that might be causing the problem.

Physical examination: The doctor bends, straightens, rotates (turns), or presses on the knee to feel for injury and to determine how well the knee moves and where the pain is located. The doctor may ask you to stand, walk, or squat to help assess the knee's function.

Diagnostic tests: Depending on the findings of the medical history and physical exam, the doctor may use one or more tests, including X-ray, computerized axial tomography (CT) scan, bone scan, magnetic resonance imaging (MRI), arthroscopy, joint aspiration, and biopsy, to determine the nature of a knee problem.

What are some common knee injuries and problems?

There are many diseases and types of injuries that can affect the knee. These are some of the most common.

Arthritis: There are some 100 different forms of arthritis, rheumatic diseases, and related conditions. Virtually all of them have the potential to affect the knees in some way; however, the following are the most common.

- **Osteoarthritis:** In this disease, the cartilage gradually wears away and changes occur in the adjacent bone. Osteoarthritis may be caused by joint injury or being overweight. It is associated with aging and most typically begins in people age 50 or older. A young person who develops osteoarthritis typically has had an injury to the knee or may have an inherited form of the disease.

- **Rheumatoid arthritis:** Rheumatoid arthritis, which generally affects people at a younger age, is an autoimmune disease. It occurs as a result of the immune system attacking components of the body. In rheumatoid arthritis, the primary site of the immune system's attack is the synovium, the membrane that lines the joint. This attack causes inflammation of the joint. It can lead to destruction of the cartilage and bone and, in some cases, muscles, tendons, and ligaments as well.

- **Other rheumatic diseases:** These include gout, systemic lupus erythematosus (lupus), ankylosing spondylitis, psoriatic arthritis, and infectious arthritis.

Chondromalacia: Chondromalacia, also called chondromalacia patellae, refers to softening of the articular cartilage of the kneecap. This disorder occurs most often in young adults and can be caused by injury, overuse, misalignment of the patella, or muscle weakness.

Instead of gliding smoothly across the lower end of the thigh bone, the kneecap rubs against it, thereby roughening the cartilage underneath the kneecap. The damage may range from a slightly abnormal surface of the cartilage to a surface that has been worn away to the bone. Chondromalacia related to injury occurs when a blow to the kneecap tears off either a small piece of cartilage or a large fragment containing a piece of bone (osteochondral fracture).

Meniscal injuries: The menisci can be easily injured by the force of rotating the knee while bearing weight. A partial or total tear may occur when a person quickly twists or rotates the upper leg while the foot stays still (for example, when dribbling a basketball around an opponent or turning to hit a tennis ball). If the tear is tiny, the meniscus stays connected to the front and back of the knee; if the tear is large, the meniscus may be left hanging by a thread of cartilage. The seriousness of a tear depends on its location and extent.

Cruciate ligament injuries: Cruciate ligament injuries are sometimes referred to as sprains. They don't necessarily cause pain, but they are disabling. The anterior cruciate ligament is most often stretched or torn (or both) by a sudden twisting motion (for example, when the feet are planted one way and the knees are turned another). The posterior cruciate ligament is most often injured by a direct impact, such as in an automobile accident or football tackle.

Medial and lateral collateral ligament injuries: The medial collateral ligament is more easily injured than the lateral collateral ligament. The cause of collateral ligament injuries is most often a blow to the outer side of the knee that stretches and tears the ligament on the inner side of the knee. Such blows frequently occur in contact sports such as football or hockey.

Tendon injuries: Knee tendon injuries range from tendonitis (inflammation of a tendon) to a ruptured (torn) tendon. If a person overuses a tendon during certain activities such as dancing, cycling, or running, the tendon stretches and becomes inflamed.

Iliotibial band syndrome: Iliotibial band syndrome is an inflammatory condition caused when a band of tissue rubs over the outer bone (lateral condyle) of the knee. Although it may be caused by direct injury to the knee, it is most often caused by the stress of long-term overuse, such as sometimes occurs in sports training and, particularly, in running.

Osteochondritis dissecans: Osteochondritis dissecans results from a loss of the blood supply to an area of bone underneath a joint surface. It usually involves the knee. The affected bone and its covering of cartilage gradually loosen and cause pain. This problem usually arises spontaneously in an active adolescent or young adult. A person with this condition may eventually develop osteoarthritis.

Plica syndrome: Plica syndrome occurs when plicae (bands of synovial tissue) are irritated by overuse or injury. Synovial plicae are the remains of tissue pouches found in the early stages of fetal development. As the fetus develops, these pouches normally combine to form one large synovial cavity. If this process is incomplete, plicae remain as four folds or bands of synovial tissue within the knee. Injury, chronic overuse, or inflammatory conditions are associated with this syndrome.

What kinds of doctors evaluate and treat knee problems?

After an examination by your primary care doctor, he or she may refer you to a rheumatologist, an orthopedic surgeon, or both. A rheumatologist specializes in nonsurgical treatment of arthritis and other rheumatic diseases. An orthopedic surgeon, or orthopedist, specializes in nonsurgical and surgical treatment of bones, joints, and soft tissues such as ligaments, tendons, and muscles.

You may also be referred to a physiatrist. Specializing in physical medicine and rehabilitation, physiatrists seek to restore optimal function to people with injuries to the muscles, bones, tissues, and nervous system.

How can people prevent knee problems?

Some knee problems, such as those resulting from an accident, cannot be foreseen or prevented. However, people can prevent many knee problems by following these suggestions:

- Before exercising or participating in sports, warm up by walking or riding a stationary bicycle, then do stretches. Stretching the muscles in the front of the thigh (quadriceps) and back of the thigh (hamstrings) reduces tension on the tendons and relieves pressure on the knee during activity.

- Strengthen the leg muscles by doing specific exercises (for example, by walking up stairs or hills or by riding a stationary bicycle). A supervised workout with weights is another way to strengthen the leg muscles that support the knee.

- Avoid sudden changes in the intensity of exercise. Increase the force or duration of activity gradually.

- Wear shoes that fit properly and are in good condition. This will help maintain balance and leg alignment when walking or running. Flat feet or over-pronated feet (feet that roll inward) can cause knee problems. People can often reduce some of these problems by wearing special shoe inserts (orthotics).

- Maintain a healthy weight to reduce stress on the knee. Obesity increases the risk of osteoarthritis of the knee.

Chapter 39

Knee Cartilage Injuries

Chapter Contents

Section 39.1

Patellofemoral Knee Pain
(Chondromalacia Patella)

What Is Patellofemoral Pain?

Pain around the front of the knee is often referred to as patellofemoral pain. This pain may be caused by soft cartilage under the kneecap (patella), referred pain from another area such as the back or hip, or soft tissues around the front of the knee.

In athletes, soft tissue pain in the retinaculum (tendon tissue) of the anterior (front of the knee) is fairly common. This may come from strain of the tendon—which connects the kneecap to the lower leg bone (patellar tendon), upper leg bone (quadriceps tendon), or the retinaculum (which supports the kneecap on both the left and right sides).

Some patellofemoral pain is caused because the kneecap is abnormally aligned. If the patella is not correctly aligned, it may come under excessive stress, particularly with vigorous activities. This can also cause excessive wear on the cartilage of the kneecap, which can result in chondromalacia (a condition in which the cartilage softens and may cause a painful sensation in the underlying bone or irritation of the synovium [joint lining]).

Treatment of Patellofemoral Pain

Treatment depends on the specific problem causing the pain. If the soft tissues (retinaculum, tendon, or muscle) are the source of the pain, stretching, particularly in the prone (face down) position, can be very helpful to make the support structures more resilient and flexible. One simple stretch is to lie prone, grab the ankle of the affected leg with one hand, and gently stretch the front of the knee. Hamstring stretching (rear thigh) can also be very helpful. It helps to warm up before doing these, or any other stretches.

Other treatments may involve exercises to build the quadriceps muscle, taping the patella, or using a specially designed brace which provides support specific to the problem. Using ice and non-steroidal anti-inflammatory medications can also be helpful. It is often necessary to temporarily modify physical activities until the pain decreases.

In more extreme situations, a specific surgical procedure may be needed to help relieve the pain. If the cartilage under the kneecap is fragmented and causing mechanical symptoms and swelling, arthroscopic removal of the fragments may be helpful. If the patella is badly aligned, however, a surgical procedure may be needed to place the kneecap back into proper alignment, thereby reducing abnormal pressures on the cartilage and supporting structures around the front of the knee.

In some people, particularly those who have had previous knee surgery, there may be a specific painful area in the soft tissue around the patella which may require resection (removal).

Controlling or Preventing Patellofemoral Pain

Good general conditioning is important. Stretching, particularly in the prone position, will keep the supporting structures around the front of the knee flexible and less likely to be irritated with exercise. Proper training, without sudden increases of stress to the front of the knee, will help avoid pain. Weight reduction and activity modification may be necessary in some people.

Section 39.2

Osteochondritis Dissecans of the Knee

An unusual cause of knee pain is that of osteochondritis dissecans (OCD). When present, OCD lesions usually become symptomatic during a child's development. The lesion, which has multiple etiologies, has as a final common pathway the loss of blood supply to a small portion of the bone. That bone becomes separated from the rest of the bone surrounding it, and the bone, with its cartilage cap, becomes loose. This can be thought of as a fragment within a crater. As the fragment becomes loose or breaks off, the symptoms escalate and direct patients to a physician's office for both diagnosis and treatment. OCD lesions most commonly occur on the medial condyle of the femur, although they can be seen both on the lateral side of the knee and within the patellofemoral joint.

Causes

Most OCD lesions occur for unknown reasons. Some believe that the lesion is genetically determined and occurs no matter what the activity level or age of the patient is. Other theories include repetitive trauma or specific trauma to the knee at a young, susceptible age. These types of injuries often go unnoticed when they occur and are recalled only after close questioning of a patient's past.

Symptoms

- Aching pain, not always made worse with activity
- Mild swelling
- Clicking and or locking as the piece becomes loose and as it becomes a free fragment

Treatment

Non-Operative

Treatment of OCD lesions is dictated by the extent of the lesion and the age of the patient at the time of diagnosis. Younger patients with minimal discomfort can be treated with rest and a period of non-weight bearing to allow the bony fragment to heal into its anatomic location.

Alternative Treatment Options

- Glucosamine

- Hyaluronic acid

- Non-steroidal anti-inflammatory medications (NSAIDs)

Operative

If the fragment is large and/or the patient is older, surgical treatment is often recommended. Surgical treatment is directed first at trying to save the fragment. If a large piece of bone is present, then use of a screw or pin can secure the fragment into its anatomic location and bony healing is allowed to occur. However, if the fragment is not large or if it is loose and displaced out of its normal site, then it is usually necessary to remove the fragment entirely and treat the defect as would be done in traumatically caused cases of a chondral (cartilage) defect.

Section 39.3

Meniscal Injuries

What is the meniscus?

The human meniscus is a wedge-shaped structure in the knee that consists of fibrocartilage, a very tough but pliable material. The medial meniscus is located on the inside of the knee (towards the middle of the body) and the lateral meniscus is located on the outside of the knee. Together, they act primarily as shock absorbers and stabilizers in the knee joint. They also help nourish the articular cartilage through their rich blood supply. This blood enhances the ability of the cartilage to repair itself.

How is the meniscus torn or injured?

In young athletes, most injuries to the meniscus are the result of trauma. The menisci are especially vulnerable to injuries in which there is both compression and twisting applied across the knee. It is also common for the meniscus to be damaged in association with injuries to the anterior cruciate ligament.

In older athletes, many meniscal tears are the result of trivial trauma, like twisting the knee, squatting, or through repetitive activities like running, which stress the knee joint. These tears happen because the meniscus has a tendency to degenerate as part of the aging process. This degeneration often takes place in conjunction with early arthritic changes in the knee joint.

How is a meniscal tear diagnosed?

When a meniscus is torn, it will often produce pain, swelling, and mechanical symptoms like catching, or locking, in the knee joint. An injury to the meniscus can be diagnosed based upon the history that the patient provides and a physical examination of the knee. The orthopaedic surgeon may also require further diagnostic studies like an MRI (magnetic resonance imaging) which provides a three-dimensional image of the interior of the knee joint. In some cases, surgeons may also recommend arthroscopic inspection of the knee joint, a minimally invasive surgical procedure.

How is a meniscal tear treated?

Certain patterns of injury, especially in younger patients, may call for repair of the meniscus. The decision to repair is based on many factors, including: location and pattern of the tear, age of the patient, and predictability of whether the injury will be able to heal.

Other patterns of tears, especially in older patients, are not suitable for repair. If the patient is symptomatic, and conservative treatment options like physical therapy are not working, surgery to remove the torn section is recommended. This surgery is called arthroscopic partial meniscectomy and is usually performed on an outpatient basis, typically in one hour or less.

Most patients ask, "What is the benefit of removing the meniscus? Isn't it an important structure in my knee?" Clearly, the meniscus does play an important role in the human knee, but once torn and unable to be repaired, many of the beneficial effects of that structure are lost. If a tear is causing pain and impaired function, removal of that tear is the treatment of choice.

Chapter 40

Knee Ligament Injuries

Chapter Contents

Section 40.1

Posterior Cruciate Ligament (PCL) Injury

© 2011 A.D.A.M., Inc. Reprinted with permission.

A posterior cruciate ligament injury is a partial or complete tearing or stretching of any part of the posterior cruciate ligament (PCL), which is located inside the knee joint.

Considerations

Your doctor will perform a physical examination to check for signs of PCL injury. This includes moving the knee joint in various ways.

Your doctor may also check for the presence of fluid in the knee joint. This test may show joint bleeding.

PCL injury may be seen using the following tests:

- Knee MRI [magnetic resonance imaging]
- Knee joint X-ray

Causes

The posterior cruciate ligament (PCL) is the strongest ligament in the knee. It extends from the top-rear surface of the tibia (bone between the knee and ankle) to the bottom-front surface of the femur (bone that extends from the pelvis to the knee).

The ligament prevents the knee joint from posterior instability. That means it prevents the tibia from moving too much and going behind the femur.

The PCL is usually injured by overextending the knee (hyperextension). This can happen if you land awkwardly after jumping. The PCL can also become injured from a direct blow to the flexed knee, such as smashing your knee in a car accident (called "dashboard knee") or falling hard on a bent knee.

Most PCL injuries occur with other ligament injuries and severe knee trauma. This injury usually occurs with a knee dislocation which has a high chance of nerve and vessel injuries. If you suspect PCL injury, it is important to be seen by a medical professional immediately.

Symptoms

- Knee swelling and tenderness in the space behind the knee (popliteal fossa)
- Knee joint instability
- Knee joint pain

First Aid

At first, a PCL injury is treated by:

- checking the pulse and circulation in the area;
- splinting;
- applying ice to the area;
- elevating the joint (above the level of the heart);
- taking nonsteroidal anti-inflammatory drugs (NSAIDs) for pain.

Limit physical activity until the swelling is down, motion is normal, and the pain is gone. Physical therapy can help you regain joint and leg strength. If the injury happens suddenly (acute) or you have a high activity level, you may need surgery. This may be either knee arthroscopy or "open" surgical reconstruction.

Age has an effect on treatment. Younger patients are more likely to have problems without surgery, because chronic instability may lead to arthritis symptoms many years later. Which patients need surgery is controversial, because many people seem to do well without surgery. Injuries in which the bone is pulled off with the ligament, or multiple ligaments are injured, need to be repaired with surgery.

PCL injuries are commonly associated with other ligament injuries or knee dislocation. It is important to have your knee examined for other injuries. Some of these injuries need to be treated urgently.

When to Contact a Medical Professional

Call your health care provider if:

- you have symptoms of PCL injury;
- you are being treated for PCL injury and you have greater instability in your knee;
- pain or swelling return after they went away;

- your injury does not appear to be getting better with time;

- you re-injure your knee;

- you have loss of sensation and decreased in circulation in your foot.

A lot of PCL injuries are associated with other ligament injuries or severe knee trauma. You should be checked early for these other conditions.

Prevention

Use proper techniques when playing sports or exercising. Many cases are not preventable.

Alternative Names

Cruciate ligament injury–posterior; PCL injury; Knee injury–posterior cruciate ligament (PCL); Hyperextended knee

References

Honkamp NJ, Ranawat AS, Harner CD. Knee: Posterior cruciate ligament injuries in the adult. In: DeLee JC, Drez D Jr, Miller MD, eds. *DeLee and Drez's Orthopaedic Sports Medicine*. 3rd ed. Philadelphia, Pa: Saunders Elsevier; 2009:chap 23, section E.

Honkamp NJ, Ranawat AS, Harner CD. Knee: Posterior cruciate ligament injuries in the child. In: DeLee JC, Drez D Jr, Miller MD, eds. *DeLee and Drez's Orthopaedic Sports Medicine*. 3rd ed. Philadelphia, Pa: Saunders Elsevier; 2009:chap 23, section E.

Section 40.2

Anterior Cruciate Ligament (ACL) Injury

Introduction

The anterior cruciate ligament (ACL) is one of the most commonly injured ligaments in the knee. Ligaments are strong non-elastic fibers that connect our bones together. The ACL crosses inside of the knee, connecting the thighbone to the leg. It provides stability to the knee joint.

ACL tears most commonly occur in very active people or athletes. The ACL can tear when people abruptly slow down from running, land from a jump, or change directions rapidly. These types of actions are frequently performed during sports, such as football, basketball, skiing, and soccer. Athletes are especially at risk for ACL tears, although they may occur in active workers and the general population as well.

The ACL can tear completely or partially. It is unable to repair itself. When the ACL is injured, it is common to see other surrounding knee structures damaged as well. Some cases of ACL tears are treated with non-surgical methods. However, there are several surgical options that successfully restore knee strength and stability.

Anatomy

The knee is structurally complex. Our knee is composed of three bones. The femur, or thighbone, sits on top of the tibia, the larger leg bone. The patella, or kneecap, glides in a groove on the end of the femur.

Large muscle groups in the thigh give the knee strength and stability. The quadriceps muscles are a large group of muscles on the front of our thigh that straighten and rotate the leg. The hamstring muscles are located on the back of the thigh and bend or flex the knee.

Four ligaments connect our knee bones together. The ligaments are strong tissues that provide stability and allow motion. The ligaments enable our knee to have the flexibility to move in various directions while maintaining balance. The medial collateral ligament is located on the inner side of our knee. The lateral collateral ligament is at the outer side of our knee. These two ligaments help the joint to resist side-to-side stress and maintain positioning.

The anterior cruciate ligament and the posterior cruciate ligament cross inside of the knee joint. These two ligaments help to keep the joint aligned. They counteract excessive forward and backward forces and prohibit displacement of the bones. They also produce and control rotation of the tibia. We rotate our tibia when we turn our leg outward to push off the ground with our foot. We use this motion to push off from the side when we skate, run, or move our body to get into a car.

Two cartilage disks, called menisci, are located on the end of the tibia. The cartilage forms a smooth surface and allows our bones to glide easily during motion. The menisci also act as shock absorbers when we walk or run.

A smooth tissue capsule covers the bones in our knee joint. A thin synovial membrane lines the capsule. The synovium secretes a thick liquid called synovial fluid. The synovial fluid acts as a cushion and lubricant between the joints, allowing us to perform smooth and pain-less motions.

Proprioceptive nerve fibers are contained in the ligaments and joint capsule. The proprioceptive nerve endings send signals about body movements and positioning. For instance, the proprioceptors in the knee send signals to let us know how far to bend our joint in order to place our foot for a step. They plan and coordinate our leg movements whenever we move.

Causes

The ACL can tear during strong twisting motions of the knee. The ACL can also tear if the knee is hyperextended or bent backwards. People frequently tear the ACL while pivoting, landing awkwardly from a jump, changing directions suddenly, or abruptly slowing down from running. ACL tears occur most frequently in young athletes. Football, basketball, skiing, and soccer are sports associated with the highest injury rates.

Researchers show that female athletes have a higher rate of ACL injury than males in certain sports. They suspect the greater angles in the female hip and leg alignment may make the knee more vul-nerable to force. Additionally, female hormones can relax ligaments and make them less stable, making some women more susceptible to knee injury.

It is common for additional injuries to result when an ACL tear occurs. Surrounding structures, such as the meniscus, cartilage, and ligaments, can be injured as well. Some people may also experience bruised or broken bones.

Symptoms

People usually experience pain, swelling, and knee instability immediately after the ACL tears. Your knee may buckle or give out on you. You may not be able to fully straighten your knee. You may have difficulty moving your knee and walking. Typically, within a few hours the swelling in the knee increases dramatically.

Diagnosis

If you suspect you have torn your ACL, you should go to your doctor or an emergency room right away. A doctor can evaluate your knee by gathering your medical history, performing a physical examination, and viewing medical images. Your doctor will ask you about your symptoms and what happened if you were injured. Your doctor will examine your knee and your leg alignment. You will be asked to perform simple movements to help your doctor assess your muscle strength, joint motion, and stability.

Doctors typically perform the Lachman test to determine if the ACL is intact. For this test, you will lie on your back and slightly bend your knees. Your doctor will place one hand on your thigh and attempt to pull your leg forward with the other hand. Your doctor will test both of your legs to compare the results. If you can move your leg three to five millimeters, the test is positive.

The pivot shift test is another test to determine if the ACL is functioning. For this test, you will straighten your leg. Your doctor will hold your leg while turning it and moving it toward your body. If your leg moves in and out of position, the test is positive for an ACL tear.

Your physician will order X-rays to see the condition of the bones in your knee and to identify fractures. Sometimes a fracture or soft tissue injury does not show up on an X-ray. In this case, your doctor may order a magnetic resonance imaging (MRI) scan. A MRI scan will provide a very detailed view of your knee structure. Like the X-ray, the MRI does not hurt and you need to remain very still while the images are taken.

Treatment

Initially following an injury, your knee will be treated with rest, ice, compression, and elevation. You should rest your knee by not placing weight on it. You may use crutches to help you walk. Applying ice packs to your knee can help reduce pain and swelling. You should apply ice immediately after injuring your knee. Your doctor will provide you with a continued icing schedule. Your doctor may provide over-the-counter or prescription pain medication. In some cases, a knee brace may be recommended to immobilize and support the knee. A knee immobilizer is used for only a short period of time. Elevating your knee at a level above your heart helps to reduce swelling.

Treatment for ACL tears is very individualized. Many factors need to be considered, such as your activity level, severity of injury, and degree of knee instability. Treatments may include physical therapy, surgery, or a combination of both. The most likely candidates for non-surgical treatments have partial ACL tears without knee instability, complete tears without knee instability, sedentary lifestyles or are willing to give up high-demand sports, or are children whose knees are still developing.

Physical therapy and rehabilitation can help restore knee functioning for some individuals. Your physical therapist will help you strengthen your knee. Special emphasis is placed on exercising the quadriceps muscles on the front of the thigh and the hamstring muscles on the back of the thigh. Eventually, you will learn exercises to improve your balance and coordination. You may need to wear a knee brace during activities. Your therapists will educate you on how to prevent further injury.

Editor's Note: A study published in the July 22, 2010, issue of the *New England Journal of Medicine* compared early surgery versus a "wait and see" strategy for young adults with acute ACL tears. It found no advantage to early surgery and that about 60% of patients did not require surgery at all after a course of physical therapy. While decisions on whether to perform surgery remain highly individualized, this study suggests that it may be reasonable for most patients with ACL tears to undergo physical therapy first, and only undergo surgery later if they have not improved. High-level athletes, however, generally have immediate surgery.

Surgery

Surgical treatment is most frequently recommended for individuals with ACL tears accompanied with other injuries. The most likely candidates for surgical treatment are active individuals in sports or jobs with heavy manual work that requires pivoting or pushing off with the knee. Surgery is also recommended for people with unstable knees or injuries combined with damage to the menisci, articular cartilage, joint capsule, or ligaments.

Prior to surgery, most people participate in physical therapy. Swelling can make the knee stiff. Immobility can cause the muscles and ligaments to shorten. Your physical therapist will help you stretch your knee to regain full movement. If your collateral ligaments are involved, you may need to wear a brace to allow them to heal prior to your surgery. These steps will help you prepare for a successful recovery after your surgery.

The goal of ACL repair is to reconstruct your knee joint to restore its function and stability, and prevent further injury. During surgery, your doctor will replace your damaged ACL with a healthy tendon, called a graft. There are several options for acquiring grafts. They may be taken from an area near your knee or from a donor cadaver.

A patellar tendon autograft uses the middle third of the patellar tendon and bone plugs from the shin and kneecap. This type of reconstruction is most often recommended for high-demand athletes and individuals that do not have to perform a lot of kneeling activities. This grafting procedure has been considered the "gold standard" for ACL repair.

A hamstring tendon autograft uses one or two tendons from the hamstring muscles at the inner side of the knee. The hamstring tendon autograft is most appropriate for lighter-weight individuals with a small patella bone and a history of pain. This method can be associated with a faster recovery.

A quadriceps tendon autograft uses the middle third of the quadriceps tendon and a bone plug from the upper end of the kneecap. The quadriceps graft is large. It is most appropriate for taller and heavier individuals. It is also used for individuals with prior failed ACL reconstructions. Because it is a large graft, this method uses a larger incision.

Allografts are tendon grafts taken from cadavers. Allografts are most appropriate for older individuals that are moderately active or those with a history of pain. It is also used for individuals with prior failed ACL reconstructions, those attempting to return to sports more quickly, and those that need more than one ligament reconstructed. Because the graft is not taken from the individual, this method is associated with less pain, smaller incisions, and a shorter surgery time.

Many ACL reconstructions are performed as outpatient procedures. You can be anesthetized for surgery or receive a nerve block to numb your knee and leg area. After you have received your anesthesia and your leg is relaxed, your doctor will examine your knee by performing similar tests that were done in your clinical examination. This provides your doctor with more information about your knee and helps to formulate the surgical plan.

Your surgeon will make one or more small incisions, about ¼" to ½" in length, near your joint. Your surgeon will fill the joint space with a sterile saline (salt-water) solution. Expansion of the space allows your surgeon to have a better view of your joint structures. Your surgeon will insert an arthroscope and will reposition it to see your joint from different angles.

An arthroscope is a very small surgical instrument. It is about the size of a pencil. An arthroscope contains a lens and lighting system that allows a surgeon to see inside of a joint. The surgeon only needs to make small incisions and the joint does not have to be opened up fully. The arthroscope is attached to a miniature camera. The camera allows the surgeon to view the magnified images on a video screen or take photographs and record videotape.

Your surgeon may make additional small incisions and use other slender surgical instruments if you are having your meniscus, cartilage, or ligaments repaired or removed. Your new graft will be attached using surgical hardware. Your surgeon will test the new graft and your knee function. Again, your doctor will examine your knee by performing similar muscle tests that were done in your clinical examination. This is to ensure that your knee is stable and has full range of motion. In addition to bandages, some surgeons apply a knee brace or a cold therapy device to help reduce swelling at the completion of your surgery.

Recovery

You will most likely go home on the same day of your surgery. You will receive pain medication to make you feel as comfortable as possible. In some cases, ice is applied to the knee throughout the day to help to reduce pain and swelling. Your doctor may prescribe blood thinning medication and special support stockings. You should keep your leg elevated and move or pump your foot and ankle. In some cases, doctors prescribe compression boots and a continuous passive motion (CPM) machine. Compression boots are inflatable leg coverings that are attached to a machine. They work to gently squeeze your legs to aid blood circulation. A CPM machine will move your leg in a cycling motion while you are in bed. The CPM machine is helpful to improve circulation, decrease swelling, and restore movement in your knee.

Walking and knee movements are very important to your recovery. Exercising will begin immediately after your surgery. You will begin physical therapy soon after your surgery. You first goals will include straightening your knee and strengthening your quadriceps muscles.

At first, you will need to use a walker or crutches while standing and walking. Your doctor may also prescribe a knee brace for you to wear during activities. Your physical therapist will help you walk and show you how to go up and down stairs. You will also learn ways to exercise to further strengthen your quadriceps and hamstring muscles and regain balance and coordination. It can take up to four to six months to restore proprioception and coordinated leg movements.

An occupational therapist can show you ways to dress and bathe within your movement restrictions. Your therapists can also recommend durable medical equipment for your home, such as a raised toilet seat or a shower chair. The equipment may make it easier for you to take care of yourself as you heal and help to prevent further injury.

The success of your surgery will depend, in part, on how well you follow your home care instructions and participate in exercise during the weeks following your ACL reconstruction. You may need a little help from another person during the first few days at home. If you do not have family members or a friend nearby, talk to your physician about possible alternative arrangements.

Recovery times differ depending on the severity of your injury, the type of procedure that you had, and your health at the time of your injury. Your doctor will let you know what to expect. Generally, you should be able to resume some of your regular activities in one to three weeks after your procedure and progress to full sporting activity in about six months. Overall, you should notice a steady improvement in your strength and endurance over the next 6 to 12 months. The majority of people are able to resume functional activities after ACL reconstruction.

Prevention

It is important that you adhere to your exercise program and safety precautions when you return home. You should stay as active as possible. It is especially important to keep your quadriceps and hamstrings very strong. You should also continue to use the durable medical equipment as advised.

It is also important to avoid injuring your ACL again. Depending on your injury, your surgeon may provide you with temporary or permanent activity or lifting restrictions. In some cases, specialized knee braces may be recommended for specific activities.

Section 40.3

Medial and Lateral Collateral Ligament Injuries

"Collateral Ligament Injuries," reproduced with permission from *Your Orthopaedic Connection*. © American Academy of Orthopaedic Surgeons (www.aaos.org), Rosemont, IL, 2007.

The knee is the largest joint in your body and one of the most complex. It is also vital to movement.

Your knee ligaments connect your thighbone to your lower leg bones. Knee ligament sprains or tears are a common sports injury.

Athletes who participate in direct contact sports like football or soccer are more likely to injure their collateral ligaments.

Anatomy

Three bones meet to form your knee joint: your thighbone (femur), shinbone (tibia), and kneecap (patella). Your kneecap sits in front of the joint to provide some protection.

Bones are connected to other bones by ligaments. There are four primary ligaments in your knee. They act like strong ropes to hold the bones together and keep your knee stable.

Cruciate Ligaments

These are found inside your knee joint. They cross each other to form an *X* with the anterior cruciate ligament in front and the posterior cruciate ligament in back. The cruciate ligaments control the back and forth motion of your knee.

Collateral Ligaments

These are found on the sides of your knee. The medial or "inside" collateral ligament (MCL) connects the femur to the tibia. The lateral or "outside" collateral ligament (LCL) connects the femur to the smaller bone in the lower leg (fibula). The collateral ligaments control the sideways motion of your knee and brace it against unusual movement.

Description

Because the knee joint relies just on these ligaments and surrounding muscles for stability, it is easily injured. Any direct contact to the knee or hard muscle contraction—such as changing direction rapidly while running—can injure a knee ligament.

Injured ligaments are considered "sprains" and are graded on a severity scale.

Grade 1 sprains: The ligament is mildly damaged in a grade 1 sprain. It has been slightly stretched, but is still able to help keep the knee joint stable.

Grade 2 sprains: A grade 2 sprain stretches the ligament to the point where it becomes loose. This is often referred to as a partial tear of the ligament.

Grade 3 sprains: This type of sprain is most commonly referred to as a complete tear of the ligament. The ligament has been split into two pieces, and the knee joint is unstable.

The MCL is injured more often than the LCL. Due to the more complex anatomy of the outside of the knee, if you injure your LCL, you usually injure other structures in the joint, as well.

Cause

Injuries to the collateral ligaments are usually caused by a force that pushes the knee sideways. These are often contact injuries, but not always.

Medial collateral ligament tears often occur as a result of a direct blow to the outside of the knee. This pushes the knee inwards (toward the other knee).

Blows to the inside of the knee that push the knee outwards may injure the lateral collateral ligament.

Symptoms

- Pain at the sides of your knee (if there is an MCL injury, the pain is on the inside of the knee; an LCL injury may cause pain on the outside of the knee)
- Swelling over the site of the injury
- Instability (the feeling that your knee is giving way)

Doctor Examination

Physical Examination and Patient History

During your first visit, your doctor will talk to you about your symptoms and medical history.

During the physical examination, your doctor will check all the structures of your injured knee, and compare them to your non-injured knee. Most ligament injuries can be diagnosed with a thorough physical examination of the knee.

Imaging Tests

Other tests which may help your doctor confirm your diagnosis include:

X-rays: Although they will not show any injury to your collateral ligaments, X-rays can show whether the injury is associated with a broken bone.

MRI: This study creates better images of soft tissues like the collateral ligaments.

Treatment

Injuries to the MCL rarely require surgery. If you have injured just your LCL, treatment is similar to an MCL sprain. But if your LCL injury involves other structures in your knee, your treatment will address those, as well.

Nonsurgical Treatment

Ice: Icing your injury is important in the healing process. The proper way to ice an injury is to use crushed ice directly to the injured area for 15 to 20 minutes at a time, with at least one hour between icing sessions. Chemical cold products ("blue" ice) should not be placed directly on the skin and are not as effective.

Bracing: Your knee must be protected from the same sideways force that caused the injury. You may need to change your daily activities to avoid risky movements. Your doctor may recommend a brace to protect the injured ligament from stress. To further protect your knee, you may be given crutches to keep you from putting weight on your leg.

Physical therapy: Your doctor may suggest strengthening exercises. Specific exercises will restore function to your knee and strengthen the leg muscles that support it.

Surgical Treatment

Most isolated collateral ligament injuries can be successfully treated without surgery. If the collateral ligament is torn in such a way that it cannot heal or is associated with other ligament injuries, your doctor may suggest surgery to repair it.

Return to Sports

Once your range of motion returns and you can walk without a limp, your doctor may allow functional progression. This is a gradual, progressive return to sports activities.

For example, if you play soccer, your functional progression may start as a light jog. Then you progress to a sprint, and eventually to full running and kicking the ball.

Your doctor may suggest a knee brace during sports activities, depending on the severity of your sprain.

Chapter 41

Patella and Patellar Tendon Injuries

Chapter Contents

Section 41.1

Patellar Tendon Ruptures

The patellar tendon attaches to the tibial tubercle on the front of the tibia (shin bone) just below the front of the knee. It also is attached to the bottom of the patella (kneecap). At the top of the patella, the quadriceps tendon is attached. At the top of the quadriceps tendon is the quadriceps muscle. The quadriceps muscle is the large muscle on the front of the thigh. As the quadriceps muscle contracts (shortens), it pulls on the quadriceps tendon, the patella, the patellar tendon, and the tibia to move the knee from a flexed (bent) position to an extended (straight) position. Conversely, when the quadriceps muscle relaxes, it lengthens. This allows the knee to move from a position of extension (straight) to a position of flexion (bent).

Injury

When the patellar tendon ruptures, the patella loses its anchoring support to the tibia. Without this anchoring effect of the intact patella tendon, the patella tends to move superiorly (towards the hip) as the quadriceps muscle contracts. Without the intact patella tendon, the patient is unable to straighten the knee. If a rupture of the patella tendon occurs, and the patient tries to stand up, the knee will usually buckle and give way because the body is no longer able to hold the knee in a position of extension (straight).

Diagnosis

The examination consists of palpating the patellar tendon and the patella. Usually, when the tendon ruptures, the patella moves upwards on the thigh. At the same time, the hole between the ends of the ruptured tendon is palpable on the front of the knee. X-rays of the knee reveal the abnormal position of the patella, indicating a rupture of the patella tendon.

When X-rays are taken, the patella (kneecap) is seen to move away from the knee and towards the mid thigh when compared to a normal knee X-ray.

Treatment

This is an injury that must be treated surgically. Since the tendon is outside of the joint, it cannot be repaired arthroscopically. Usually, the repair is done as an outpatient or overnight stay.

An incision is made on the front of the knee, overlaying the tendon. The site of the tendon rupture is identified.

The tendon ends are retracted to allow inspection of the underlying joint and femur.

The tendon ends are identified and then sewn together. Afterwards, a cast or brace is often used to protect the repair. The length of time required for casting or bracing is usually a minimum of six weeks followed by several weeks of rehabilitation.

Problems

The usual risks of surgery are involved including: infection, stiffness, suture reaction, failure of satisfactory healing, risks of anesthesia, phlebitis, pulmonary embolus (blood clot in the lungs), and persistent pain or weakness after the injury and repair.

Section 41.2

Patellar Tendonitis

Jumper's knee—also known as patellar tendonitis or patellar tendinopathy—is an inflammation or injury of the patellar tendon, the cord-like tissue that joins the patella (kneecap) to the tibia (shin bone). Jumper's knee is an overuse injury (when repeated movements cause tissue damage or irritation to a particular area of the body).

Constant jumping, landing, and changing direction can cause strains, tears, and damage to the patellar tendon. So athletes who regularly play sports that involve a lot of repetitive jumping—like track and field (particularly high-jumping), basketball, volleyball, gymnastics, running, and soccer—can put a lot of strain on their knees.

Jumper's knee can seem like a minor injury that isn't really that serious. Because of this, many athletes keep training and competing and tend to ignore the injury or attempt to treat it themselves. But it's important to know that jumper's knee is a serious condition that can get worse over time and ultimately require surgery. Early medical attention and treatment can help prevent continued damage to the knee.

How the Knee Works

To understand how jumper's knee happens, it helps to understand how the knee works. The knee, which is the largest joint in the body, provides stability to the leg and allows it to bend, swivel, and straighten. Several parts of the body interact to allow the knee to function properly:

- Bones like the femur (thighbone), the tibia (shinbone), and the patella (kneecap) give the knee the strength needed to support the weight of the body. The bones that meet at the knee allow it to bend smoothly.

- Muscles provide the tug on the bones needed to bend, straighten, and support joints. The muscles around the knee include the quadriceps (at the front of the thigh) and the hamstring (on the back of the thigh). The quadriceps muscle helps straighten and extend the leg, and the hamstring helps bend the knee.

- Tendons are strong bands of tissue that connect muscles to bones. The tendons in the front of the knee are the quadriceps tendon and the patellar tendon. The quadriceps tendon connects to the top of the patella and allows the leg to extend. The patellar tendon connects to the bottom of the kneecap and attaches to the top of the tibia.

- Similar to tendons, ligaments are strong bands of tissue that connect bones to other bones.

By working together, bones, muscles, tendons, and ligaments enable the knee to move, bend, straighten, provide strength to jump, and stabilize the leg for landing.

About Jumper's Knee

When the knee is extended, the quadriceps muscle pulls on the quadriceps tendon, which in turn pulls on the patella. Then, the patella pulls on the patellar tendon and the tibia and allows the knee to straighten. In contrast, when bending the knee, the hamstring muscle pulls on the tibia, which causes the knee to flex.

In jumper's knee, the patellar tendon is damaged. Since this tendon is crucial to straightening the knee, damage to it causes the patella to lose any support or anchoring. This causes pain and weakness in the knee, and leads to difficulty in straightening the leg.

Symptoms

Common symptoms of jumper's knee include:

- pain directly over the patellar tendon (or more specifically, below the kneecap);

- stiffness of the knee, particularly while jumping, kneeling, squatting, sitting, or climbing stairs;

- pain when bending the knee;

- pain in the quadriceps muscle;

- leg or calf weakness.

417

Less common symptoms include:

- balance problems;

- warmth, tenderness, or swelling around the lower knee.

Treatment

Jumper's knee is first evaluated by a grading system that measures the extent of the injury (grades range from 1 to 5, with grade 1 being pain only after intense activity and grade 5 being daily constant pain and the inability to participate in any sporting activities).

While examining the knee, a doctor or medical professional will ask the patient to run, jump, kneel, or squat to determine the level of pain. In addition, an X-ray or MRI [magnetic resonance imaging] might be recommended. Depending on the grade of the injury, treatment can range from rest and icepacks to surgery.

For mild to moderate jumper's knee, treatment includes:

- resting from activity or adapting a training regimen that greatly reduces any jumping or impact;

- icing the knee to reduce pain and inflammation;

- wearing a knee support or strap (called an intrapatellar strap or a Chopat strap) to help support the knee and patella; the strap is worn over the patellar tendon, just beneath the kneecap (a knee support or strap can help minimize pain and relieve strain on the patellar tendon);

- elevating the knee when it hurts (for example, placing a pillow under the leg);

- anti-inflammatory medications, like ibuprofen, to minimize pain and swelling;

- massage therapy;

- minimum-impact exercises to help strengthen the knee;

- rehabilitation programs that include muscle strengthening, concentrating on weight-bearing muscle groups like the quadriceps and calf muscles;

- specialized injections to desensitize nerve endings and reduce inflammation.

On rare occasions, such as when there's persistent pain or the patellar tendon is seriously damaged, jumper's knee requires surgery.

Surgery includes removing the damaged portion of the patellar tendon, removing inflammatory tissue from the lower area (or bottom pole) of the patella, or making small cuts on the sides of the patellar tendon to relieve pressure from the middle area.

After surgery, a rehabilitation program involving strengthening exercises and massage is followed for several months to a year.

Recovery

Recovering from jumper's knee can take a few weeks to several months. It's best to stay away from any sport or activity that can aggravate the knee and make conditions worse.

However, recovering from jumper's knee doesn't mean that someone can't participate in any sports or activities. Depending on the extent of the injury, low-impact sports or activities can be substituted (for instance, substituting swimming for running). Your doctor will let you know what sports and activities are off-limits during the healing process.

Preventing Jumper's Knee

The most important factor in preventing jumper's knee is stretching. A good warm-up regimen that involves stretching the quadriceps, hamstring, and calf muscles can help prevent jumper's knee. It's always a good idea to stretch after exercising, too.

Section 41.3

Dislocated Patella

"Patella Dislocations," by David Edell, MEd, ATC, LAT, CSCS.
© 2010 David Edell. Reprinted with permission from
www.AthleticAdvisor.com.

The patella (knee cap) is a sesamoid bone. A sesamoid bone is one that is encased in tendon or ligament. The patella is located inside the quadriceps tendon. The patella acts as a fulcrum to increase the strength of the quad muscle. It is held in place by the quadriceps tendon above, the patellar tendon below, and very thin ligaments on either side. The patellofemoral joint is formed by the patella and trochlear groove of the femur.

Due to the twisting nature of sports, the patella can dislocate (come out of joint) with an awkward twist of the femur (thigh) on the tibia (shin). A twisting motion causes the patella to shift to the side. Usually, the patella moves laterally (to the outside). This occurs because the quadriceps muscle contracts to maintain the stability of the body. The shin has shifted so that the line of pull of the quads causes the patella to shift laterally. The patella is pulled laterally because it wants to remain in line with the muscle.

The patella can dislocate more easily in some people than others. Individuals with a greater "Q-angle" are at a greater risk for patellar dislocations. The "Q-angle" is formed by envisioning a circle around the patella, the line of pull of the quad muscle forms the tail of the "Q." If the tail of the "Q" is more than 25 degrees off of the center of the quad-patella-patellar tendon line of pull, it is considered an abnormally high "Q-angle."

This places the patella at a greater risk to slide off of the femur. The quad-patella-patellar tendon mechanism wants to form a straight line when the quad muscle contracts; due to this, the patella is pulled laterally. This places a person with a high "Q-angle" at a greater risk for patellar dislocations.

Another risk factor for patellar dislocations is a malformed patella or trochlear groove (the groove located between the two heads of the femur). The back side of the patella should have a peak, like an inverted mountain top. The trochlear groove should look like the valley between mountains. If either the mountain or the groove are not large enough, the patella is more prone to dislocate.

Females seem to have a greater risk for patellar dislocations than males. This may be due, in part, to the shape of their hips. A female's hips are shallower and wider to accommodate pregnancy. This tends to cause genu valgum ("knock-kneed" appearance); in other words, their knees are closer together than their ankles. This can result in a greater "Q-angle," thus making patellar dislocations more probable.

Patella alta (the patella rides too high in the trochlear groove) is also another predicting factor for patellar dislocations. If the patella rides too high in the trochlear groove, it may be prone to dislocating more easily. Often this is present on both knees, so comparing one to the other may not make this symptom easy to find. Most often, this is seen on X-ray by a physician.

If an athlete suffers a patella dislocation that does not spontaneously reduce (go back into place), it is rather obvious to detect. The patella will be lying near the outside of the knee joint. However, it is quite common for the patella to spontaneously reduce. Many times the athlete will straighten his/her leg inadvertently after the injury, causing the patella to reduce.

If the patella has been reduced, the athlete will present with increased pain, swelling, and a decrease in range of motion of the knee. The swelling may be great enough as to make the patella "disappear." Due to the swelling, the patella may also feel, when pressed straight down, as if it is a boat floating in water.

The swelling is due to tearing of the ligaments on the medial side of the patella. This swelling is located inside of the joint, accounting for the patella feeling like a floating boat. Since this injury usually results from a twist, and the swelling is located inside of the joint, an orthopaedic surgeon should be consulted to differentiate between a dislocated patella and an ACL tear.

An apprehension test is used to determine if a patellar dislocation has occurred. The athletic trainer or physician will push the patella laterally (outside); if this elicits pain or apprehension, it is a positive test.

Any athlete who suffers a dislocated patella should consult with an orthopaedic surgeon for X-rays, protective bracing, and appropriate rehabilitation. X-rays are necessary to rule out a fracture of the patella. In some cases the mountain peak of the patella will be "knocked off" when it impacts with the femur. This piece of bone can cause severe damage to the joint if it is not properly addressed.

Appropriate rehabilitation should concentrate on pain control, swelling reduction, return of full range of motion, and return to normal strength.

The vastus medialis muscle should be targeted during the rehabilitation. This muscle helps to place a medial pull on the patella, reducing the lateral, dislocating force. This is especially important in those individuals with a high "Q-angle" or genu valgum.

Surgery is not indicated unless dislocations are recurrent. The surgical interventions center around correcting improper alignment. They are often viewed as "salvage" or "last resort" procedures.

Chapter 42

Other Overuse Knee Injuries

Chapter Contents

Section 42.1

Iliotibial (IT) Band Friction Syndrome

What Is Iliotibial Band Syndrome?

Iliotibial band syndrome (ITBS) is the most common cause of knee
pain in runners, by some estimates accounting for 12% of all running-
related injuries. While ITBS is most prevalent in runners, it can potentially happen to any athlete who runs in the course of their sport.
Although ITBS is not as common in cyclists, it does occur, and at the
very least the multi-sport athlete who develops it with running may
continue to aggravate it on the bike. ITBS is commonly labeled as an
"overuse" injury. However, this is really a misnomer, as it is generally
not the fact that the knee is being used too much but rather that there
are predisposing biomechanical factors causing injury with even appropriate levels of training.

The iliotibial band (IT band) is essentially a long tendon, connecting
the hip abductor muscles (tensor fascia latae [TFL] and the gluteus
minimus, medius, and portions of the maximus) to the outer part of the
knee. ITBS occurs when the IT band is excessively tight and frictions
against the outside edge of the knee joint (lateral tibial or femoral
condyle.) With continued use over time, the IT band becomes inflamed,
painful, and eventually develops adhesions (scar tissue).

The pain is typically most pronounced when running, especially when
going downhill. Often for a given individual the pain will begin at a
certain distance or time from one run to the next (e.g., consistently after
30 minutes of running). During a run the pain is classically felt on the
outside of the knee about one inch above the crease. However, pain can
be felt anywhere on the outside of the hip down to the knee and still
technically be called ITBS. Rest almost always helps but is frequently
only temporary; when training resumes the pain will often return.

ITBS usually responds well to appropriate conservative (non-surgical) treatment. However, if the condition is not treated and the athlete were to allow it to progress, ITBS can become more disabling with time and require further intervention such as cortisone injections or in extreme cases even surgery.

What Causes ITBS?

ITBS sometimes relates to ergonomic issues in running or biking. This can include, for example, prolonged running on cantered surfaces such as the side of the road (the left leg is usually affected when running against traffic). Running on a track consistently in the same direction creates asymmetrical forces in the lower extremities, so excessive track training can be an issue. On the bike, two common issues are riding in clipless pedals that force the foot to toe-in (more of a problem with older-style pedals that don't float) and/or an improper seat height.

In the absence of (or in addition to) ergonomics, ITBS most often originates with biomechanical problems above the knee in the hip and/or below in the foot. In terms of the hip, in almost all cases of ITBS the tightness of the IT band stems from shortening of the hip abductor muscles. Again, the IT band itself is the collective tendon of these muscles. In recently developed cases of ITBS it is not uncommon to find that the IT band itself isn't particularly tight, but rather is being tensioned by the shortened hip abductors and has become inflamed. This point is relevant in treatment as soft-tissue measures such as stretching and foam rolling directed solely at the IT band (but not including the hip abductors) will often fail to fully resolve the problem. It is not uncommon for athletes to train through this injury for years with locally directed measures without ever being able to fully overcome the pain.

In these more chronic cases the IT band itself becomes shortened and additionally accumulates adhesions (scar tissue.) Self-managing (or ignoring) ITBS without true resolution leads to repeated cycles of inflammation in the body's attempts to heal. Anytime there is long-standing inflammation in the musculoskeletal system adhesion formation occurs. In ITBS this tends to be most pronounced in the lower third of the tendon and especially where the tendon frictions at the knee. Frequently the IT band adheres to the adjacent lateral portions of either the quadriceps (vastus lateralus) or hamstrings (biceps femoris).

Sometimes ITBS is straightforward: the hip abductors and IT band are tight, and stretching and releasing these tissues resolves the problem. This might be true for instance in a runner who participates in other sports that develop strong but tight musculature, such as rock climbing. However, in the vast majority of cases of ITBS severe enough to require treatment, there is an underlying weakness of the gluteus medius which precipitates tightening of the abductors. (In fact it is uncommon to find hip abductors tight enough to cause ITBS without gluteus medius weakness.) The hip abductors stabilize the pelvis during the stance phase of gait (when the foot contacts the ground), with the gluteus medius providing the bulk of that support. When the gluteus medius is weak, it essentially over-works with otherwise appropriate levels of training and over time tends to shorten. Often the two other smaller hip abductors (the TFL and gluteus minimus) attempt to over-compensate and also tighten.

As previously stated, IT band tightness often stems from hip abductor tightness. Because a weak gluteus medius equals tight hip abductors, it can be said that gluteus medius weakness is the underlying cause of most cases of ITBS. Since gluteus medius strength is such an integral part of the prevention and treatment of most cases of ITBS, it is important to investigate why the muscle is weak in the first place.

Of course in some cases the hips and other supporting muscles are just plain weak. Running in and of itself doesn't necessarily strengthen the gluteal muscles, particularly with the common form deficiencies evidenced by many athletes (i.e., heel-striking, poor pelvic/core control, excessive forward-leaning at the waist). Therefore, a runner with poor form, who does no other specific cross-training, and especially one who has an occupation where they sit for long periods, is likely to have weak gluteals in general. This type of athlete may experience chronic low-grade IT band tightness on both sides, but often not to the degree that they seek professional help. Most cases of ITBS pronounced enough to require treatment are unilateral and most of these athletes will have an obvious discrepancy in gluteus medius strength with the affected side being weaker.

Expanding the biomechanical picture further, most individuals with a unilaterally weak gluteus medius have other issues further down the kinetic chain in the foot/ankle. During gait the gluteus medius receives its signal to fire from nerve endings in the foot as that side is hitting the ground. If there are biomechanical issues in the foot/ankle complex interfering with this signal, the gluteus medius may not be engaging fully, and over time becomes weak. Problems in the foot can stem from such things as prior injuries (i.e., ankle sprains), leg-length discrepancies, or improper footwear. ITBS sufferers who otherwise have good running form and adequate hip and core strength will invariably have an issue in the foot/ankle weakening the gluteus medius, leading to tightness of the hip abductors and subsequent affecting the IT band.

Another way in which the lower extremity can factor into ITBS is when the foot/ankle isn't strong enough to support the body during gait. This tends to lead to excessive rolling in of the ankle, or over-pronation. The tibia sits on top of the ankle, so when the ankle over-pronates the tibia follows. This inward rotation pulls the lateral tibial condyle into position to friction the IT band. It is less common for over-pronation to cause ITBS in and of itself, but is frequently a contributing factor, and can overlap with the other causative factors. For example, someone with residual ankle weakness after a past injury may over-pronate on that side in addition to having a weak gluteus medius and tight hip abductors. In this case the over-pronation will hamper full recovery unless addressed.

Treatment

While diagnosing ITBS isn't difficult it is important to obtain an understanding of the entire biomechanical picture, and not just direct treatment to where it hurts. Evaluation might include hands-on palpation, gait analysis, movement screens, and/or muscle testing to reveal what's weak and what's tight. Determination is made as to which portions of the hip abductor and IT band are affected, the degree to which adhesions are present, and also to what extent the surrounding musculature is involved. Examination of the relevant joints helps to uncover joint dysfunction along the kinetic chain.

Once an overall picture is obtained, treating ITBS would usually include elements of the following:

1. **Acute care measures to reduce inflammation:** Icing applied locally reduces inflammation and should be done after training that aggravates the pain. Non-steroidal anti-inflammatory drugs like ibuprofen can be taken, although using them to mask pain to allow further training is not a good idea.

2. **Training modification:** Rest almost always helps, although depending on the severity of the condition, an athlete may not need to cease training altogether. The biggest effect will be on running and can range from a slight decrease in miles and intensity to complete cessation for an appropriate period. Athletes who can continue to run will often find symptoms begin at a certain time or distance, for example consistently after around 40 minutes of running. In this case the injury might allow for running up to 30–35 minutes as often as every other day (but this should be discussed with the treating provider).

When running, any downhill sections encountered should be walked. Taping, such as McConnell and Kinesio taping, and/or IT band supports might help to reduce pain when running, although these should be viewed as temporary adjuncts and not a stand-alone treatment. Pool running is generally pain-free and can maintain fitness for the dedicated runner. Cycling and elliptical machines are other means of training, provided they don't increase pain levels.

Cycling usually won't aggravate ITBS, and if it does there are modifications available to possibly allow for unaltered training. For example, spacers can be inserted between the pedal and the crank, which effectively puts the tibia in external rotation. Fortunately for triathletes, swimming generally doesn't affect ITBS, so training in the pool may continue. Overall the earlier in the process treatment is sought, the less training will be affected.

3. **Increasing flexibility of the tight tissue:** Any number of soft-tissue release techniques can be helpful. Active Release Technique® (A.R.T.) is particularly effective at lengthening the shortened hip abductors and IT band. Instrument assisted soft-tissue modalities such as Graston Technique work well in locating and removing adhesions, especially along the lower portion of the IT band. Home stretching exercises will also typically be given. In addition, the same factors that lead to ITBS will also frequently cause other issues, including tight hip flexors and adductors and pelvic and lower back joint dysfunction. These may need to be addressed as well with further soft-tissue work, stretching, and joint manipulation/mobilization.

4. **Strengthening the weak supporting muscles:** For those with an identified gluteus medius weakness, building strength is key. It is important to utilize exercises that isolate this muscle; likely the body has adapted to over-compensate with other muscles and needs to be retrained to make sure the gluteus medius is engaging. Since core strength is also integral in stabilizing the pelvis during gait, core muscles weakness should be screened for and addressed as well. Squats and lunges should be minimized or avoided during the early stages of treatment as the mechanics are very similar to running. An athlete with a unilaterally weak gluteus medius performing a more complicated motion such as a one-legged squat will likely just continue to use their same faulty mechanics and

perpetuate inflammation. Taking time in the beginning to rebuild gluteus medius strength and then progressing to multi-joint exercises that engage the entire kinetic chain is generally a good strategy.

Prevention of ITBS

Of course, prevention is the best medicine. As discussed, gluteus medius and core muscle weakness is a common finding with ITBS (and in fact can be implicated in many other low back, hip, and knee issues as well.) Therefore a consistent gluteal- and core-strengthening program can be considered mandatory for any athlete.

Stretching and foam rolling are also important self-maintenance tools. It should be noted, however, that an individual without major biomechanical issues, good running form, and adequate hip and core strength should not be developing noticeable IT band tightness. An athlete feeling the continued need to stretch the IT bands usually indicates problems elsewhere. At the very least a stretching routine should include the hip abductors as well as the IT band itself. An athlete with ongoing tightness in one IT band likely has an underlying biomechanical issue affecting that side such as ankle weakness or a leg length discrepancy.

It is worth investing some time into running form, especially if this hasn't been addressed. The most common form flaw is heel-striking, which accentuates pronation and allows more jarring forces to translate up through the leg. Heel-striking is usually the result of over-striding: allowing the foot to land too far out in front of the center of gravity. A quick cadence or turnover helps to minimize over-striding. (While beyond the scope of this section, there is a growing awareness of the importance of good form and a large body of information on this topic available in books and websites.) Note that making changes to running form takes time and practice. An individual with an established case of ITBS might not be advised to make changes until their injury is less acute. On the other hand, a recently returned runner who was totally out of commission for an extended period may find this an ideal time to revamp running form as they work their way back up through distances.

Running ergonomic awareness can help prevent ITBS as well as other running injuries. Large jumps or sudden increases in training should be avoided. Running exclusively on cantered surfaces or asphalt isn't ideal. If possible frequent track runners should alternate direction from time to time.

Footwear is important: ensure that running shoes are appropriate for your running style (over-pronation being by far the most common issue), supportive enough, and not too worn down. A generally accepted number for the life span of a running shoe is 500 miles. For an athlete logging consistent miles, alternating between two pairs of shoes will increase the life span of both. Technical running stores are more knowledgeable about matching up particular gait mechanics with the right shoe.

On the bike, fit is everything. In particular make sure that the pedal and shoe cleats are properly aligned and that the seat height and fore/aft positioning are correct. Most bike shops have fitting services and can assist making these measurements.

ITBS is largely preventable. When it does occur, it generally responds well to appropriate treatment. An athlete starting to develop pain on the outside of the knee or hip shouldn't wait too long before seeking assistance. The earlier it is treated the quicker it will respond, and the less training time will be lost.

Section 42.2

Plica Syndrome

"Plica Syndrome," by David Edell, MEd, ATC, LAT, CSCS.
© 2010 David Edell. Reprinted with permission from
www.AthleticAdvisor.com.

A plica is a thin wall of fibrous tissue that are extensions of the synovial capsule of the knee. During fetal development, the knee is divided into three separate compartments. As the fetus develops these compartments develop into one large protective cavity (synovial membrane). The majority of people have remnants of these three cavities, referred to as a plica. Most often the plica is on the medial (inside) of the knee at the level of the medial femoral condyle. Most individuals are not adversely affected by the presence of plicas.

The plica only becomes a problem when the knee is irritated, causing an inflammation in the synovial sack. When the synovium is inflamed, the area of the plica becomes thicker. This thickened area then begins to catch on the femur as the knee moves. This in turn keeps the plica inflamed resulting in a vicious cycle.

The plica can be located anywhere in the knee. The exact symptoms will be determined by the plica's location. The most common location is along the medial (inside) side of the knee. The plica can tether the patella to the femur, be located between the femur and patella, or be located along the femoral condyle. Regardless of location the pain is due to the plica catching or being pinched between the patella and femur. If the plica connects the patella to the femoral condyle, symptoms will mimic patellofemoral syndrome.

Without a complete clinical examination, the plica may be missed, resulting in an inappropriate rehabilitation plan. For example, if the patella is tethered by the plica, the clinician may design a rehab plan to address a patellofemoral disorder. This may only exacerbate the condition. If the plica is truly tethering the patella, the rehab should focus on decreasing the inflammation, and increasing the overall strength of the quad muscles.

Treatment of Plica Syndrome

The first concern is to decrease the inflammation of the synovial capsule. This can be attacked with numerous methods. First, the orthopaedic surgeon may prescribe a non-steroidal anti-inflammatory medication. Examples of these medications are Motrin®, DayPro®, Naprosyn®, Celebrex®, and Indocin®. These medications act systemically to slow the inflammation process. Therapeutic exercises and modalities may also be used to treat the plica. To attack the inflammation, modalities such as iontophoresis (utilizing low intensity electric current to transport medications through skin), phonophoresis (using ultrasound to transport medications through skin), and ice are most commonly utilized.

Rehabilitative exercises should be instituted when the inflammation has been controlled and pain levels are falling. These exercises should focus on increasing overall quadriceps, hamstring, and calf strength, as well as increasing overall muscular flexibility. Examples of appropriate exercises are: pain-free squats that progress to one-leg squats, side step-ups, closed chain terminal knee extension, and applicable sport-specific exercises. Care should be taken to avoid deep squats as this can increase pain and inflammation.

The exercises should be performed utilizing PRE (progressive resistance exercises) principles, gradually increasing load and intensity as pain and inflammation allows.

Case Study

An 18-year-old male football player presents with a history suspicious of a medial meniscal tear. This was confirmed by MRI [magnetic resonance imaging]. Surgery was performed to repair the medial meniscal tear. Upon arthroscopic evaluation the plica was found. The MRI did not visualize the plica. This plica was located on the medial synovial lining, running superiorly into the suprapatellar pouch. The plica was distending the synovial lining into the knee joint. With the plica removed, the synovial lining is no longer pulled into the joint. The torn meniscus was also addressed.

The athlete was seen in the training room for five total visits in a two-week span. Treatment emphasized basic quadriceps strength and range of motion. Following his 10-day post-op physician's visit, the athlete was released to normal strength training (10-day gradual return to previous routine) in the weight room.

Part Eight

Injuries to the Lower Legs, Ankles, and Feet

Chapter 43

Leg Injuries

Chapter Contents

Section 43.1

Stress Fractures

© 2007 American College of Sports Medicine (www.acsm.org). Reprinted with permission of the American College of Sports Medicine, "ACSM Current Comment: Stress Fractures," written for the American College of Sports Medicine by Belinda R. Beck, Ph.D.

Stress fractures comprise between 0.7% and 15.6% of all athletic injuries. Athletes particularly at risk of stress fracture are runners and jumpers, gymnasts and dancers. Stress fracture incidence among U.S. military recruits is also high, ranging from approximately 1% to 20%, with higher rates reported for women than for men. In general, the bones most commonly injured are the metatarsals, fibula, and tibia.

Etiology

Normal physiological loading provokes a range of deformation reactions (strains) in bone, including compression, tension, shear, torsion, and vibration. Bone exhibits an intrinsic ability to adapt to alterations in chronic loading to withstand future loads of the same nature, a phenomenon commonly referred to as Wolff's Law. Adaptation of bone to load changes occurs via increased modeling and/or remodeling. Modeling is a process whereby bone tissue is either deposited or removed to modify the shape and size of a bone. Remodeling describes a process of bone resorption, followed (after a delay of roughly one month) by deposition of new bone (for approximately six months). While some level of remodeling is constantly occurring in normal bone, in bone undergoing adaptation to altered loading, the degree of remodeling increases substantially. The initial increase in resorption will render a bone relatively porous until the process of deposition can replace the lost tissue in full. During this prolonged replacement phase, bone is more susceptible to stress fracture by virtue of increased porosity.

Risk Factors

The following factors contribute to the incidence of stress fracture either directly or indirectly via their influence on bone strain and commensurate relationship to bone remodeling:

- Training changes (e.g., terrain, shoes, activity, training intensity)
- Running and jumping activities
- Inappropriate footwear
- Muscle inflexibility
- Muscle weakness
- Excessive muscle strength
- Lower extremity alignment anomalies
- Poor running technique
- Previous history of injury
- Low bone mineral density (in women, often secondary to inadequately circulating estrogen)

Diagnosis

Positive symptoms of stress fracture include local tenderness, pain with direct and/or indirect percussion, and pain with weight bearing (particularly hopping on the affected limb). Signs of swelling at the injury site may be present. Confirmation of clinical diagnosis may be obtained via triple-phase Technetium 99 bone scans (often considered the standard diagnostic tool) and magnetic resonance imaging (MRI). Plain X-rays are normally inadequately sensitive for the purposes of early diagnosis. Generally, historical symptoms and physical signs are enough for diagnosis.

Management Recommendations

Because stress fractures are pathological expressions of the normal adaptive response of bone to modified loading, unloading (rest) remains an effective treatment under most conditions.

Prevention is, however, undoubtedly the best management approach. Coaches must be cognizant of stress fracture risk factors when designing training programs. Recommendations that minimize the risk of stress fracture and promote recovery include the following:

DURING Training

- Wear lightweight, activity-specific athletic shoes and replace them after approximately 500–700 kilometers of running.

- Increase training intensity gradually over a period of weeks, introducing hills, interval training, jumping exercises, and high-strain, sport-specific activities only after approximately six weeks of graduated training.

- If various surfaces will be encountered during training and competition, begin training on surfaces that absorb shock well, such as level asphalt. Then progress to man-made track, grass, sand, or uneven terrain, thereafter varying the training surface.

- Maintain adequate dietary calcium intake (at least 1,200 mg/day for those younger than 25 years; 800 mg/day for those older) to allow healthy bone mineralization during remodeling.

- Female athletes should maintain normal concentration of circulating estrogen, using menstrual dysfunction as a warning flag.

When INJURED

- Maintain aerobic fitness when injured via reduced weight-bearing exercise such as pool running and bicycling.

- Resume training gradually, incorporating pool running during the latter stages of healing and early stages of return, building rest days into the regimen. Ask for light-intensity training guidelines from your therapist or exercise physiologist.

- If a particularly fast return to activity is necessary, use protective devices, e.g. a pneumatic tibia brace, to splint bones from strain during weight bearing.

DO NOT

- excessively stretch adjacent muscles when acutely injured;
- perform local muscle-strengthening exercises when acutely injured;
- engage in pain-producing activities when injured;
- train on unusually soft or uneven surfaces when injured.

New Directions

Preliminary evidence suggests that the application of electric and electromagnetic fields or sound waves may enhance the healing of stress fractures. A number of bone stimulatory devices are currently on the market, and research in the field of stress fracture application is ongoing.

Summary

Stress fractures are a recognized complication of the chronic, intensive, weight-bearing training familiar to athletic, dance, and military populations. Bones are most susceptible to stress fracture when weakened by remodeling-related porosity, a primary stage in the adaptive response of bone to changes in patterns of loading. Prevention is the most appropriate management approach, best achieved through graduated training increments. The goal of stress fracture treatment is to facilitate the natural progression of bone remodeling by reducing loads on the injured site to the greatest extent. Thus, rest from pain-provoking activities remains the most effective, if often prolonged, intervention approach at this time.

Section 43.2

Tibia (Shinbone) Fractures

Introduction

The tibia, commonly called the shinbone, is located in your lower leg. A tibia fracture is a common injury. A fracture is a broken bone. Vehicle crashes, falls, and sports injuries are frequent causes of tibia fractures. Depending on the location and type of fracture, treatment involves casting or surgery.

Anatomy

The tibia is the larger of the two long bones in your leg. The smaller bone next to the tibia is the fibula. The top of the tibia is part of the knee joint. The long length of bone is called the shaft. The lower part of the tibia helps form the ankle joint.

439

Causes

Tibia fractures can result from vehicle crashes and or falls. Tibia fractures can occur in people that have been hit by a car. Jumping or rotating during sports, such as gymnastics, basketball, and football, can cause tibia fractures. Stress fractures result from prolonged impact from jogging, running, or other repetitive activities.

Symptoms

Tibia fractures can cause pain and swelling. You may not be able to put weight on your leg or walk. In some cases, the nearby fibula bone is fractured as well.

Diagnosis

Your doctor can diagnose a tibia fracture by examining your leg and taking X-rays. Tests that show more detail, such as a computed tomography (CT) scan or magnetic resonance imaging (MRI) scan, may be used as well. Your doctor will evaluate the nerves and blood vessels in your leg.

Treatment

Casting can be used to treat tibia shaft fractures if the bones are in good alignment. Casting is also used for people that are not good candidates for surgery. A long leg cast that covers the knee and ankle is used to provide support and stability while the bones heal.

Surgery

There are various types of surgery to treat fractures with bones that have moved out of position or are otherwise unstable. Intramedullary fixation involves inserting a rod (intramedullary nail) into the center of the bone. The rod is secured with surgical screws. The rod provides support while the fracture heals.

Other tibia surgeries include plating and external fixation. Plating involves securing a plate and screws into the bone to keep it in proper position while it heals. Plating is useful for tibia fractures around the ankle or knee. External fixation uses a frame that is aligned on the outside of the leg and secured with surgical pins to keep the bones from moving while they heal. External fixation is useful if there are severe skin wounds associated with a fracture.

Recovery

The tibia can take a long time to heal, ranging from about four months to over nine months for severe fractures. Physical therapy may follow casting or surgery. You will need to use crutches or a walker for a period while you heal. Your doctor will check your progress with X-rays and gradually increase the amount of weight that you can put on your leg.

Section 43.3

Medial Tibial Stress Syndrome (Shin Splints)

"Medial Tibial Stress Syndrome (Shin Splints)," by Kayla Fulghum, ATC. © Georgia High School Association (www.ghsa.net). Reprinted with permission. Reviewed by David A. Cooke, MD, FACP, September 2011.

What Are They?

Medial tibial stress syndrome, or shin splints, is a term that has been used to refer to pain in the lower leg. Conditions such as muscle strains and stress fractures have been given the term shin splints. Most people who develop shin splits are involved in sports which involve running. Shin splints are more commonly seen in sports such as track, cross country, basketball, and gymnastics, as the athletes run or pound on hard surfaces both during competition and at practice.

How Common Are They and What Leads to Shin Splints?

Shin splints account for about 10% to 15% of all running injuries. It has also been found that up to 60% of all conditions that cause leg pain in athletes have contributed to shin splints. There are many factors that can contribute to shin splints.

- Having weakness in the muscles of the leg

441

- A tight heel cord
- Having shoes that provide little support or cushioning
- Training errors such as running on hard surfaces or overtraining
- Abnormal foot pattern (could be slightly tilted in or out when walking)

Signs and Symptoms

There are different categories to classify shin splits depending on when the pain arrives. The different grades are as follows:

- **Grade 1:** Pain occurring after athletic activity
- **Grade 2:** Pain occurring before and after athletic activity, but does not affect the performance of the individual
- **Grade 3:** Pain occurring before, during, and after athletic activity and does affect the performance of the individual
- **Grade 4:** Pain that is so severe that performance in activity is impossible

Treatment/Management

Immediate management for an individual with shin splints is to have a physician rule out a possible stress fracture in the bone, which can cause serious consequences if left untreated. Next, it is imperative to modify activity. For example, a cross-country runner can do cardiovascular exercises in the pool to take pressure off of the legs. Most of the time, a break in activity or modification of training techniques will help eliminate the problem.

If the problem is occurring from an abnormal foot pattern, custom made foot orthotics (insoles) will aid in correcting it. Another treatment technique that can be utilized is stretching. Stretching the calf muscles is a good way to help relieve tightness that may be causing the pain in the front of the leg.

In addition to stretching, all athletes with lower leg pain can use ice massage. The ice along with the massaging technique helps deliver cold to the area and allows for pain management by numbing the area and reducing inflammation (or swelling). The best way to make an ice massage tool is to do the following:

1. Take a small or medium paper cup (i.e., Dixie cup).
2. Fill the cup with water but do not overflow the cup.

3. Put the cup of water in the freezer.

4. Remove the cup of water after it has frozen.

5. Peel away the top of the cup until the ice is exposed.

6. Take the exposed ice and gently massage the area on the front of the leg.

7. Massage the area for 5–15 minutes until the area is numb.

   a. Cold creams or gels (i.e., Biofreeze or Mineral Ice) can also be used in conjunction with the ice massage and allow for deeper treatment.

8. Repeat steps 1–7 every hour or when pain occurs.

References

Prentice, William. "Arnheim's Principles of Athletic Training: A Competency-Based Approach" 2003 McGraw-Hill.

Chapter 44

Achilles Tendon Injuries

David Beckham is one of the many athletes who suffered from a torn Achilles tendon injury. The torn Achilles tendon requires surgical repair and rehabilitation that likely requires six to nine months before return to competitive play.

While an Achilles tendon injury can be seen in almost all levels of competitive athletes, they have been historically linked with the "weekend warrior" athlete who may be somewhat de-conditioned. Recognition and treatment of an Achilles tendon injury is very important, as neglected or unrecognized ruptures can cause many future problems with both daily activities and sports competition.

What is the anatomy and function of the Achilles tendon?

The Achilles tendon connects the muscles of the calf and to the heel bone. The tendon is large and must be able to withstand and transmit the large forces generated by these powerful muscles to move the foot. These forces can be many times our own body weight. The tendon is particular active with pushing down (plantar flexion) of the foot, and is therefore critical to perform in all sports, especially those in which jumping is critical. Correspondingly, sports such as basketball, track and field, and volleyball place high stresses on the Achilles tendon with jumping and landing and are likely the highest risk for tendon injury. However, a torn Achilles tendon has been reported with virtually every sport.

The Achilles tendon is located just beneath the skin and can be palpated just above the heel bone. It is nourished by a blood supply from an enveloping sheath of tissue (paratenon), although an area approximately two to four centimeters above the tendon's insertion into the heel bone is the least well-perfused ("watershed" area). For this reason, this area of limited healing potential is a common location for tendon ruptures. The location of the tendon directly beneath the skin is also an important consideration for wound healing in the surgical treatment of ruptures.

What is an Achilles tendon injury?

An Achilles tendon injury is a disruption in the integrity of the tendon somewhere between the muscle bellies and the heel bone (calcaneus). Most commonly, tears occur at the muscle-tendon junction two to four centimeters above the insertion into bone, but they can occur as avulsions directly from the calcaneus.

Tears can result from trauma or transection injuries which extend through the skin and underlying tendon. More commonly, however, athletes suffer these injuries during sporting activities. Up to one-third of the athletes who suffer a rupture complained of some injury or symptoms in the tendon in the preceding weeks, suggesting that a preceding event may place the Achilles tendon at risk for rupture. Chronic inflammation or irritation of the tendon for repetitive activities ("Achilles tendinitis") can also weaken the tendon and render it vulnerable to rupture as well.

What places me at higher risk for an Achilles tendon injury as an athlete?

Virtually anyone can suffer an Achilles tendon injury, but certain pre-existing factors can place an athlete at greater risk and should be considered. These include:

- de-conditioning with weakness of the calf muscles, a common problem in "weekend" athletes who have not been training;

- injections of steroid in or around the Achilles tendon—these can weaken the tendon and increase the risk of rupture with provocative activities, and should generally be avoided;

- pre-existing Achilles tendinitis (inflammation of the tendon) with secondary degeneration and weakening of the tendon over time;

- certain antibiotics (fluoroquinolones—Ciprofloxacin, Levofloxacin, Ofloxacin, etc) can place tendon at higher risk of injury;

- gout;

- hyper-parathyroidism;

- diabetes.

How does an Achilles tendon injury occur in athletes?

Most of the time, athletes will suffer an Achilles tendon injury when a significant force is placed on the leg with the knee extended and foot pulled up (dorsi-flexed). This usually happens when awkwardly landing from a jump and stresses the tendon when it is maximally stretched. This is a common occurrence on the basketball court.

Although Achilles tendon ruptures have been classically associated with the "weekend" athlete that is over the age of 30, they are certainly not restricted to them. Professional, well-conditioned athletes have suffered from them as well. These include NFL players Vinny Testaverde and Takeo Spikes, tennis champion Boris Becker, and many all-star NBA players, including Dominique Wilkins, Elton Brand, and Christian Laettner.

What are the symptoms of an Achilles tendon rupture in athletes?

The symptoms of an Achilles tendon rupture are generally not subtle. The athlete will usually complain about a "popping" that could be heard and felt when jumping or landing on the court or field. Up to one-third of the time, the athlete will have complained of some pain or symptoms in the Achilles in the prior weeks—it is thought that this inciting event may render it vulnerable to injury. The athlete will immediately complain of weakness with pushing off on the foot (plantar-flexion), reflected in difficulty walking and an inability to jump with the involved leg. Often there is a palpable defect at the location of rupture just above the heel bone, with loss of integrity of the "taut band" just deep to the skin. Examination of the opposite, normal side will help to detect these differences.

Some classic findings of an Achilles tendon injury have been described. These include:

- **Thompson test:** Normally, squeezing the calf muscle in the seated athlete will cause the foot to flex down (plantar-flex). In the setting of an Achilles rupture, however, no movement of the foot will occur.

447

- **Hyper-dorsiflexion sign:** With the athlete lying on their stomach, both knees are flexed up. The injured foot can be pushed down (dorsi-flexed) further than the normal side.

Are imaging studies useful?

Imaging studies can be useful as confirmatory tests for the diagnosis and to determine the location of the Achilles tendon injury. Plain X-rays can help to rule out a "bony" avulsion fracture but are of limited utility. Magnetic resonance imaging (MRI) and ultrasound are the most common imaging modalities used to visualize an Achilles tendon injury. Ultrasound (US) not only allows visualization of the tear, but is also dynamic and permits examination with active attempts at plantar-flexion and dorsi-flexion of the foot. MRI is more than 98% sensitive in diagnosing Achilles tendon rupture and can accurately be used to determine the location of rupture and severity of tendon retraction. This information can be helpful in planning for an Achilles tendon surgery repair.

What are my treatment options for an Achilles tendon injury as an athlete?

Treatment options for a Achilles tendon injury are quite simple: operative or nonoperative. Some prompt treatment is important, however, as a torn Achilles tendon will seldom heal on its own. With rupture, the muscle belly and tendon retract proximally into the calf and leave a large "gap" defect that cannot heal. Furthermore, waiting for a long time before seeking medical attention ("chronic" rupture) or failing to recognize the injury can compromise treatment options—the tendon becomes stiff and scarred and sometimes cannot be repaired primarily ("end-to-end").

Nonsurgical options offer the advantage of avoiding the complications of surgery. Typically, the foot is kept in a down position (plantar-flexed) to approximate the ruptured tendon ends as close as possible and immobilized in a cast or rigid boot until healing occurs. The major limitation of nonoperative treatment, however, remains the risk of incomplete or no healing and is a significant concern when there is significant tendon retraction. Correspondingly, the risk of recurrent rupture is higher with nonoperative treatment. This option is generally *not* pursued by athletes, given their desire to return to sporting and at-risk activities, and to therefore have the strongest repair possible.

Achilles tendon surgery offers the benefits of an immediate and secure "end-to-end" repair of the ruptured tendon. This allows for a predictable course of recovery and decreased risk of repeat rupture. The main risk of Achilles tendon surgery, however, relates to the surgical wound and healing. The Achilles tendon is directly beneath the skin, and the skin flaps for a repair can have a tenuous blood supply that can place healing of the both the skin and tendon at risk. For this reason, meticulous handling of the skin and surrounding tendon sheath ("paratenon") with a surgical repair is of critical importance.

What is nonoperative treatment and what outcome can I expect as an athlete?

Nonoperative treatment may be reasonable with Achilles tendon injuries that (i) have minimal retraction and gapping between the tendon ends, or (ii) older, low-demand patients with multiple medical comorbidities that are at greater risk for surgical complications. Athletes who expect to return to competitive, jumping sports typically will not elect this option due to the greater risk of recurrent rupture.

The foot is immobilized in the "down position" (equinus or plantar-flexed) to approximate the tendon edges as close as possible. The leg can be held in this position in a short arm cast or rigid boot. Weight bearing on the leg is protected early and gradually initiated after healing ensues typically at four to six weeks. The plantar-flexed position is gradually corrected to neutral over time. Rehabilitation to strengthen the muscles of the leg and calf is pursued after significant healing has occurred.

The results of nonoperative treatment are not perfect. Athletes cannot expect to fully return to competitive sports for one year or more. Furthermore, the risk of recurrent rupture can range from 4% to 30%. In addition, the tendon edges are often not completely approximate, resulting in a tendon that has healed in a "longer" position. This can reduce both the strength and endurance by as much as 30% compared to the normal, uninjured tendon.

What does Achilles tendon surgery involve?

Surgical repair is typically the treatment of choice for athletes. Surgical repair usually allows for:

- a more predictable postoperative course of healing;
- secure "end-to-end" repair of the tendon;
- earlier return to sports;
- lower risk of recurrent tendon rupture;
- earlier and more predictable return of muscle power.

Both percutaneous and open repair techniques to repair the tendon have been described. The motivation for percutaneous techniques has been to avoid the surgical wound and associated risks of wound infection or dehiscence at this location just above the heel bone. The blood supply of the skin in this location is tenuous and can be at risk for sloughing if not carefully handled during open Achilles tendon surgery. While percutaneous techniques may protect the skin, they can place the adjacent nerves and vessels at greater risk of injury. The sural nerve is particularly at risk as it lies just lateral the Achilles tendon.

Open surgery is typically performed by making an incision just medial to the tendon. A medial incision avoids risk to the sural nerve and protects it from the risk of abrasion immediately on the back side of the Achilles tendon. The skin flaps are handled very gently to avoid trauma and injury to its blood supply. The enveloping sheath of the Achilles tendon (paratenon) is identified below and incised longitudinally over the tendon defect. The paratenon is also carefully handled and preserved so that it can be closed after tendon repair—this sheath nourishes the healing tendon and provides a protective layer between the tendon and overlying skin. A collection of blood (hematoma) from the trauma is typically encountered and irrigated away to visualize the ends of the ruptured tendon. The proximal end can sometimes "recoil" deep into the calf and may need to retrieved into the wound. Any scar and adhesions of the ruptured tendon ends should be broken to allow full mobilization and "end-to-end" approximation of the tendon under minimal tension. Grasping sutures are then placed into both tendon ends and tied together to approximate the tendon to re-create its native, resting length. While various techniques and suture configuration have been described, the ultimate common goal is to resist gap formation and confer sufficient strength to the repair until interval healing of tendon occurs.

Repair of chronic or neglected ruptures is more difficult. In certain cases, the tendon stumps can be so retracted, stiff, and scarred that they cannot be brought "end-to-end" for a primary repair. In these circumstances, augmentation with other tissue or tendon transfer from another muscle may be required and is usually associated with a less optimal result.

What is involved in postoperative rehabilitation?

A plaster splint is typically used to protect the wound for the first one to two postoperative weeks. After satisfactory wound healing is confirmed, the athlete is transitioned to a short leg cast or protective boot and protected weight bearing with crutches is allowed for the next six to eight weeks. No active plantar flexion and passive stretching of the Achilles tendon repair is encouraged during this time. Roll-a-bouts can be useful during this period to improve mobility and completely protect the healing tendon from weight bearing. At approximately six weeks, gentle active plantar flexion and tendon stretching is initiated. Isotonic dorsi-flexion and full weight bearing in the protective boot are gradually allowed as well. By three months, muscle strengthening and proprioceptive training are initiated. These exercises can include:

- isotonic plantar and dorsi-flexion exercises;
- isokinetics;
- balance board and perturbation training;
- Stairmaster or Versiclimber.

How long will it take for me to get back to my sport?

Return to sport is highly variable, and depends upon the type and severity of the Achilles tendon injury, associated comorbidities, strength and rehabilitation, as well as treatment pursued. In general, healthy athletes who choose nonoperative treatment cannot expect a full return to sports for one year. On the other hand, an uncomplicated surgical repair in a healthy athlete often permits return to sport at six to nine months.

Can I prevent an Achilles tendon injury?

Unfortunately, it is hard to anticipate and therefore "prevent" an Achilles tendon rupture. However, there has been some evidence to support that de-conditioning, loss of proprioception, and weakness of the calf musculature may increase the vulnerability to injury during exertion in sports. For this reason, staying well-conditioned and balanced with a steady training program is the most effective way to minimize the risk of an Achilles rupture. Nonetheless, even an athlete in "tip-top" condition can suffer an unfortunate, high-load Achilles tendon injury!

It is also advisable to avoid fluoroquinolone antibiotics which can predispose to risk of tendon injury with provocative activities.

If you suspect that you have an Achilles tendon injury, it is critical to seek the urgent consultation of a local sports injuries doctor for appropriate care.

References

Inglis A, Scott W, Sculco T, Patterson A. Ruptures of the tendoachilles. An objective assessment of surgical and non-surgical treatment. *J Bone Joint Surg Am* 1976 Oct; 58(7): 990–3.

Nistor L. Conservative treatment of fresh subcutaneous rupture of the Achilles tendon. *Acta Orthop Scand*. 1976 Aug;47(4):459–62.

Nistor L. Surgical and non-surgical treatment of Achilles Tendon rupture. A prospective randomized study. *J Bone Joint Surg Am*. 1981 Mar;63(3):394–9.

Chapter 45

Ankle Injuries

Chapter Contents

Section 45.1

Ankle Sprains

There's a good chance that while playing as a child or stepping on an uneven surface as an adult you sprained your ankle—some 25,000 people do it every day.

Sometimes, it is an awkward moment when you lose your balance, but the pain quickly fades away and you go on your way. But the sprain could be more severe; your ankle might swell and it might hurt too much to stand on it. If it's a severe sprain, you might have felt a "pop" when the injury happened.

A sprained ankle means one or more ligaments on the outer side of your ankle were stretched or torn. If it is not treated properly, you could have long-term problems.

You're most likely to sprain your ankle when you have your toes on the ground and heel up (plantar flexion). This position puts your ankle's ligaments under tension, making them vulnerable. A sudden force like landing on an uneven surface may turn your ankle inward (inversion). When this happens, one, two, or three of your ligaments may be hurt.

Tell your doctor what you were doing when you sprained your ankle. He or she will examine it and may want an X-ray to make sure no bones are broken. Depending on how many ligaments are injured, your sprain is classified as Grade I, II, or III.

Treating Your Sprained Ankle

Treating your sprained ankle properly may prevent chronic pain and instability. For a Grade I sprain, follow the R.I.C.E. guidelines:

- Rest your ankle by not walking on it.
- Ice it to keep the swelling down.
- Compressive bandages immobilize and support your injury.

454

- Elevate your ankle above your heart level for 48 hours.

- The swelling usually goes down within a few days.

For a Grade II sprain, follow the R.I.C.E. guidelines and allow more time for healing. A doctor may immobilize or splint your sprained ankle.

A Grade III sprain puts you at risk for permanent ankle instability. Surgery may rarely be needed to repair the damage, especially in competitive athletes. For severe ankle sprains, your doctor may also consider treating you with a short leg cast for two to three weeks or a walking boot. People who sprain their ankle repeatedly may also need surgical repair to tighten their ligaments.

Rehabilitating Your Sprained Ankle

Every ligament injury needs rehabilitation. Otherwise, your sprained ankle might not heal completely and you might re-injure it. All ankle sprains, from mild to severe, require three phases of recovery:

- Phase I includes resting, protecting, and reducing swelling of your injured ankle.

- Phase II includes restoring your ankle's flexibility, range of motion, and strength.

- Phase III includes gradually returning to straight-ahead activity and doing maintenance exercises, followed later by more cutting sports such as tennis, basketball, or football.

Once you can stand on your ankle again, your doctor will prescribe exercise routines to strengthen your muscles and ligaments, and increase your flexibility, balance, and coordination. Later, you may walk, jog, and run figure eights with your ankle taped or in a supportive ankle brace.

It's important to complete the rehabilitation program because it makes it less likely that you'll hurt the same ankle again. If you don't complete rehabilitation, you could suffer chronic pain, instability, and arthritis in your ankle. If your ankle still hurts, it could mean that the sprained ligament(s) has not healed right, or that some other injury also happened.

To prevent future sprained ankles, pay attention to your body's warning signs to slow down when you feel pain or fatigue, and stay in shape with good muscle balance, flexibility, and strength in your soft tissues.

Section 45.2

High Ankle Sprain

A high ankle sprain is an injury to the ligaments that connect the
tibia and fibula (the lower leg bones) just above the ankle joint. There
are five ligaments that connect the tibia to the fibula, and together
these are called the syndesmosis. Compared to lateral ankle sprains
which affect the lower part of the ankle joint, high ankle sprains are
much less common and take longer to heal.

A grade I sprain to the syndesmosis is the mildest form of injury
and consists of a stretch to the ligaments. A grade II sprain is a partial
tear of the ligaments, and a grade III sprain is a complete tear of the
ligaments.

How It Occurs

A high ankle sprain is caused by a twisting injury to the ankle,
usually while it is flexed with the foot turned out excessively.

Signs and Symptoms

Symptoms include pain, swelling, bruising, limited ankle motion,
and difficulty walking. Some people describe feeling a snap, pop, or
tearing sensation at the time of the injury. Grade I sprains have little
to no swelling. Grade III sprains can have significant swelling and
bruising over a large area of the lower leg and ankle. Pain is located
in the front of the ankle and is worse with walking.

Diagnosis

Your doctor will ask you to describe how your injury happened and
to list your symptoms. After examining your ankle, your doctor may
order X-rays to determine the grade of your injury and the amount of
instability at the joint.

Treatment

Treatment will depend on the grade of injury. For the first 24–48 hours after any high ankle sprain, treatment is focused on reducing the pain and swelling. Wrap the ankle in an elastic bandage, elevate it as often as possible, and apply ice packs for 15 minutes every two to four hours. An anti-inflammatory medication such as ibuprofen can be helpful. Crutches are recommended until you can walk without pain. Your doctor may recommend a supportive brace, air stirrup, or walking boot to help you walk sooner without crutches.

For grade I sprains, physical therapy should begin as soon as possible. Most grade II sprains usually require a short period of immobilization in a cast or boot before physical therapy can begin. In addition to helping control pain and swelling, physical therapy is necessary to regain ankle mobility, strength, and balance. Physical therapy allows the ankle heal faster and reduces your risk of re-injury.

Grade III sprains and some grade II sprains will require surgery to stabilize the ankle joint, followed by physical therapy.

Returning to Activity and Sports

Return to sports will depend on the grade of injury and method of treatment. You should be able to return to sports and activities when you have regained full strength and mobility of the ankle joint and can walk and jog without pain or a sensation of instability. High ankle sprains can take much longer to heal than typical lateral ankle sprains. For grade I and II sprains treated without surgery, it may take up to six weeks or longer until you are able to resume athletic activities. For grade II and III sprains treated with surgery, return to sports can take several months.

Preventing High Ankle Sprains

Since the syndesmosis remains looser than normal after a high ankle sprain, you are vulnerable to spraining this ankle again in the future. The best way to protect your ankle and reduce your chances of re-injury is to keep the muscles that support the ankle joint strong. This means continuing to perform ankle strengthening and balance exercises two or three times a week, even after your physical therapy has ended and you have been cleared to return to sports. Taping the ankle or wearing a supportive brace during sports can provide some added protection but should not replace the strengthening exercises.

Section 45.3

Ankle Instability

Recurring or persistent (chronic) pain on the outer (lateral) side of the ankle often develops after an injury such as a sprained ankle. However, several other conditions may also cause chronic ankle pain.

Signs and Symptoms

- Pain, usually on the outer side of the ankle (the pain may be so intense that you have difficulty walking or participating in sports; in some cases, the pain is a constant, dull ache)
- Difficulty walking on uneven ground or in high heels
- A feeling of giving way (instability)
- Swelling
- Stiffness
- Tenderness
- Repeated ankle sprains

Possible Causes for Chronic Lateral Ankle Pain

The most common cause for a persistently painful ankle is incomplete healing after an ankle sprain. When you sprain your ankle, the connecting tissue (ligament) between the bones is stretched or torn. Without thorough and complete rehabilitation, the ligament or surrounding muscles may remain weak, resulting in recurrent instability. As a result, you may experience additional ankle injuries. Other causes of chronic ankle pain include:

- an injury to the nerves that pass through the ankle (the nerves may be stretched, torn, injured by a direct blow, or pinched under pressure [entrapment]);

458

- a torn or inflamed tendon;
- arthritis of the ankle joint;
- a break (fracture) in one of the bones that make up the ankle joint;
- an inflammation of the joint lining (synovium); or
- the development of scar tissue in the ankle after a sprain (the scar tissue takes up space in the joint, thus putting pressure on the ligaments).

Evaluation and Diagnosis

The first step in identifying the cause of chronic ankle pain is taking a history of the condition. Your doctor may ask you several questions, including:

- Have you previously injured the ankle? If so, when?
- What kind of treatment did you receive for the injury?
- How long have you had the pain?
- Are there times when the pain worsens or disappears?

Because there are so many potential causes for chronic ankle pain, your doctor may do a number of tests to pinpoint the diagnosis, beginning with a physical examination. Your doctor will feel for tender areas and look for signs of swelling. He or she will have you move your foot and ankle to assess range of motion and flexibility. Your doctor may also test the sensation of the nerves and may administer a shot of local anesthetic to help pinpoint the source of the symptoms.

Your doctor may order several X-ray views of your ankle joint. You may also need to get X-rays of the other ankle so the doctor can compare the injured and noninjured ankles. In some cases, additional tests such as a bone scan, computed tomography (CT) scan, or magnetic resonance image (MRI) may be needed.

Treatment

Treatment will depend on the final diagnosis and should be personalized to your individual needs. Both conservative (nonoperative) and surgical treatment methods may be used. Conservative treatments include:

- anti-inflammatory medications such as aspirin or ibuprofen to reduce swelling;

- physical therapy, including tilt-board exercises, directed at strengthening the muscles, restoring range of motion, and increasing your perception of joint position;

- an ankle brace or other support;

- an injection of a steroid medication; or

- in the case of a fracture, immobilization to allow the bone to heal.

If your condition requires it, or if conservative treatment doesn't bring relief, your doctor may recommend surgery. Many surgical procedures can be done on an outpatient basis. Some procedures use arthroscopic techniques; other require open surgery. Rehabilitation may take 6 to 10 weeks to ensure proper healing.

Surgical treatment options include:

- removing (excising) loose fragments;

- cleaning (debriding) the joint or joint surface;

- repairing or reconstructing the ligaments or transferring tendons.

Prevention

Almost half of all people who sprain their ankle once will experience additional ankle sprains and chronic pain. You can help prevent chronic pain from developing by following these simple steps:

1. Follow your doctor's instructions carefully and complete the prescribed physical rehabilitation program.

2. Do not return to activity until cleared by your physician.

3. When you do return to sports, use an ankle brace rather than taping the ankle. Bracing is more effective than taping in preventing ankle sprains.

4. If you wear hi-top shoes, be sure to lace them properly and completely.

Section 45.4

Ankle Fractures

During the past 30 years, doctors have noted an increase in the number and severity of broken ankles, due in part to an active, older population of "baby boomers." More than 1.3 million people visited emergency rooms in 1998 because of ankle problems. The ankle actually involves two joints, one on top of the other. A broken ankle can involve one or more bones, as well as injuring the surrounding connecting tissues (ligaments).

Anatomy of the Ankle

The top ankle joint is composed of three bones:

- The shinbone (tibia)
- The other bone of the lower leg (fibula)
- The anklebone (talus)

The leg bones form a scooped pocket around the top of the anklebone. This lets the foot bend up and down.

Right below the ankle joint is another joint (subtalar), where the anklebone connects to the heel bone (calcaneus). This joint enables the foot to rock from side to side. Three sets of fibrous tissues connect the bones and provide stability to both joints. The knobby bumps you can feel on either side of your ankle are the very ends of the lower leg bones. The bump on the outside of the ankle (lateral malleolus) is part of the fibula; the smaller bump on the inside of the ankle (medial malleolus) is part of the shinbone.

When a Break Occurs

Any one of the three bones that make up the ankle joint could break as the result of a fall, an automobile accident, or some other trauma to the ankle.

461

Because a severe sprain can often mask the symptoms of a broken ankle, every injury to the ankle should be examined by a physician. Symptoms of a broken ankle include:

- immediate and severe pain;
- swelling;
- bruising;
- tender to the touch;
- inability to put any weight on the injured foot;
- deformity, particularly if there is a dislocation as well as a fracture.

A broken ankle may also involve damage to the ligaments. Your physician will order X-rays to find the exact location of the break. Sometimes, a CT scan or a bone scan will also be needed.

Treatment and Rehabilitation

If the fracture is stable (without damage to the ligament or the mortise joint), it can be treated with a leg cast or brace. Initially, a long leg cast may be applied, which can later be replaced by a short walking cast. It takes at least six weeks for a broken ankle to heal, and it may be several months before you can return to sports at your previous competitive level. Your physician will probably schedule additional X-rays while the bones heal, to make sure that changes or pressures on the ankle don't cause the bones to shift. If the ligaments are also torn, or if the fracture created a loose fragment of bone that could irritate the joint, surgery may be required to "fix" the bones together so they will heal properly. The surgeon may use a plate, metal or absorbable screws, staples, or tension bands to hold the bones in place. Usually, there are few complications, although there is a higher risk among diabetic patients and those who smoke. Afterwards, the surgeon will prescribe a program of rehabilitation and strengthening. Range of motion exercises are important, but keeping weight off the ankle is just as important. A child who breaks an ankle should be checked regularly for up to two years to make sure that growth proceeds properly, without deformity or uneven leg length.

Section 45.5

Osteochondritis Dissecans of the Talus

This section excerpted from "Osteochondritis Dissecans - Talus" by Rick Hammesfahr, M.D. © 2010 The Center for Orthopaedics and Sports Medicine. All rights reserved. Reprinted with permission. For additional information, visit www.arthroscopy.com.

Anatomy and Function

The ankle is a joint which is formed by the tibia and fibula (bones above the ankle in the foreleg) and the talus (below the ankle joint). The ankle joint allows for the upwards (dorsiflexion) and downwards (plantarflexion) motion. The end of the shin bone (tibia) forms the inner bony prominence of the ankle called the medial malleolus. The outer bony prominence is called the lateral malleolus and is formed by the small outer bone in the foreleg called the fibula.

Osteochondritis dissecans is an injury to the talus bone of the ankle joint. Because the ankle joint is so small, the amount of force that goes across the joint, with each step, has been estimated to be approximately 5–10 times a person's body weight. As a result of this tremendous force that occurs in the ankle joint, relatively small injuries to the articular surface of the talus often result in chronically painful injuries.

Osteochondritis dissecans is the result of the isolated loss of blood flow to a portion of the talus bone. Usually this occurs in conjunction with a history of trauma. It is sometimes also known as an osteochondral fracture of the talus, chip fracture of the articular surface, or a chondral fracture of the talus.

The development of osteochondritis may be very slow. Initially, a person may sustain a twisting injury to the ankle. As the ankle is injured, the talus bone twists within the space between the tibia and fibula. As this twisting occurs, the ligaments around the ankle may be stretched (ankle sprain). Unfortunately, in some people, as the twisting injury occurs, not only are the ankle ligaments stretched, but the talus bone strikes the tibia or fibula. When this occurs, some type of injury to the talus, tibia, or fibula happens. Typically, the majority of the damage occurs to the talus at the articular surface.

463

The articular surface (articular cartilage) is normally nice and smooth. It has no blood supply. Without a blood supply, the potential for healing damage to the articular cartilage is minimal. Therefore, when this tissue is damaged, it may slowly deteriorate with the passage of time. As the articular surface deteriorates, the surface changes from a nice smooth frictionless surface to a rough cobblestone-like surface. This rough degenerative surface is a form of arthritis.

When the ankle is twisted, and the talus impacts the tibia or fibula, the talar articular surface may be merely bruised, or a more serious injury may occur. If the twisting injury results in a shearing force to the talus as it impacts the tibia or fibula, then a chip fracture may occur. This "chip fracture" may either be complete, or incomplete, and it may be detached (loose body), partially detached, or non-displaced.

To further confuse things, the bone injury may not become visible on X-ray for several months.

When the chip becomes detached, then it floats freely inside the ankle joint. When this occurs, patients may develop a definite catching sensation that is associated with a loss of motion. In addition, the joint may become swollen and painful. Later, when the chip slips out of the way, the symptoms may improve, swelling decrease, and even may disappear—only to reappear at another time.

If the fragment is partially detached, then similar problems may occur.

However, if the fragment is not detached, then the only complaints may be pain and discomfort.

The location of the injury is on the articular surface of the talus. It may be located on either side of the talar dome. The talar dome is that semicircular portion of the talus that sits beneath the tibia. On this dome, the osteochondritis dissecans may occur on either the medial or lateral sides of the talar dome (articular surface of the talus).

Diagnosis

Initially, a physical exam should be done to try to determine the site of tenderness and the cause of the patient's complaint. During this process, the stability of the ligaments and tendons around the ankle is usually checked along with the range of motion of the joint. Palpation is used to determine the areas of tenderness and to check for signs of an effusion (collection of fluid within the joint).

Sometimes, it is necessary to aspirate (remove) the joint fluid collection to determine the type of fluid present. If the fluid is bloody with fat globules present (lipohemarthrosis), then some type of injury to the bone may be the cause.

X-rays are taken to evaluate the talus, tibia, and fibula. With the X-rays, it is possible to check for signs of arthritis, loose bodies, chip fractures, fractures, and other bone abnormalities. Unfortunately, because the ankle bones overlap on X-rays, it is necessary to take multiple views from different angles in order to try to completely evaluate the bones. Even with multiple views, it is still possible for the overlapping bone images to hide abnormalities. For that reason, if patients fail to improve, it is often necessary to obtain more sophisticated imaging studies such as MRIs, CT scans, bone scans, or tomograms. Unfortunately, none of these studies are 100% accurate.

With osteochondritis, sometimes, the initial imaging studies are normal. Only by repeating the imaging studies is the abnormality ever found. This is related to the fact the osteochondritis may take time to develop. Initially, the damage may be great enough to cause very mild intermittent symptoms, but too small to be visualized on X-ray. With the passage of time, as the osteochondritis worsens, then changes begin to appear on the imaging studies.

Imaging Studies

The classification of osteochondritis dissecans is important because the prognosis (expected outcome) and treatment options are often linked to the severity of the osteochondritis dissecans. Typically, the injury classification is from stage 1 through stage 4. As the severity of the injury progresses, the stage increases with stage 4 osteochondritis dissecans being the worst. Although the classification is often based upon the X-ray appearance, the abnormalities noted on X-ray may not always be completely accurate.

Treatment

The treatment depends on the age of the patient, the circumstances of the injury, and the type of bone damage. A simple bone contusion (bruise) would be treated differently then a detached bone fragment. The treatment options may vary from simply being on crutches to being casted to having surgery. The surgical procedures used to treat osteochondritis dissecans may involve removing the fragment, attempting to reattach the fragment, drilling the underlying bone to promote blood flow, or some combination of these procedures. Obviously, the exact treatment and procedure needs to be individualized to the patient, the type of bone injury, and the location of the bone injury.

Chapter 46

Injuries to the Feet

Chapter Contents

Section 46.1

Plantar Fasciitis (Heel Spurs)

Introduction

With increasing numbers of people participating in sports and the general population becoming more health conscious, problems with the feet are becoming more common. A very common problem seen in the foot is often referred to as a heel spur. Usually, this is actually plantar fasciitis, though sometimes a heel spur (an overgrowth of bone on the heel) may develop as part of this condition.

Anatomy

Plantar fasciitis is an inflammatory stress syndrome of the plantar fascia or plantar aponeurosis. The plantar fascia connects the toes to the heel and makes up part of the arch of the foot. Microtears and inflammation of the plantar fascia are a result of repeated traction of the plantar fascia at its insertion into the calcaneus (heel bone). The stress on the plantar fascia from the weight transfer up onto the toes causes a "whiplash" effect.

The plantar fascia is an important structure which stabilizes and locks the foot in supination prior to push-off in running. It is usually stressed with extensive foot pronation as the medial longitudinal arch collapses. Therefore this condition is seen most often in people who have a "flat foot" and/or roll in as they walk or run.

Also attached to the calcaneus is the heel cord, or Achilles tendon. This pulls in the opposite direction of the plantar fascia, and any restriction of movement will increase the stress on the plantar fascia.

Signs and Symptoms

Symptoms usually begin very gradually and are tolerated until they begin to affect one's activities. Typical symptoms include burning pain at the inside of the calcaneus on the sole of the foot, stiffness and pain in the morning or after prolonged inactivity, and pain as the athlete walks on the toes, runs hills or stairs, pushes off from a crouched position, or does cutting motions in field sports. Pain may increase with continued activity.

Some tenderness on palpation of the calcaneus is also present in a very localized area.

Other conditions that can cause similar symptoms are calcaneal stress fracture and plantar nerve entrapment (including tarsal tunnel syndrome), medial calcaneal nerve neuroma, and subtalar joint arthritis. If symptoms persist, the athlete should consult a physician to rule out these other conditions.

Management

Treatment is aimed at reduction of the inflammation, decrease of the tension on the plantar fascia, restoration of tissue strength and mobility, and controlling any biomechanical abnormality. Inflammation can be controlled with the use of ice, particularly immediately after activity. Ice can be applied as a pack for 20 minutes, or as an ice massage directly on the painful area and along the plantar fascia. Anti-inflammatory medication may help but should be taken over prolonged periods of time with caution. In cases that fail to respond to earlier treatment, a local corticosteroid injection is a treatment option. It is vital that this is done into the correct area by a qualified professional.

Stretching is important to increase flexibility and to prevent the foot from going into increased pronation to compensate for the lack of ankle movement. It is important to stretch the two muscle groups which attach to the Achilles tendon (soleus and gastrocnemius) as well as the plantar fascia itself. Stretches should be held for 30 seconds so that the soft tissues are not springing back with an elastic band effect, which happens with short, fast stretches. Strengthening exercises for the intrinsic muscles which flex the foot are important to provide increased muscle support for the arch.

Taping of the arch to prevent pronation can also help to relieve stress to the plantar fascia. Correct footwear and possibly an orthosis will help to prevent excessive pronation when walking and running. If the heel has one very tender spot, a "donut" may be used to reduce direct pressure on this point.

Rest from the repetitive activity that is causing the problem should also be part of the management. Athletes do not find this easy, but a short break from activity with other treatments will often mean a faster return to full activity. Overall fitness can be maintained through pool running, cycling, and swimming for cardiovascular training and weight lifting for maintaining strength. Running is restored through the use of a run-walk progression with hopping, skipping, and jumping activities to follow. If morning stiffness persists, the use of a night splint to maintain the foot in dorsiflexion may be helpful.

When all else has failed, and usually after 12 months of conservative care, surgery may be considered. Surgery involves the release of the plantar fascia at its origin, heel spur removal, and exploration for nerve entrapment in scar tissue.

Shoe Selection

It is important to select the correct type of shoe to minimize stress to the plantar fascia. As the problem is mostly associated with overpronation, the shoe selected should be for this type of foot. The shoe should be either board- or straight-lasted. It should have maximum rearfoot stability, substantial medial and lateral support, and the firmest midsole possible. Generally, these shoes are heavier than less supportive shoes.

Section 46.2

Metatarsalgia

Metatarsalgia describes a wide group of conditions that cause general pain to the ball of the foot. The word metatarsalgia means pain in the metatarsals, which are long bones located along the length of the foot. These long bones begin in the middle of the foot, and end at the bases of the toes. Each bone corresponds with a toe, so there are five total. Any pain that is felt in the ball of the foot, where these bones meet the toes, is often grouped together into the general condition of metatarsalgia.

Metatarsalgia can be caused by numerous separate conditions, but nearly all of them have one thing in common: the foot structure. Simply put, those with flat feet and those with high arches have a much higher chance of developing metatarsalgia than those with a more normal foot structure. Flat feet and high arches lead to increased pressure and strain to the ball of the foot. Flat feet over-stretch, leading to strain under the ball of the foot. High arched feet are much more rigid, with increased pressure to the ball of the foot the result of an inability to relax the foot structure sufficiently. Eventually, the simple daily act of walking and standing on a flat or high arched foot will lead to pain under where the metatarsals meet the toes under the ball of the foot. This area contains several structures that can become inflamed and painful as a result of this increased strain and pressure. The area where the metatarsal meet the toe is actually a joint, and the tissue that covers the joint and keeps it in place can become inflamed. This condition is called capsulitis, named after inflammation of the joint "capsule." The joint itself can also become arthritic and inflamed due to long-term wear and tear. Sometimes, the metatarsal bone is abnormally angled downward due to genetics or backwards pressure from the toe, which can lead to abnormal joint stress. Next to each joint is a nerve that can often become inflamed, and can contribute to metatarsalgia. If one is older or has certain diseases involving collagen or skin, the fat pad

471

underneath the metatarsals can be thin or displaced away from the bones it is padding. This can result in bone bruising due to abnormal pressure. The skin overlying this area on the bottom of the foot can become callused, further causing pain and discomfort. Finally, certain poorly fitting shoes can actually lead to more pressure to the ball of the foot, worsening a foot that is at risk for metatarsalgia.

Treatment for metatarsalgia revolves around addressing the specific conditions that are causing the pain. Some of this treatment, however, is universal, and applies to multiple conditions. Techniques like reducing the inflammation with icing and medication, as well as providing further foot support for the underlying foot structure problem, are usually effective. This support comes in the form of better shoes for one's specific foot structure, as well as orthotic inserts to control a flat foot or cushion a high arch. Depending on the underlying condition, other treatment may be needed, including injections, immobilization of the foot, or surgery. There is not one specific answer for this group of conditions, and multiple types of treatment is usually necessary.

Section 46.3

Sesamoiditis and Sesamoid Fracture

Introduction

The sesamoids are two small bones near the base of the big toe. They help to bear weight and act as pulleys to help move your big toe when you walk. Too much repetitive pressure, force, or tension can cause sesamoiditis, an inflammatory condition. If the impact is great enough, the bones can break (fracture). The majority of people with sesamoiditis or sesamoid fracture heal well with non-surgical treatment.

Anatomy

The sesamoids are two very small bones. They are located at the joint at the base of the big toe on the bottom of the foot. The sesamoid bones sit in two small grooves and are stabilized by a triangular shaped ligament. The sesamoid bones help form a pulley system (sesamoid apparatus) for the muscles that move the toe towards the ground when you walk. They also work with the big toe to bear the forces associated with walking.

Causes

Sesamoiditis and sesamoid fractures are most frequently caused by significant repetitive pressure and force on the ball of the foot. Ballet dancers and catchers in baseball are prone to the condition. However, it may occur from other sources of constant tension and pressure on the forefoot, such as walking, or a strong immediate force, such as falling or jumping from a height.

Symptoms

Symptoms of sesamoiditis tend to develop gradually and then intensify over time. You may experience aching increasing to intense pain located beneath your big toe and in the ball of your foot. Your pain may increase with movement. It may be difficult to bend or straighten your big toe and to walk. You may or may not experience redness and swelling in the affected area.

A sesamoid fracture causes immediate pain. You may develop a large bruise under your toe. Significant swelling throughout the forefoot may make it difficult to bend your toes or walk.

Diagnosis

Your podiatrist can diagnose sesamoiditis or a sesamoid fracture by reviewing your medical history and examining your foot. You should tell your doctor about your activities or any falls or accidents. X-rays or a bone scan will be taken to help identify a fracture.

Treatment

Sesamoiditis and sesamoid fractures are most frequently treated without surgery. Rest, over-the-counter pain medication, and ice can help reduce pain and swelling. You should wear low-heeled shoes. Your podiatrist may recommend a specific type of shoe or padding to help relieve pressure. Tape or athletic strapping may be used to keep your big toe from moving while it heals.

Steroid injections are used for severe cases of sesamoiditis. The medication relieves inflammation. Some people may need to use crutches and wear a removable short leg fracture brace or a below the knee walking cast for several weeks. Fractures require immobilization and zero weight bearing for six to eight weeks.

Surgery

Surgery is rarely used for sesamoid fractures, but in some cases it may be necessary if symptoms fail to respond to non-surgical treatments. A sesamoidectomy is a surgical procedure to remove the sesamoid bone. The toe joint may be weaker following sesamoidectomy, making it at risk for bunion formation.

Recovery

Recovery is individualized and depends on the severity of your condition, whether you have a fracture or sesamoiditis, and the treatment that you receive. Your podiatrist will let you know what to expect.

Section 46.4

Fifth Metatarsal Fracture (Jones Fracture)

"5th Metatarsal Fractures and Treatment" by David Edell, MEd, ATC, LAT, CSCS. © 2010 David Edell. Reprinted with permission from www.AthleticAdvisor.com.

Fractures of the fifth metatarsal (shaft of the small toe) are common in athletics. The method of injury is similar to that of an ankle sprain. The athlete will invert and dorsiflex the foot; this can result in a twisting force about the base of the fifth metatarsal. Do not discount pain at the base of the foot when evaluating an ankle sprain to avoid missing a fracture of the fifth.

There are four basic types of fractures that can occur to the fifth metatarsal.

- Avulsion fracture of the tuberosity of the fifth

- Jones fracture

- Shaft fracture of fifth metatarsal

- Stress fracture

All of these fractures need to be treated appropriately to avoid long-term problems.

The diagnosis of a Jones fracture has been used to describe several injuries. The true Jones fracture is a transverse fracture at the junction of the diaphysis and metaphysis of the fifth metatarsal.

This is potentially the worst fracture of the fifth metatarsal. The area in question has a very limited blood supply. Due to this healing is very slow and many times healing may not occur.

In an athlete, surgical fixation may be the first treatment option. Non-surgical treatment can consist of 6 to 16 weeks in a cast. Since this area does not heal well, many athletes treated without surgery experience recurrent fractures of this bone.

During surgery, the physician will drill a hole in the bone from the tuberosity (bump on the outside of the base of the fifth metatarsal) into the shaft of the bone. The surgeon then inserts a screw into the hole to hold the two fragments of the bone together.

The athlete is then placed in a cast, non-weight bearing for four to six weeks. During this time, the athlete is performing light range of motion and strength training exercises. After weight bearing is allowed, the athlete can begin more difficult strength training, proprioception (balance and coordination) exercises, and finally sport specific drills.

Avulsion fractures happen, most often, in a skeletally immature athlete. The peroneus brevis tendon attaches near the growth plate at the base of the fifth metatarsal. The mechanism of injury is similar to an ankle sprain. The ankle "rolls over," the peroneal muscles contract to prevent the sprain, and the growth plate is fractured.

Treatment for this injury is usually conservative. The young athlete will be casted for four to six weeks. The athlete then begins rehabilitation exercises for range of motion, strength, and proprioception. These injuries heal with little or no long-term disabilities; return to full athletic competition is normal.

Fractures to the shaft of the fifth metatarsal are the next group of injuries. Fractures can happen along the entire shaft of the bone. Treatment depends upon the location of the fracture.

Treatment can range from conservative casting and non-weight bearing to internal fixation with a screw.

Chronic pain on the outside of the foot following an acute injury can be indicative of a fracture that was missed on the initial evaluation. If the athlete continues to have low-grade pain on the outside of the foot three to six weeks after the initial injury, repeat X-rays should be taken to rule out a stress fracture.

Again, a fracture in this area may or may not heal. The bone near the fracture site is changing; this is indicative of the fracture failing to heal. A recurrent stress fracture may respond to internal fixation with better healing results than conservative treatment (casting) only.

Pain in the outside of the foot, especially after an ankle sprain, needs to be investigated. The differential evaluation should include the fifth metatarsal. Skeletally immature athletes should be evaluated by an orthopedic surgeon to rule out fractures, especially avulsion fractures of the ankle and to the base of the fifth metatarsal. Chronic pain should also be investigated to rule out a chronic stress fracture.

Section 46.5

Stress Fractures of the Foot

A stress fracture is a break in a bone caused by an accumulation of a large number of small stresses, such as occurs with repeated running and jumping. Stress fractures most commonly occur in bones of the lower leg (tibia and fibula) and feet (metatarsals). There are five metatarsal bones in the foot. Ninety percent of metatarsal stress fractures occur in the second, third, and fourth metatarsals, with the second metatarsal being the most commonly affected. Metatarsal stress fractures were first described in 1855 and termed "march fractures" since they commonly occurred in military recruits.

How It Occurs

Bones are in a continuous natural cycle of breakdown and rebuilding. High-impact, weight-bearing activities (such as running, jumping, and dancing) generate stress to the bone, causing small areas of bone breakdown. Bone rebuilding occurs naturally during the rest periods between these stressful activities. When there is repetitive stress without sufficient rest, or when there is an abrupt increase in duration or intensity of activity, bone rebuilding is not able to keep up with bone breakdown. This imbalance results in a stress fracture, a collection of tiny cracks in the bone.

Risk Factors

- Rapid increase in volume, intensity, or duration of activity
- Repeated bouts of activity with insufficient time for rest and recovery
- Change in shoes or inappropriate shoes for the activity
- Change in playing/running surface (e.g., grass to concrete)
- Change in running terrain (e.g., flat to hills)

- Inflexible or weak muscles
- High-arched feet or flat feet
- Low bone density
- Family history of osteopenia or osteoporosis

Signs and Symptoms

The main symptom is gradually worsening pain on the top of the foot. Initially the pain may only be felt with sports. Eventually it progresses to pain with daily activities such as walking. Swelling or bruising may also be present.

Diagnosis

Your doctor will review your symptoms and examine your foot. X-rays may reveal the fracture, but are not the most sensitive test. If your X-rays are normal but your signs and symptoms suggest a stress fracture, an MRI [magnetic resonance imaging] or bone scan can confirm the diagnosis.

Treatment

Treatment of a metatarsal stress fracture requires a period of rest from your activity, usually at least three to four weeks. If there is pain with daily activities you may need to use crutches or a walking boot for a short period of time, until you can walk comfortably without pain. Ice can be helpful in reducing pain. Anti-inflammatory medications are not recommended in the treatment of stress fractures. This initial period of rest is followed by a gradual return to activity over the next two to four weeks. Depending on your individual risk factors, your doctor may prescribe a change in shoewear, inserts for your shoes, or a course of physical therapy to correct any imbalances in muscle strength and flexibility. It is important that you maintain a healthy diet, with an adequate amount of calories and calcium (1,300 mg/day if you are 9–18 years old; 1,000 mg/day if you are 19–50 years old). Most metatarsal stress fractures heal completely with this non-operative treatment. Rarely, they will require surgical repair.

Returning to Activity and Sports

The goal is to return you to your sport or activity as quickly and safely as possible. If you return to activities too soon or play with pain, the stress fracture may not heal. An unhealed stress fracture can lead to chronic pain, may require surgery, and/or may result in difficulty returning to sports. Everyone recovers from injury at a different rate. Return to your sport or activity will be determined by how soon your stress fracture recovers, not by how many days or weeks it has been since the injury occurred. In general, the longer you have symptoms before starting treatment the longer it will take to get better. You will be able to safely return to your sport/activity when your pain is resolved and the doctor's examination of your foot is normal. Remember that return to your sport will be gradual, starting at a very low level, and building by small amounts each week. This gradual increase conditions the bone, allowing it to become even stronger, which protects it from reinjury.

Preventing Metatarsal Stress Fractures

- Increases in activity should happen in small, incremental steps (no more than 10%–15% increase in volume, duration, or intensity of activity per week).

- Changes to playing/running surface or terrain should be done gradually.

- Rest from your activity for at least one to two days each week.

- Wear shoes that are appropriate for the activity (e.g., run in running shoes, play basketball in basketball shoes). Runners should replace their shoes every 300–500 miles.

- Stay physically fit.

- Eat a well-balanced diet with an adequate amount of calcium (1,300 mg/day if you are 9–18 years old; 1,000 mg/day if you are 19–50 years old).

- Stretch muscles that are tight. Your doctor can show you how to stretch your calf and thigh muscles. The best time to stretch is after a warm-up or at the end your workout.

- Do not play through pain. Pain is a sign of injury, stress, or overuse. Rest is required to allow time for the injured area to heal. If pain does not resolve after a couple days of rest, consult your physician. The sooner an injury is identified, the sooner proper treatment can begin. The result is shorter healing time and faster return to sport.

Chapter 47

Toe Injuries

Chapter Contents

Section 47.1

Turf Toe

Turf toe is a sprain of the metatarsophalangeal (MTP) joint of the first toe. That is, the joint of the toe to the foot is sprained. The injury usually results from a hyperflexion mechanism; the toe is bent too far upward. This can result from a hard push off on a rigid surface, having the toe forcibly flexed while being tackled, or by stopping short allowing the toe to jam in the toe box of the shoe. These mechanisms cause damage to the ligaments of the joint and the joint capsule.

The first MTP joint is instrumental in all sports that involve foot contact with the ground. The great toe is the final structure in contact with the ground on push-off. Due to this, up to eight times a person's body weight may be transferred through the first MTP joint. Contact sport athletes are at a greater risk of injury of the first MTP due to the possibility that during contact, the joint may be forcibly hyperflexed.

The joint is comprised of four bones, nine ligaments, and three muscular attachments. This makes for a very complex joint. Of the four bones, two are sesamoid bones that are encapsulated within tendon. A common example of a sesamoid is the patella, or kneecap. Sesamoids serve as fulcrums to increase the power of the muscles that cross them.

The sesamoids are contained within the flexor hallucis brevis tendon and are connected to the under side of the toe by a ligament. Other muscles of the great toe are the adductor hallucis and abductor hallucis. The ligaments of the first MTP are comprised of two collaterals (located on either side of the joint) and two plantar (on the underside) ligaments. Their attachments combined with the muscular attachments make the great toe a strong yet flexible structure.

It is the amount of flexibility that may lead to easier injuries. The great toe usually has approximately 80 degrees of flexion. It is when this normal range is passed that injury occurs. Another factor in the injury process is the amount of support offered by the athlete's shoes.

Worn out shoes allow too much freedom of motion in the forefoot area. This lack of support will assist in transference of forces from the shoe to the foot, increasing the likelihood of injury.

The amount of force is directly proportional to the extent of the injury. The grades of injury are listed in Table 47.1.

Table 47.1. Grades of Turf Toe Injury

Grade	Signs and Symptoms	Tissue Damage
1	Plantar or medial pain, minimal swelling, negative X-rays	Stretched joint capsule and ligaments
2	General tenderness, moderate swelling, loss of motion, bruising	Partially torn capsule and ligaments, with no joint surface injury
3	Severe pain, severe swelling and bruising, loss of motion	Ruptured ligaments, joint surface injury, possible joint dislocation

Treatment of the injury begins with proper assessment of the extent of the injury. Determining if it is a first-, second-, or third-degree sprain is instrumental in returning the athlete to play that day or scheduling a physician's appointment.

The immediate treatment for all grades of sprains is the same: rest, ice, compression, and elevation. This is the standard for acute care of any athletic injury.

First-Degree Sprains

A first-degree sprain usually results in very little time loss. The athlete must be able to run and change direction properly prior to return to competition. Application of ice and taping the toe may be enough treatment for return to competition on the day of the injury. Also, spring steel shoe inserts can be of great benefit to reduce the forces applied to the joint.

Second-Degree Sprains

This type of injury often leads to time loss. This is due to the greater amount of tissue damage suffered. This athlete may need crutches for walking and should be seen by a physician to rule out a bony fracture. When the athlete can run and change direction without pain and loss of mobility, he/she may return to participation with the toe taped and a steel shoe insert.

Third Degree Sprains

These injuries are severe and may be a season ending injury. It must be determined if the joint surfaces have been damaged. If so, early return to participation may result in severe degenerative arthritis and the loss of a career. Surgery may be required to repair the torn ligaments and tendons.

Rehabilitation

Rehabilitation for this injury is fairly simple. Acutely, ice and restriction of motion of the joint is critical in the healing process. As mentioned previously, crutches for walking may be necessary for a period of one to two weeks.

After the acute stage, it is necessary to return full strength and range of motion to the toe, foot, and ankle. During the acute phase lower body strength and endurance will decrease. Utilizing a stationary bicycle for aerobic conditioning is advised. Strength training in a non-weight-bearing fashion for the affected limb is also appropriate. The strength of the foot and ankle should be addressed with Theraband® and range of motion exercises.

For the first MTP itself, gentle range of motion exercises should be instituted as pain allows. These are necessary to prevent hallux rigidus, a condition that arises when the joint is not moving properly. This can also result in degenerative arthritis of the MTP. Have the athlete bend the toe gently within the limits of pain. As the pain decreases, the amount of motion increases.

As mentioned, toe taping and spring steel shoe inserts will assist in supporting the toe and allow the athlete to return to participation sooner.

Section 47.2

Toe and Forefoot Fractures

"Toe and Forefoot Fractures," reproduced with permission from *Your Orthopaedic Connection*. © American Academy of Orthopaedic Surgeons (www.aaos.org), Rosemont, IL, 2001. Reviewed by David A. Cooke, MD, FACP, October 2011.

Nearly one-fourth of all the bones in your body are in your feet, which provide you with both support and movement. A broken (fractured) bone in your forefoot (metatarsals) or in one of your toes (phalanges) is often painful but rarely disabling. Most of the time, these injuries heal without operative treatment.

Types of Fractures

Stress fractures frequently occur in the bones of the forefoot that extend from your toes to the middle of your foot. Stress fractures are like tiny cracks in the bone surface. They can occur with sudden increases in training (such as running or walking for longer distances or times), improper training techniques, or changes in training surfaces. Most other types of fractures extend through the bone. They may be stable (no shift in bone alignment) or displaced (bone ends no longer line up). These fractures usually result from trauma, such as dropping a heavy object on your foot, or from a twisting injury. If the fractured bone does not break through the skin, it is called a closed fracture.

Several types of fractures occur to the forefoot bone on the side of the little toe (fifth metatarsal). Ballet dancers may break this bone during a misstep or fall from a pointe position. An ankle-twisting injury may tear the tendon that attaches to this bone and pull a small piece of the bone away. A more serious injury in the same area is a Jones fracture, which occurs near the base of the bone and disrupts the blood supply to the bone. This injury may take longer to heal or require surgery.

Symptoms

Pain, swelling, and sometimes bruising are the most common signs of a fracture in the foot. If you have a broken toe, you may be able to walk, but this usually aggravates the pain. If the pain, swelling, and discoloration continue for more than two or three days, or if pain interferes with walking, something could be seriously wrong; see a doctor as soon as possible. If you delay getting treatment, you could develop persistent foot pain and arthritis. You could also change the way you walk (your gait), which could lead to the formation of painful calluses on the bottom of your foot or other injuries.

Diagnosis

The doctor will examine your foot to pinpoint the central area of tenderness and compare the injured foot to the normal foot. You should tell the doctor when the pain started, what you were doing at the time, and if there was any injury to the foot. X-rays will show most fractures, although a bone scan may occasionally be needed to identify stress fractures. Usually, the doctor will be able to realign the bone without surgery, although in severe fractures, pins or screws may be required to hold the bones in place while they heal.

Treatment

See a doctor as soon as possible if you think that you have a broken bone in your foot or toe. Until your appointment, keep weight off the leg and apply ice to reduce swelling. Use an ice pack or wrap the ice in a towel so it does not come into direct contact with the skin. Apply the ice for no more than 20 minutes at a time. Take an analgesic such as aspirin or ibuprofen to help relieve the pain. Wear a wider shoe with a stiff sole.

Rest is the primary treatment for stress fractures in the foot. Stay away from the activity that triggered the injury, or any activity that causes pain at the fracture site, for three to four weeks. Substitute another activity that puts less pressure on the foot, such as swimming. Gradually, you will be able to return to activity. Your doctor or coach may be able to help you pinpoint the training errors that caused the initial problem so you can avoid a recurrence.

The bone ends of a displaced fracture must be realigned and the bone kept immobile until healing takes place. If you have a broken toe, the doctor will "buddy-tape" the broken toe to an adjacent toe, with a gauze pad between the toes to absorb moisture. You should replace the gauze and tape as often as needed. Remove or replace the tape if swelling increases and the toes feel numb or look pale. If you are diabetic or have peripheral neuropathy (numbness of the toes), do not tape the toes together. You may need to wear a rigid flat-bottom orthopaedic shoe for two to three weeks.

If you have a broken bone in your forefoot, you may have to wear a short-leg walking cast, a brace, or a rigid, flat-bottom shoe. It could take six to eight weeks for the bone to heal, depending on the location and extent of the injury. After a week or so, the doctor may request another set of X-rays to ensure that the bones remain properly aligned. As symptoms subside, you can put some weight on the leg. Stop if the pain returns.

Surgery is rarely required to treat fractures in the toes or forefoot. However, when it is necessary, it has a high degree of success.

Part Nine

Diagnosis, Treatment, and Rehabilitation of Sports Injuries

Chapter 48

Imaging and Diagnostic Tests

Chapter Contents

Section 48.1

Arthrogram

This section excerpted from "Arthrogram: Consumer Information." Contributors: Associate Professor Howard Galloway, MBBS, FRANZCR, Ms. Ann Revell, Dr. Christine Walker, and Professor Stacy Goergen. © 2009 Royal Australian and New Zealand College of Radiologists. Reprinted with permission from InsideRadiology (www.insideradiology.com.au). This material was written to provide information for health consumers. This information is of a general nature only and is not intended as a substitute for medical advice. It is designed to support, not replace, the relationship that exists between a patient and his/her doctor. It is recommended that any specific questions regarding your procedure be discussed with your family doctor or medical specialist.

What is an arthrogram?

An arthrogram is a diagnostic test which examines the inside of a joint (e.g., shoulder, knee, wrist, ankle) to assess an injury or a symptom you may be experiencing.

The test is done by first injecting contrast medium (or "dye" as it is sometimes called) which outlines the soft tissue structures in the joint (e.g., ligaments and cartilage) and makes them clearer to see on the images or pictures that will be taken of the joint. This is usually done using fluoroscopy. Fluoroscopy uses X-rays to transmit moving images onto a screen to guide the placement of the needle containing the contrast medium. This may also be done using computed tomography (CT) or ultrasound for guidance.

The exact technique will vary from doctor to doctor and also depend on the joint being injected.

This is then followed by a magnetic resonance imaging (MRI) or CT scan.

While an MRI or CT scan without the use of contrast medium can provide information on the soft tissue structures, using contrast medium with MRI or CT (an arthrogram) may provide more information about what is wrong with the joint.

How do I prepare for an arthrogram?

Generally no specific preparation is required.

Normally you should have already had at least a plain X-ray of the joint and often an ultrasound, CT scan, or MRI to assess any pain or other symptom you may be experiencing. If so you should bring these scans with you to your arthrogram appointment.

It may be best to wear comfortable clothing with easy access to the joint being examined.

What happens during an arthrogram?

Generally you will be asked to lie down and the skin over the joint being examined will be cleaned with an antiseptic solution. Following this a local anesthetic may be injected into the skin to numb the area where the contrast medium will be injected. You may feel a slight stinging sensation.

Then using X-ray, ultrasound, MRI, or CT for guidance, a needle will be placed into the joint and after ensuring the needle is in the right place the contrast medium will be injected into the joint.

The injection may be accompanied by a feeling of fullness in the joint but should not be painful.

The contrast medium used depends on the exact nature of the arthrogram and the specialist doctor performing the arthrogram. This is generally iodinated contrast medium.

If you are having an MRI arthrogram, this will be followed by a very dilute mixture of MRI contrast (gadolinium chelates) together with sterile saline (mildly salty water). If you are having a CT arthrogram, occasionally air is injected either on its own, or with a small amount of X-ray contrast prior to the scan.

Following the injections you will be taken to either the MRI suite (for an MRI arthrogram), or the CT suite (for a CT arthrogram), where the scan of the joint will be performed.

Are there any after effects of an arthrogram?

Many people have a sore joint as the reason for the examination. Most patients feel some mild to moderate increase in soreness in the joint for 24–48 hours following the injection. The joint will then return to feeling the way it was before the examination.

How long does an arthrogram take?

The arthrogram itself usually takes about 15 minutes. You may then have to wait a short time before having the scan performed. A subsequent MRI scan may take 30–45 minutes and a CT scan may take

15 minutes, depending on the joint and the number of scans that have to be done. You should allow approximately two hours from arrival at the radiology department.

What are the risks of arthrography?

Arthrography is a very safe procedure and complications are unusual.

The most serious complication is an infection of the joint. This is usually caused by organisms from the patient's skin being transferred into the joint and for this reason the procedure should not be carried out if there is broken or infected skin overlying the joint.

The risk of infection is not precisely known but the best available information suggests that it is in the order of 1 in 40,000 people having the test.

Occasionally people may be allergic to the contrast medium that is injected, and this most commonly results in a rash but may be more serious. The risk of minor reaction (e.g., hives) has been reported in 1 in 2,000 having the test. More serious reactions appear to be very rare.

Complications of gadolinium contrast medium used in an MRI have not been reported in the very small amounts used in arthrography.

What are the benefits of an arthrogram?

The injection of contrast medium into the joint makes the subsequent scan more sensitive in detecting damage to the internal structure of the joint.

Some common reasons for an arthrogram in addition to the scan are:

- in the shoulder (where the joint is unstable or if an ultrasound or plain MRI has not shown a suspected tendon tear);

- in the hip (to show any tear of the cartilage labrum, or rim of the joint);

- in the wrist (to show any tear of the small ligaments of the wrist).

There are many other individual situations where your referring doctor may feel that the additional information obtained by an arthrogram may help to determine the best course of treatment.

Who does the arthrogram?

A radiologist (specialist doctor) will perform the arthrogram, injecting the contrast medium into the joint. The radiologist is also responsible for ensuring that the appropriate scans are performed following the injection and for analyzing the scans and preparing a formal report of the findings, which is sent to the doctor who referred you for the test.

Either a nurse or a radiographer may assist the radiologist in the arthrogram. The radiographer is responsible for taking the pictures in the arthrogram and the subsequent scan under the radiologist's direction.

Where is an arthrogram done?

An arthrogram is performed in the diagnostic imaging department of most public and private hospitals and at private radiology practices.

When can I expect the results of my arthrogram?

The time that it takes your doctor to receive a written report on the test or procedure you have had will vary, depending on:

- the urgency with which the result is needed;

- the complexity of the examination;

- whether more information is needed from your doctor before the examination can be interpreted by the radiologist;

- whether you have had previous X-rays or other medical imaging that needs to be compared with this new test or procedure (this is commonly the case if you have a disease or condition that is being followed to assess your progress);

- how the report is conveyed from the practice or hospital to your doctor (in other words, email, fax, or mail).

Please feel free to ask the private practice, clinic, or hospital where you are having your test or procedure when your doctor is likely to have the written report.

It is important that you discuss the results with the doctor who referred you, either in person or on the telephone, so that they can explain what the results mean for you.

Section 48.2

Bone Scan

"Bone Scan," Clinical Center, National Institutes of Health (www.cc.nih
.gov), 2000. Reviewed by David A. Cooke, MD, FACP, September 2011.

A bone scan helps your doctor find out if there is a tumor, infection,
or other abnormality in your bone. This scan is a safe, effective, and
painless way to make pictures of your bones. For the scan, you will
be given a compound containing a small amount of radioactivity. This
compound is used only for diagnostic purposes. The scan is done in the
nuclear medicine department.

Preparation

There is no special preparation for the scan. You may eat and drink
whatever you like.

Procedure

- In the morning, a small amount of the compound (radioisotope)
  will be given to you by vein. You will then go back to your room.

- After the injection, try to drink extra glasses of water over the next
  few hours. This will help your body rid itself of the radioactivity.

- You will return to the diagnostic imaging section at the time
  scheduled for you by the appointment clerk: about 2½ to 3 hours
  after the injection.

- Once you are in the imaging room, you will rest on a firm table
  with your head flat. During the scan, you will lie on your back.

- While you are in this position, a sensitive machine (called a
  scanner) will record the radiation given off by the radioisotope.
  Many pictures will be taken as the scanner moves from your
  head to your toes. After the scan, more pictures will be taken of
  your head and hands. You will need to stay very still while these
  pictures are being taken.

After the Procedure

There are no side effects, and the scan is painless. The only sensation you will feel will be the injection of the radioisotope in your vein. If you have questions about the procedure, please ask. Your nurse and doctor are ready to assist you at all times.

Special Instructions

- Because it uses radioactivity, this scan is not performed in pregnant women. If you are pregnant or think you might be pregnant, please inform your doctor immediately so that a decision can be made about this scan.

- Also, please inform your doctor immediately if you are breast-feeding. Some scans can be performed in breast-feeding women if they are willing to stop breast-feeding for a while.

Section 48.3

Computed Tomography (CT) Scan

This section excerpted from "Computed Tomography (CT): Questions and Answers," National Cancer Institute (www.cancer.gov), September 8, 2003. Reviewed by David A. Cooke, MD, FACP, August 2011.

What is computed tomography?

Computed tomography is a diagnostic procedure that uses special X-ray equipment to obtain cross-sectional pictures of the body. The CT computer displays these pictures as detailed images of organs, bones, and other tissues. This procedure is also called CT scanning, computerized tomography, or computerized axial tomography (CAT).

What can a person expect during the CT procedure?

During a CT scan, the person lies very still on a table. The table slowly passes through the center of a large X-ray machine. The person might hear whirring sounds during the procedure. People may be asked to hold their breath at times, to prevent blurring of the pictures.

Often, a contrast agent, or "dye," may be given by mouth, injected into a vein, given by enema, or given in all three ways before the CT scan is done. The contrast dye can highlight specific areas inside the body, resulting in a clearer picture.

Computed tomography scans do not cause any pain. However, lying in one position during the procedure may be slightly uncomfortable. The length of the procedure depends on the size of the area being X-rayed; CT scans take from 15 minutes to one hour to complete. For most people, the CT scan is performed on an outpatient basis at a hospital or a doctor's office, without an overnight hospital stay.

Are there risks associated with a CT scan?

Some people may be concerned about the amount of radiation they receive during a CT scan. It is true that the radiation exposure from a CT scan can be higher than from a regular X-ray. However, not having the procedure can be more risky than having it. People considering CT must weigh the risks and benefits.

In very rare cases, contrast agents can cause allergic reactions. Some people experience mild itching or hives (small bumps on the skin). Symptoms of a more serious allergic reaction include shortness of breath and swelling of the throat or other parts of the body. People should tell the technologist immediately if they experience any of these symptoms, so they can be treated promptly.

What is spiral CT?

A spiral (or helical) CT scan is a new kind of CT. During a spiral CT, the X-ray machine rotates continuously around the body, following a spiral path to make cross-sectional pictures of the body. Benefits of spiral CT include the following:

- It can be used to make three-dimensional pictures of areas inside the body.

- It may detect small abnormal areas better than conventional CT.

- It is faster, so the test takes less time than a conventional CT.

What is total or whole body CT? Should a person have one?

A total or whole body CT scan creates images of nearly the entire body—from the chin to below the hips. This test has not been shown to have any value as a screening tool. ("Screening" means checking for signs of a disease when a person has no symptoms.)

The American College of Radiology (as well as most doctors) does not recommend scanning a person's body on the chance of finding signs of any sort of disease. In most cases abnormal findings do not indicate a serious health problem; however, a person must often undergo more tests to find this out. The additional tests can be expensive, inconvenient, and uncomfortable. The disadvantages of total body CT almost always outweigh the benefits.

Where can people get more information about CT?

Additional information about CT is available from the CT Accreditation Department of the American College of Radiology, 1891 Preston White Drive, Reston, VA 20191-4397. The toll-free telephone number is 800-227-5463 (800-ACR-LINE). The CT Accreditation Department can be reached by e-mail at ctaccred@acr.org. The American College of Radiology website is located at www.acr.org.

Information about diagnostic radiology, including CT, is also available on the Radiology Info website at www.radiologyinfo.org. Radiology Info is the public information website of the Radiological Society of North America and the American College of Radiology.

Section 48.4

Magnetic Resonance Imaging (MRI)

Magnetic resonance imaging or MRI is a technique for creating pictures of the organs inside your body to help doctors with your medical evaluation. MR imaging uses special properties of magnetic fields and atoms inside the body to allow a computer to create pictures in a different process from the way X-rays, CT scans, and ultrasound images are made.

The MRI machine is basically a large magnet with a central opening. A computer uses the signals sent by this magnet and radio waves to make a picture of the body appear on a screen. There are no known harmful effects from exposure to the magnetic fields or radio waves used in making MR images.

Due to the strong magnetic field produced by the MRI, it cannot be used on patients who have cardiac pacemakers. Most patients with vascular clips, eye implants, heart valves, or implanted electronic devices cannot undergo MR examination. The presence of metal in your body may affect a portion of the MR image but please be sure to inform me or the radiologist if you have any metallic prostheses, magnets in your dentures, cochlear implants, artificial heart valves, or if you are pregnant.

Preparing for MR Examination

Unless given other instructions you may eat before the test and should continue to take your usual medications. When you arrive for your MR examination you will be given a hospital gown and robe to wear. You will be asked to remove your jewelry, watches, keys, hair pins, hearing aids, wallet, and any other accessories. This is necessary so that metallic objects in these items will not affect the quality of the MR picture. This includes wigs and dentures.

During the Examination

Once you are in the scan room you will be placed on a motorized table, usually lying on your back. This table slides into the opening of the magnet and depending on the parts of your body to be examined, a small device may be placed around a portion of your body. It is very important that you are as comfortable as possible at the beginning of the examination as it is essential that you lie still during the exam. The scan is very safe and there is nothing to be afraid of and the technologist will monitor you from another room. You will be able to talk to the technologist by microphone and you will not feel the magnetic field or see any moving parts around you. You will hear repetitive tapping, thumping sounds or other noises during the MR scan. These sounds come from the internal part of the magnet and will be dampened by the ear plugs you are given prior to the exam. Occasionally patients will require some sedation if they become claustrophobic.

Each examination consists of a number of scans to get the information required and the examination can take between 30 and 90 minutes. While the scan is taking place, you should breathe quietly but comfortably and not move your head or body. Most people find that after several minutes of imaging they become quite relaxed and have few problems lying still for the required period of time. Often the radiologist will need images made after a special contrast agent has been given. These contrast agents are only used in MR imaging and are different from those used in kidney tests or CT scanning because they do not contain iodine. This can be injected either through a small needle into a vein in your arm or for orthopedic purposes usually directly into the joint itself. There is a very small risk of allergic reaction or infection to these injections but the information gained by using this dye is extremely important in determining your treatment.

When the Examination Is Over

When your examination is finished you may leave. A radiologist will review the images made during your examination and report the findings.

The MRI is a high quality medical examination. It is expensive and the federal government has restricted which scanners can give a rebate for this examination. Please note that the magnetic field interferes with your credit cards and may ruin the timing mechanism in some watches.

Section 48.5

Ultrasound

Overview

Ultrasound is the name given to high frequency sound waves which are out of the range of human hearing. In medicine, an ultrasound scanner uses the sound waves to make a television image of many structures within the body. There are no known harmful effects from exposure to diagnostic ultrasound waves and they do not involve the use of X-ray or radiation.

The ultrasound scanner is a sophisticated machine; the examination is simple and painless and usually requires much less than one hour of time.

A handheld instrument called a transducer is placed against your skin after applying a lubricant and slowly passed over the area to be examined. The lubricant helps the transducer keep close contact with the skin and it will be necessary that your clothes be removed and a gown worn instead.

The majority of your scan is usually done by an ultrasound technician who has several years of education and training in the use of ultrasound. The result will be interpreted by a radiologist and a careful review of your ultrasound pictures and medical history are necessary with this interpretation.

The technologist will not give the results to you and the findings will be reported to your referring doctor.

Chapter 49

Medications for Sports Injuries

Chapter Contents

Section 49.1

Medications to Treat Sports-Related Injuries

"The Role of Medications in the Treatment of Sports-Related Injuries," by George B. Batten, MD. © 2009 Tri-Valley Orthopedic Specialists, Inc. All rights reserved. Reprinted with permission. For additional information, visit www.trivalleyorthopedics.com.

As a sideline observer, I have frequently witnessed coaches, first aid providers, and anxious parents reaching into their training bags and purses and medicating the acutely injured athlete. As an orthopedic surgeon interested in sports medicine I treat athletes who were initially prescribed medications by their primary care physicians, emergency room personnel, or have self-medicated with over-the-counter (OTC) medications or those found left over in their medicine cabinets. It is important to understand the role of medication in the treatment of sports related injuries, particularly in regards to their efficacy and, most importantly, their potential side effects. The purpose of this section is to review the classes of medications commonly used in this environment and to provide guidelines for their rational usage. While other classes of medication may be mentioned, this discussion will be focused on the most commonly used classes of drugs, pain relievers (analgesics) and anti-inflammatory medications.

Analgesics: Analgesics are used specifically for their pain-relieving property. Two subcategories exist, narcotic and non-narcotic preparations. Narcotics exist in both injectable and oral forms. Injectables include morphine, Demerol, and Dilaudid. These are almost exclusively used in emergency rooms and hospitals for the treatment of moderate to severe pain associated with acute musculoskeletal injuries or following surgical treatment. The oral forms commonly prescribed are Tylenol with codeine, Vicodin, Norco, and Lortab. Each is combined with acetaminophen to enhance its pain relieving properties. They should likewise be reserved for the treatment of moderate to severe pain. Side effects of narcotics include GI [gastrointestinal] upset, nausea, and altered consciousness. They also have the capacity for recreational drug abuse and physical addiction. Acute injuries and chronic musculoskeletal conditions requiring their usage under almost all circumstances should preclude the athlete from returning to his or her sport until the medical condition has evolved to the point where these medications are no longer necessary. One particular injury requiring special consideration is the treatment of head trauma. Because of narcotics' effect on the central nervous system, including sedation and potential mental status changes, they may interfere with the need for monitoring an injured player who has sustained this type of injury, including even minor concussions. This is particularly important in the first 24 to 48 hours following injury.

The most common non-narcotic analgesic is acetaminophen. This is marketed under its generic name, as well as the popular Tylenol brand. It has long been recognized as safe and effective in the treatment of mild to moderate pain. It is usually well tolerated and has minimal side effects or interactions with other medications. It can be safely used to supplement the pain relieving properties of nonsteroidal anti-inflammatories. Available in a liquid form, it may be useful in youth athletes who have difficulty swallowing tablets or pills. It does, however, have the potential for causing liver damage when used in dosages which exceed the maximum recommended daily dosage. In an adult, the maximum dosage should not exceed 4,000 mg (4 grams) in a 24-hour period. When used in children, parents should follow the recommended dosages included on the product's packaging. As noted, acetaminophen is frequently combined with oral narcotics. Therefore, the patient needs to be careful that this be figured into their maximum daily dosage. As will be discussed in more detail, acetaminophen has no effect on blood clotting. Whether or not an injured athlete using acetaminophen should continue to compete ultimately depends on the specific condition requiring its use.

Anti-inflammatory medications: The other class of drugs commonly used in the treatment of athletes are the anti-inflammatory medications. These exist as steroid and nonsteroidal anti-inflammatories. Anti-inflammatory steroids, however, should not be confused with the anabolic steroids recently publicized as being abused by athletes. Anti-inflammatory steroids are available only through prescription. They include the commonly prescribed oral form, prednisone, and the various preparations that are the main ingredient of "cortisone shots." Neither form has much value in the treatment of acute athletic injuries with the possible exception of severe head or spinal trauma. They may be utilized in such conditions as exercise-induced asthma, or allergic reactions to environmental substances or insect bites. When used in the proper setting under a physician's care, anti-inflammatory steroids can be extremely beneficial in the treatment of chronic athletic conditions involving inflammation such as tendinitis, bursitis, and low back pain.

Nonsteroidal anti-inflammatory medications (NSAIDs) have been available for decades. All initially came to market as prescription medication. As they lose patent protection, many are sold over the counter. The only difference between those prescribed and those sold OTC is that of dosage. The most recognized NSAIDs are ibuprofen and naproxen sodium. Ibuprofen is marketed under its generic name, as well as various brand names including Advil and Motrin. Naproxen sodium is the main ingredient of Aleve and Naprosyn. Additionally, they are commonly included in OTC cold and allergy preparations. These medications have two properties which make them useful in the treatment of sports injuries. Much like acetaminophen, they provide a direct analgesic effect. As their name implies, they are also useful in reducing inflammation most commonly associated with non-traumatic or more chronic musculoskeletal conditions. Their frequent use, therefore, in the treatment of acute athletic injuries is worth some additional attention. While soft tissue swelling is oftentimes associated with chronic inflammatory conditions, the swelling associated with acute injuries will probably be little affected by anti-inflammatory medication.

The majority of anti-inflammatory medications have an influence on the body's blood clotting system. This side effect has been publicized as being useful in the prevention of heart attacks in adult patients. While a benefit in this instance, the "blood-thinning" side effects of anti-inflammatory medications may have negative consequences in many acute sports-acquired injuries by increasing the risk of additional bleeding. This is particularly the case in those injuries such as fractures, significant muscle tears, contusions often acquired in contact sports, and even the more severe ligament sprains about the knee and ankle. In fractures and deep contusions, bleeding may cause potentially limb-threatening complications because of the buildup of excessive pressure within the tissues involved. In contusions, most notably those sustained by soccer players to the lower leg, excess bleeding may result in the formation of hematomas, localized areas of blood accumulation which the body may have difficulty resorbing, ultimately requiring surgical drainage. At the very least, excessive bleeding following these types of injuries will certainly lengthen the athlete's recovery period and prolong the time prior to return to sports. Their use following head injury is also potentially dangerous in causing additional cerebral bleeding. It is important to remember that the anticoagulation effects of anti-inflammatory medications will persist for a period of 7 to 10 days following discontinu-ation of their use. If an athlete has been taking these medications, it is possible sustaining an acute injury during that time frame might lead to undesirable increased bleeding and bruising.

When used in the proper setting, oral anti-inflammatory medica-tions can be of great benefit in the treatment of specific sports related injuries and other conditions affecting the musculoskeletal system. Aside from the specific side effect involving blood coagulation, other common side effects include gastrointestinal upset, gastrointestinal bleeding, fluid retention, and for those patients on high-dose long-term usage, the risk of liver or kidney damage. Patients using these medi-cations chronically need to be monitored. Remember that these side effects are present in both over-the-counter and prescribed forms.

Recently the lay press has highlighted the potential complications of increased risk of heart attack and stroke in patients being prescribed the newer generation of anti-inflammatory medications referred to as COX-2 inhibitors. These include the highly marketed Celebrex, Vioxx, and Bextra brands. These complications have primarily been seen in older patients with a history of pre-existing cardiac disease, taking higher doses over longer periods of time. They may still be a beneficial in patients who are at high risk for gastrointestinal complications. Of note is that the COX-2 inhibitors do not share the increased bleeding risk associated with the earlier generations of NSAIDs. Their use may therefore be of benefit in the treatment of certain athletic injuries where additional bleeding would be detrimental. This, however, must be an informed decision made between patient and physician.

Antibiotics: Antibiotics may be required in the treatment of sports-sustained lacerations and abrasions which become secondarily infected. Recently there has been concern raised over the growing incidence of infections caused by an antibiotic-resistant strain of the very common bacteria, *Staphylococcus aureus*. This is referred to as methicillin-resistant *Staphylococcus aureus* (MRSA). Infections caused by this bacteria apparently can develop without an obvious open skin wound. Many times it will be mistaken for an infected hair follicle, "pimple," or insect or spider bite. It can appear rather innocuous in the first several days following its presentation but can quickly develop into a more sig-nificant infection which can be limb- and even life-threatening. While often seen in athletes participating in close contact sports such as football and wrestling, it has been reported in almost every sport and its incidence seems to be growing at an alarming rate. Any athlete who exhibits such a condition should seek immediate medical attention.

When antibiotics have been prescribed they should be continued for the full treatment course. If an infection does not seem to be responding or certainly worsening while under treatment, this should be reported to the treating physician.

Miscellaneous OTC medications: These include the highly publicized glucosamine and chondroitin sulfate, MSM [methylsulfonylmethane], a large variety of herbal-based medications, as well as nutritional and mineral supplements. Athletes should be aware that these are poorly monitored and controlled substances. Despite the fact that they are sold OTC and marketed as containing "natural" ingredients, many of these substances can have significant side effects and drug interactions. It is important to remember that their efficacy, content, and purity are not monitored by the FDA [Food and Drug Administration]. Their value in the treatment of acute and chronic sports injuries is usually anecdotal and rarely supported by investigational or clinical studies.

Conclusion: In summary, medications can be an important part of treatment programs designed for the management of both acute and chronic sports injuries and musculoskeletal conditions. Their use and value must, however, be considered on a case-by-case basis. Potential side effects must be recognized and understood.

Analgesics are valuable in the management and control of pain associated with injury. They should not, however, be used to allow an athlete to return to sports participation prematurely. This is especially true when narcotic analgesics are required. The use of narcotic analgesics should also be avoided in acute head trauma under most circumstances, especially in the critical first 24 to 48 hours. Nonsteroidal anti-inflammatory medications are of considerable usefulness, particularly in the treatment of those conditions associated with inflammation or chronic in nature. They are probably over-prescribed, however, in the acute injury setting. Because of their potential for increased bleeding, they should be used with caution in injuries where significant bleeding may occur. Athletes and parent care providers for younger sports participants need to be aware that even OTC medications have potential side effects that can be detrimental and even dangerous when used in an improper fashion. Aside from the minor bumps and bruises that most athletes sustain during their playing careers, the utilization of medications in the treatment of athletic injuries should be discussed with physicians familiar and comfortable with their management.

Section 49.2

Injections for Pain Management

You may not like the idea of getting a shot, but injections often help relieve pain and inflammation and help improve joint movement. To control your pain, your doctor can inject medication directly into the problem area instead of prescribing pills to be taken by mouth. Injections are not a cure, but they can help you through a period of intense pain. Often, injections offer an alternative to patients whose only other choice to relieve pain is surgery. Injections also offer relief to patients for whom surgery is not a viable option because of other health conditions. Injections are used to relieve knee pain, low back pain, hip pain, and many other conditions resulting from acute injuries, overuse injuries, and medical conditions such as arthritis.

What Are Injections Used For?

Injections can be used to diagnose as well as to treat injuries and illnesses. Injections are sometimes used to learn more about what is causing your pain and how it can be treated. For example, if an injection provides pain relief in the area that is injected, it is likely that the area is the source of the problem. On the other hand, if the injection does not relieve the pain at the injection site, the pain could be the result of nerve damage, which can mean the pain traveled to that area of the body from another area. Therapeutic injections are used as treatments for temporary relief from pain and are typically divided into three categories based on the part of the body that is injected. Joint injections, soft tissue injections, and nerve block injections are common treatments for the relief of inflammation and pain.

Joint Injections

An adult over age 45 often experiences arthralgia or joint pain. Many types of injuries or conditions can cause joint pain. For example, rheumatoid arthritis is an autoimmune disorder that causes pain and stiffness in the joints, and osteoarthritis involves the growth of bone spurs and degeneration of cartilage at the joint, causing severe pain. An injection of corticosteroid medication is often prescribed to help relieve the pain caused by different types of arthritis, or it can be prescribed after an injury or surgery.

Corticosteroid medications imitate the effects of the hormones cortisone and hydrocortisone, which are produced by your adrenal glands. Corticosteroids can be injected into affected joints, such as the shoulder, elbow, hip, or knee, and can relieve pain for four to six months.

Injections are often given in the hip joint to relieve pain resulting from arthritis. The most common disease that affects the hip, arthritis is a degenerative disease that can cause pain, stiffness, inflammation, and damage to the joint cartilage (the smooth tissue at the ends of bones that allows them to glide against one another). Such damage can lead to joint weakness, instability, and visible deformities that can interfere with basic daily tasks such as walking, climbing stairs, sitting, rising from a chair, or getting out of bed.

Usually, three injections of a corticosteroid are given over a three-week period. The procedure is performed under fluoroscopy (visual diagnostic examination on a screen or monitor) while the patient lies on his or her back on the fluoroscopic table. After the hip is cleaned with iodine and alcohol, the needle is advanced into the hip joint. Often, a small amount of water-soluble contrast (dye) is injected to confirm proper needle location. Then, the needle is slowly withdrawn. The entire procedure only takes minutes, but the benefits can last for months.

Soft Tissue Injections

Bursitis, or inflammation of the bursa, causes nagging joint pain. You have more than 150 bursae (small, fluid-filled sacs) in your body, which cushion the pressure points between your bones and the tendons and muscles near your joints. When a bursa becomes inflamed, movement or pressure on the affected joint can be painful. Bursitis most often affects the shoulder, elbow, or hip. Injections of corticosteroid can help reduce the inflammation and pain.

Trigger Point Injections

Trigger point injections are prescribed when your muscles are sensitive and painful to the touch. Depending on the medication used, trigger point injections can reduce pain and inflammation in your muscle or can relax a muscle. A combined injection of anesthetic and corticosteroid medication can reduce pain and promote increased range of motion. Because the corticosteroid can take three to four days to begin reducing the inflammation and providing relief, anesthetic is also given for the pain until the inflammation can be controlled. Sometimes an anesthetic alone is used if there is little or no inflammation and the goal is to relax the muscle for effective stretching.

Nerve Block Injections

A nerve block prevents pain messages from traveling along a nerve pathway and reaching your brain. Nerve blocks are often used to relieve pain for a short period, such as during surgery. If there is inflammation around a nerve, an injection of corticosteroid medication in conjunction with the nerve block anesthetic can provide longer relief.

There are three major types of nerve blocks, peripheral, spinal, and sympathetic. Peripheral injections are used for localized pain and are injected away from the spine. For pain that affects a broad area, an anesthetic is injected in or near the spine. An injection directly into the spinal fluid is called an intrathecal injection. An intrathecal injection is often used during surgery on the abdomen or legs.

The sympathetic nervous system controls circulation and perspiration and is part of your autonomic nervous system. An injection of an anesthetic to block the sympathetic nerves can relieve chronic pain caused by diseases such as complex regional pain syndrome, which affects your sympathetic nervous system.

Side Effects

You can experience side effects after an injection, such as an infection, an allergic reaction, local bleeding, or skin discoloration. Not everyone develops side effects, and symptoms vary from person to person. Side effects rarely occur if injections are given less than every three to four months. However, if injections are given more frequently you could experience weakened ligaments, tendons, and bones.

Some people simply don't like shots, while others have serious phobias about injections. Despite any fear you may have, if your doctor recommends an injection, you should consider the benefits. You may experience some pain initially during the procedure, but that only lasts minutes. On the other hand, if you have the injection, you could get a shot of relief that lasts for months.

Chapter 50

Specialized Surgical Treatments and Therapy

Chapter Contents

513

Section 50.1

Arthroscopic Surgery

What is arthroscopy?

Surgeons use arthroscopy as a means of seeing inside joints. Initially used as a diagnostic tool, Japanese surgeon Watanabe developed the technique of knee arthroscopy in the 1960s. More extensive procedures were popularized in the 1980s. Each year orthopaedic surgeons perform more than five million arthroscopies.

During an arthroscopic procedure a small device called an arthroscope is inserted into a joint through a small cut. The tiny lens and fiber optic light of the arthroscope is connected to a camera and monitor that allows the orthopaedic surgeon to see inside the joint and perform a variety of different procedures.

When do you need arthroscopy?

While many different conditions in many kinds of joints can be treated with an arthroscopic procedure, it is not right for every problem or every patient. A surgeon can tell if the problem can be treated with arthroscopy or if a more invasive approach may be better. Surgeons sometimes still use arthroscopy as a diagnostic tool, occasionally performing both arthroscopy and an open procedure afterward. Knee arthroscopy for a torn meniscus remains one of the most common orthopaedic procedures. The knee and the shoulder are the most common arthroscopy areas with more than 4 million knee arthroscopies and 1.4 million shoulder arthroscopies performed annually, worldwide. Most large or medium sized joints, such as knees and shoulders, can be repaired using arthroscopic approaches.

What are the advantages of arthroscopy?

With the small incisions needed for arthroscopic procedures, these surgeries are typically less painful than similar open procedures. Arthroscopy also affords the surgeon an outstanding view of the inside of the joint with many different specialized techniques, procedures, and instruments. In most cases, surgery that years ago was done through an open approach now can be done via an arthroscopic approach, with similar long-term outcomes, decreased post-operative pain, and shorter hospital stays. Additionally, most arthroscopies are outpatient procedures.

What kind of anesthesia is available?

Many arthroscopic surgeries are done using regional anesthesia during which only the area or extremity that is being operated on is anesthetized. General anesthetic may be preferred in some cases. A surgeon and anesthesiologist will work with you prior to surgery to determine the best solution.

What are the potential complications of arthroscopy?

Complications during or after most arthroscopic surgeries are rare; however, every surgery has risks. The complications which can occur during or following an arthroscopic procedure include:

- blood clots;
- infection;
- joint stiffness;
- damage to nerves or blood vessels.

What can be expected following surgery?

Healing is different from patient to patient and from procedure to procedure. Even though the incisions are small, a surgeon may have done a large amount of work inside the joint. This can include tendon repair and reconstruction or joint articular cartilage surgery. The procedure performed will dictate a rehabilitation schedule much more than the size of the incisions. Every person is different, so be sure to ask the surgeon what to expect and when various activities are allowed post-operatively.

Section 50.2

Meniscal Repair

Function

The meniscus is a soft rubbery structure between the femur and tibia. There is one on both sides of the knee, medial and lateral. Meniscal tears are very common. The meniscus is often incorrectly referred to as cartilage in the community. Cartilage is the smooth lining of the joint at the ends of the bone.

The meniscus acts as a...

- shock absorber to take some of the force within the knee;

- stabilizer of the knee;

- assists with lubrication

Once a meniscus is torn, it no longer functions as it should and, if symptomatic, is best partially removed. Because the meniscus has a very poor blood supply it is unlikely it will heal itself. Tears are described according to the type of tear as simple or complex. Without the meniscus, there is an increased risk of osteoarthritis in the long term. The severity and timing of arthritis depends on numerous factors such as your age, activity levels, weight, and degree of meniscal damage. This is usually a very slow process.

History of Injury

There does not need to be a specific injury. Athletes usually but not always tear their meniscus with a specific injury, usually a twisting force, but in older people it can result from minimal or no trauma. Some people will feel a pop or something go in the knee. The pain is not usually severe, and most people can continue with sports or at least can walk around without too much pain.

Symptoms and Signs

- Swelling usually begins the next day and is usually not severe.

- Pain is usually localized to the side of the knee where the tear is.

- Locking of the knee is when the knee gets stuck so you can't move it, usually it can't be straightened. This is because a fragment of the meniscus gets stuck between the bones.

- Giving way is usually caused by pain.

- Clicking can be a symptom.

Diagnosis

This can usually be made on the history and examination. An MRI [magnetic resonance imaging] test may be ordered to confirm the diagnosis and to exclude other pathology but this is not always necessary and may delay treatment.

Treatment

Initial treatment involves rest, ice, elevation, and bandaging. There is no urgency to be seen by a surgeon unless you have a locked knee, in which case you can damage the meniscus as it gets caught between the bones of the knee joint.

Most meniscal tears require an arthroscopy (see "Arthroscopy" at www.orthosports.com.au/Content_Common/pg-knee-arthroscopy.seo). The torn meniscus can be partially removed or repaired.

Meniscal Repair

Because the meniscus has a poor blood supply it has a limited potential to heal. Only tears in the outer half of the meniscus have the potential to heal. The decision to attempt a repair is based on age, activity levels, occupation, and sporting demands.

Most patients with a repairable meniscus are under 45 years of age and up to 80% of these are associated with a tear of the anterior cruciate ligament. An MRI scan helps determine the extent of the tear, but the final decision to repair cannot be made until the time of surgery as it depends on the size, site, and the quality of the remaining meniscus. There is no point in repairing a meniscus which is unlikely to heal.

Repair can usually be performed arthroscopically without any separate incisions using special devices, but occasionally one or two other incisions in the skin may be required. There are advantages and disadvantages of meniscal suture.

Advantages

- Maintain protective role of meniscus
- Reduces the risk of arthritis

Disadvantages

- Longer rehabilitation period
- Longer restriction of work and sport activities
- Failure of the meniscus to heal (15%–20%) due to its poor blood supply
- Slightly increased risk to neurovascular structures
- Damage to articular surface from some of the devices used

Overall, if a meniscus can be repaired (in the right patient with the right type of tear), it is best to do so as it protects the knee from premature arthritis.

Post-Op

The post-op instructions will vary from one knee to another depending on the extent of the repair and damage to other structures. Usually the surgery is done as a day-only procedure. You may require crutches and a splint. Your weight bearing and bending may be restricted again depending on the extent of the repair. Time required off work varies from a few days to a few months depending on your occupation. Sporting activities can resume at three to six months.

If your meniscus does not heal, you may develop ongoing symptoms and require further arthroscopic surgery to remove the torn portion of the meniscus which has not healed.

Complications

Any surgical procedure has a risk of complications. These are rare with an arthroscopy; however, they can occur. Every precaution is taken to minimize the risk. Complications can be related to the anesthetic, general in nature as can happen with any surgery or specific to knee arthroscopy.

Surgical Complications

- **Bleeding:** Bleeding into the joint can occur as a result of the surgery. A small amount of bleeding is not uncommon; however, if your knee becomes swollen and tight, you should rest, elevate, and ice it. The knee may need to be drained in the rooms and occasionally a repeat arthroscopy is needed.

- **Oozing:** Oozing from incisions can occur and is usually not a problem. You can change the dressing yourself using antiseptic or have your local doctor do it if you are concerned.

- **Infection:** Infection is rare. If you become unwell, or the knee becomes increasingly swollen or red, you should be assessed as soon as possible. It can cause damage to the surfaces of the joint and result in stiffness. Treatment involves antibiotics and often further surgery.

- **Damage to vessels or nerves:** Damage to vessels or nerves can occur, particularly with meniscal suturing. This can result in numbness in the skin and weakness in the lower leg. Some numbness, tingling, or irritation around the skin cuts can occur but significant damage to major structures is extremely rare.

- **Reflex sympathetic dystrophy:** This is a condition resulting from overactivity of the nerves around the operative site. Its cause is not well understood by the medical profession and it is difficult to treat. Fortunately it is very rare after arthroscopy.

- **Deep venous thrombosis:** DVT or blood clots in the leg can cause calf pain and swelling, which damage vessels or nerves. These are also rare after arthroscopy. If they do occur you may require blood-thinning medication in the form of injections or tablets.

- **Failure to relieve pain:** This is not common but unfortunately some operations may not be entirely successful in relieving pain. Some knees may require further investigation or even a repeat arthroscopy.

- **Allergic reactions:** Allergic reactions to medications or materials used in the operating room.

- **Joint stiffness:** Joint stiffness can occur no matter what the procedure; this is minimized and treated with physiotherapy.

- **Pressure:** Pressure on areas of the body in the operating theater causing nerve damage.

519

- **Diathermy burns:** Diathermy burns from cautery device used in most open operations (very rare).

- **Limp:** Limp can occur from muscle weakness.

Any medical complication you have heard about can occur, especially if you already have a pre-existing medical problem. Such complications include heart attack, stroke, kidney failure, pneumonia, bowel obstruction, bladder infection or obstruction, etc. Serious medical problems can lead to ongoing health concerns, prolonged hospitalization, or rarely death.

Section 50.3

ACL Repair

Introduction

The anterior cruciate ligament (ACL) is one of the major stabilizing ligaments in the knee. It is a strong ropelike structure located in the center of the knee running from the femur to the tibia.

The anterior cruciate ligament prevents the femur moving forward and rotating abnormally on the tibia. The ACL is required for normal function of the knee. One of the main functions of the ACL is to provide stability during rotational movements such as turning, twisting, and sidestepping.

When it ruptures it does not heal itself and the knee often becomes unstable or gives way. Repeated giving way can lead to damage to other structures of the knee and eventually arthritis. Since the knee "dislocates" when the ligament ruptures there is often damage to other structures in the knee such as bone, cartilage, or meniscus. These injuries may also need to be addressed at the time of surgery.

History of Injury

Usually there is a significant injury involving a twisting force to the knee. It can also occur after landing from a jump, stopping rapidly, or direct contact such as in a tackle. It is particularly common in sports such as football, soccer, basketball, netball, and skiing but can occur in many other activities.

When the ACL ruptures the patient often feels something giving way in the knee or hears a popping sound. Most people cannot continue with their activity and the knee generally swells up within hours.

Initial Management

The knee should be treated with ice, elevation, and a compressive bandage. Crutches and analgesics usually are required. An X-ray is necessary to exclude an associated fracture. Physiotherapy is helpful to reduce swelling and regain motion.

Most patients will be referred to an orthopedic surgeon for diagnosis and assessment of the injury. Careful clinical examination is required to detect damage to the ACL, other ligaments, and structures in the knee such as the meniscus or articular cartilage. It is quite common to damage some of these other structures.

Diagnosis

This can usually be made on history and clinical examination. An MRI scan, which is a special imaging test, is often ordered to confirm the diagnosis in patients where the examination is not conclusive. It also demonstrates damage to other structures such as the menisci or articular cartilage. The diagnosis can also be made with an arthroscopy.

Treatment Recommendations

Most patients who tear their ACL during sport will elect to have it surgically reconstructed, to enable them to return to full activities with a stable knee. Other patients choose to modify their activities and give up sport to avoid further episodes of instability.

In general, the younger and more active you are then the stronger the recommendation for reconstruction. It is generally recommended to have surgery if you wish to get back to sports which involve twisting and pivoting. Many patients who do not have surgery find that their knee becomes more loose over time. This can lead to a knee that gives way during ordinary activities of daily living. These patients should strongly consider surgery to stabilize the knee.

Repeated instability or abnormal movement in the knee can cause ongoing damage leading to stretching of other structures around the knee, meniscal tears, or arthritis in the long term. If you do not elect to have surgery it is strongly advised that you give up sports that involve pivoting, sidestepping, or rotation.

It is also recommended that people with dangerous occupations such as policemen, firemen, roof tilers, and scaffolders have surgery. This is a safety issue to prevent instability in "at risk" situations.

There is no urgency in performing this operation and in fact it is sometimes better to allow the knee to settle down and regain close to full motion prior to surgery. Your surgeon will advise you on the timing in your particular case.

Pre-Op Instructions

- Cease aspirin and anti-inflammatory medications (e.g., voltaren, feldene) 10 days prior to surgery as they can cause bleeding.

- Cease any naturopathic or herbal medications 10 days before surgery as these can also cause bleeding.

- Continue with all other medications unless otherwise specified.

- Notify your surgeon if you have any abrasions or pimples around the knee.

- Please bring any X-rays, MRI scans, or other investigations you have had done which may be relevant to your surgery.

- Bring a list of medications with you to give to the anesthetist.

You are advised to stop smoking for as long as possible prior to surgery.

The hamstring tendons are harvested through a small incision just below the knee and are fashioned into a new graft which takes the place of your old cruciate ligament. Tunnels (holes) are then drilled in the tibia and femur (the two bones making up the knee joint) and the graft is passed trough this tunnel. The graft is then fixed with various devices at each end to stabilize it and allow it to heal to the bone. The fixation devices vary and are surgeon specific.

This surgery is mainly done using an arthroscope using small incisions approximately one centimeter each. The inside of the knee is thoroughly visualized and any other problems such as meniscal tears or damage to the joint lining (articular) cartilage are treated at the same time.

After Surgery

During surgery local anesthetic is injected into the knee to reduce the amount of pain you will feel. Pain-relieving medication will be provided for you both in hospital and at home.

There may be a drain in your knee which will be removed prior to discharge. You will have a dressing on your wound and a compressive wrap.

Most patients go home the day following surgery but some may go home the same day.

You will be seen by a physiotherapist prior to discharge who will teach you how to use crutches and show you some simple exercises to do at home. Your dressing should be left intact until your first post-operative visit.

Ice packs should be used regularly to reduce swelling.

Your graft is strong enough to put all your weight on your operated leg. You can walk around but rest as much as possible for the first week and elevate your leg when sitting. Most patients require crutches for a week or so.

Pain is variable and prescription painkillers may be required for a week or two.

You may shower but not bathe or swim prior to your review. It is normal to have blood under the dressing. If there is excessive ooze the dressings can be changed by someone experienced in wound care. If concerned please contact your surgeon.

You will be followed up in the rooms about 10 days after your operation when the dressings will be removed and the wounds inspected. The surgery and any other findings will be explained to you.

If there is any redness, increased swelling, or you have temperatures you should contact the rooms or the hospital where the surgery was performed so they can contact your surgeon.

Time off work depends on your work requirements and is very variable. Office workers usually require two weeks off work and manual laborers two to three months or longer.

Rehabilitation

Physiotherapy is an integral part of the treatment and is recommended to start as early as possible. Preoperative physiotherapy is helpful to better prepare the knee for surgery. The early aim is to regain range of motion, reduce swelling, and achieve full weight bearing.

The remaining rehabilitation will be supervised by a physiotherapist and will involve activities such as exercise bike riding, swimming, proprioceptive exercises, and muscle strengthening. Cycling can begin at four weeks; jogging can generally begin at around three months. The graft is strong enough to allow sport at around six months; however, other factors come into play such as confidence, fitness, and adequate fitness and training.

Professional sportsmen often return at 6 months but recreational athletes may take 10–12 months depending on motivation and time put into rehabilitation.

The rehabilitation and overall success of the procedure can be affected by associated injuries to the knee such as damage to meniscus, articular cartilage, or other ligaments.

Complications

Despite advances in surgical technique and the utmost care being taken during surgery, complications can still occur. It is very important for patients undergoing this operation to understand the reasons for the procedure and to have a major role in making an informed choice to proceed with surgery rather than nonsurgical treatment.

Conclusion

In general this procedure is very successful but complications can occur with any surgical procedure. Other rare or unexpected complications can occur. This is an elective procedure and as the patient you need to make an informed decision on whether or not to proceed with surgery.

Section 50.4

Cartilage Transfer

What Are Cartilage Lesions?

Articular or hyaline cartilage is the specialized tissue lining joints allowing smooth pain-free motion of a joint. A lot of people refer to the meniscus as cartilage but this is incorrect. Articular cartilage is normally extremely smooth and is able to absorb shock and the extreme loads placed upon it. When damaged it is not able to repair itself. When the damage is severe it results in pain, catching, swelling, and eventually arthritis.

There are continual advances in techniques to repair localized injuries to articular cartilage before arthritis occurs. One such advance is a chondrocyte or cartilage transfer procedure. This process has been developing over the last 10 years and is currently a viable alternative for certain patients with cartilage lesions.

Who Is Suitable for a Chondrocyte Transfer Procedure?

- Pain well localized to a specific part of the knee

- Young patients 15–50 years

- Well-localized lesion, i.e., lesions in one area rather than all over the knee

- No instability of the joint (i.e., no significant ligament damage)

- Normal limb alignment—not too knock kneed or bow legged

- Well motivated for rehabilitation as lots of physiotherapy required (approx three months)

- No inflammatory arthritis, i.e., rheumatoid arthritis, gout

- Body weight less than 1.5 times ideal body weight

What Is Done?

A piece of normal cartilage is taken from your knee at the time of arthroscopy from an area it is not needed. This is then sent to a laboratory where it is cultured (i.e., the cartilage cells are grown) and stored for later use. At a second operation, six weeks to six months later, the knee joint is opened up, the lesion is debrided to make a smooth defect, and the cells which are on a special membrane much like a piece of felt are placed into the defect.

Post-Op

This procedure requires prolonged and well-coordinated physiotherapy.

Hospitalization varies from two to five days depending on the size and position of the lesion.

You will usually be none or partial weight bearing for 6 weeks and then increase to full weight bearing by 12 weeks.

The cartilage takes 6–12 months to mature fully and it can be this long before the full benefits of the procedure are realized and you can return to normal activities.

You will require a knee brace to limit the degree of flexion post operatively. A graduated exercise program will be instituted but will vary from patient to patient.

When Can I Return to Sport?

Return to sporting activities and work also is variable and needs to be coordinated with your surgeon and physiotherapist. As a general rule it is not advisable to return to sports involving running and twisting for 12 months.

When Can I Return to Work?

This is a difficult question as it depends exactly what you do at work. If someone drives you and your job involves predominantly sitting then you could go back at two weeks. Physical jobs particularly those involving lifting may take six months or longer.

Complications

Any surgical procedure has a risk of complications. These are rare with this procedure; however, they can occur. Every precaution is taken to minimize the risk. Complications can be related to the anesthetic, general in nature as can happen with any surgery, or be specific to this procedure.

Surgical Complications

- **Excessive swelling and bruising of the leg:** This is due to bleeding in the joint and surrounding tissues. It can cause short-term pain and make it difficult to bend the knee. To avoid this, ice the leg and elevate it as much as possible for the first week or so. In this procedure a drain is not used as it may damage the graft.

- **Bleeding:** Small amounts of bleeding in the joint are normal. Large amounts of bleeding can occur but are more common in patients with bleeding disorders or those taking anti-inflammatory medications. These should be ceased two weeks prior to surgery. Excessive bleeding can require aspiration of the knee or occasionally a repeat arthroscopy.

- **Infection:** The procedure is done using antibiotic prophylaxis and in a sterile operating environment to reduce the risk of infection, but it still can occur. Treatment involves either oral or intravenous antibiotics and may involve further operations to wash out the joint. Occasionally this can lead to joint stiffness, destruction of the normal cartilage within the joint, or failure of the graft.

- **Ongoing pain:** This can be unpredictable but is more common in knees with more severe initial damage. If pain does continue then another arthroscopy may be recommended. This procedure if performed is usually to shave part of the graft which may be sitting too proud or has partially lifted off.

- **Joint stiffness:** Joint stiffness can result from scar tissue within the joint resulting in loss of motion. Treatment consists of physiotherapy or occasionally further surgical procedures. Full range of motion can not always be guaranteed.

- **Damage to nerves or vessels:** There are small nerves under the skin which cannot be avoided and cutting them can lead to areas of numbness in the skin below or around the knee. This numbness generally reduces in size with time and doesn't cause any functional disability. You can get also get areas of hypersensitivity or tingling around the scars. This usually settles with time.

- **Anterior knee pain:** Some patients develop pain around the kneecap. This is a result of muscle wasting and inactivity following surgery and usually resolves over time with appropriate physiotherapy and a conscientious exercise program continued at home.

- **Reflex sympathetic dystrophy:** This is a rare condition, the mechanism of which is not fully understood. It involves an overactivity of the nerves in the leg causing unexplained and excessive pain which can go on for many months and may never settle fully.

- **Deep venous thrombosis:** This condition is caused by clots in the leg which may require medical management in the form of injections or tablets to thin the blood. Very rarely these can travel to the lungs (pulmonary embolus) causing respiratory difficulties or even be life threatening.

- **Allergic reactions:** Allergic reactions to medications or materials used in the operating room.

- **Wound breakdown:** This occurs when small areas of the wound may not heal and may need to be resutured. This can sometimes result from reaction to the sutures just under the skin.

- **Instrument breakage**

- **Unsightly or thickened scar**

- **Pressure:** Pressure on areas of the body in the operating theater causing nerve damage.

- **Diathermy burns:** Burns from cautery device used in most open operations (very rare).

- **Limp:** Limp can occur from muscle weakness.

Any medical complication you have heard about can occur especially if you already have a pre-existing medical problem. Such complications include heart attack, stroke, kidney failure, pneumonia, bowel obstruction, bladder infection or obstruction, etc. Serious medical problems can lead to ongoing health concerns, prolonged hospitalization, or rarely death.

Rehabilitation Summary

Rehabilitation varies greatly between patients as it depends on the size and site of the lesion. No two knees are exactly the same. The weight bearing and degree of flexion depends in particular on the location of the lesion. If the lesion is non-weight bearing then the whole process can be accelerated.

Week 1

- Allow wound healing
- Weight bearing: nil
- Motion: nil or slight flexion except if on CPM [continuous passive motion] machine
- Brace: locked as appropriate
- Ambulation: crutches
- Physio: rest

Week 2–6

- Weight bearing: none to partial
- Motion: passive up to 90 degrees
- Brace: limited flexion
- Ambulation: crutches usually non-weight bearing
- Physio: reduce swelling, closed chain, isometric quads, gentle cycling, walking or treading water in a pool

Week 6–12

- Weight bearing: progress to full
- Motion: progress to full
- Brace: discard
- Ambulation: wean off crutches
- Physio: open chain, proprioceptive exercises, resisted cycling, swimming avoiding breaststroke

Week 12–52

- Gradual increase in all exercises to strengthen quads and hamstring muscles, jogging at 6 months, sport by 12 months

Summary

This procedure has good results for localized articular cartilage lesions. Without treatment a lot of these lesions progress to arthritis. It does involve quite a lot of rehabilitation and commitment to physiotherapy but once this is over the majority of patients are happy with their outcome.

Section 50.5

Physical Therapy

"Physical Therapy," by Jonathan Cluett, M.D., © 2011.
Used with permission of About, Inc. which can be found
online at www.about.com. All rights reserved.

Learning about Physical Therapy

A physical therapist is a specialist trained to work with you to restore your activity, strength, and motion following an injury or surgery. Physical therapists can teach specific exercises, stretches, and techniques and use specialized equipment to address problems that cannot be managed without this specialized physical therapy training.

Physical Therapy and Rehabilitation

Physical therapists are trained to identify deficiencies in the biomechanics of the body. Working with a physical therapist can target specific areas of weakness in the way our bodies work. They can relieve stress and help the body function without pain.

Physical therapists are knowledgeable about surgical procedures and treatment goals, and can tailor their efforts to improve your wellbeing. After surgical procedures, it is important that therapy is guided by the surgical procedure. Physical therapists are knowledgeable about your body's limitations after surgery and can help ensure a successful outcome.

Stretching Tight Muscles and Joints

Stretching is vital in maintaining good range of motion with joints and the flexibility of muscles. If you have stiff joints or tight muscles, normal activities, such as climbing stairs or reaching overhead, can be severely affected. With proper stretching, these functions can be preserved.

After an injury or surgery, scar tissue forms and soft tissue contracts. It is important to regularly stretch in these situations to ensure that scar formation does not get in the way of your rehabilitation.

Exercises to Strengthen Your Body

Strengthening exercises are performed to help you improve the function of your muscles. The goal is to improve strength, increase endurance, and maintain or improve range of motion.

Post-operative exercises should always be guided by your doctor and physical therapist, as there may be specific restrictions for your injury. The following guidelines can help you along your way:

- **Exercises for knee injuries:** http://orthopedics.about.com/od/physicaltherapy/p/kneerehab.htm

- **Exercises for shoulder injuries:** http://orthopedics.about.com/od/shoulderelbowtreatments/p/exercises.htm

- **Exercises for back injuries:** http://exercise.about.com/library/blbackexercises.htm

- **Exercises for neck injuries:** http://exercise.about.com/library/blseatedstretch.htm

Core Strengthening and Stability

One of the most recent developments in physical therapy is the emphasis on core strengthening and stability. The core of your body is like the foundation of your house. If you were to build your house on a weak foundation, you could risk damage and collapse. Similarly, bodies with a weak core are susceptible to acute injury and chronic overuse syndromes.

Core strengthening emphasizes the muscles of the back and pelvis. Some exercise programs, especially Pilates, are fantastic at increasing the body's core stability. That is the reason many professional athletes do regular Pilates workouts.

Ice and Heat Application

Ice and heat are useful in warming up and cooling off muscles. In addition, these methods can stimulate blood flow and decrease swelling. These can be important aspects of the therapeutic process. The key to proper ice and heat treatment is knowing when to ice and heat an injury.

Ultrasound

Ultrasound uses high frequency sound waves (not within the range we can hear) to stimulate the deep tissues within the body. By passing an ultrasound probe over your body, deep tissues are stimulated by the vibration of the sound wave. This leads to warming and increased blood flow to these tissues.

Electrical Stimulation

Electrical stimulation is a therapy that passes an electrical current to an affected area. Nerve conduction within the region is altered, which can in turn alter muscle contractility. Blood flow to these tissues is also increased with electrical stimulation. Patients often experience diminished pain after this electrical stimulation of treatment.

Part Ten

Sports Injuries in Children and Young Athletes

Chapter 51

Children and Sports Injuries

Chapter Contents

Section 51.1

Sport and Recreation Safety for Children

Key Facts

The American Academy of Pediatrics recommends that every child should have an opportunity to participate in sports or any recreational activity that promotes regular physical activity. Participation can be related to health benefits as well as health risks. Although deaths among children playing organized sports are rare, sports injuries are a common occurrence among children.

- Brain injury is the leading cause of sports-related death to children.

- Each year, more than 3.5 million children ages 14 years and under receive medical treatment for sports injuries.

- Approximately two out of five traumatic brain injuries among children are associated with participation in sports and recreational activities.

- More than 30 million children participate in sports each year in the United States.

- Nearly three-quarters of U.S. households with school-age children have at least one child who plays organized sports.

- The most common types of sport-related injuries in children are sprains (mostly ankle), muscle strains, bone or growth plate injuries, repetitive motion injuries, and heat-related illness.

Sport

- A recent survey found that among athletes ages 5 to 14 years, 15% of basketball players, 28% of football players, 22% of soccer players, 25% of baseball players, and 12% of softball players have been injured while playing their respective sports.

- In 2004, nearly 391,800 children ages 5 to 14 years were treated in hospital emergency rooms for either football- or basketball-related injuries.

Winter Sports

- Each year, children ages 0–14 years sustain nearly 52,000 injuries involving snowmobiles, sleds, snow skis, or snowboards.

- Children ages 5–14 years are at a higher risk of winter sports injuries; each year, approximately 49,000 injuries are sustained among this age group involving skiing, snowboarding, or sledding.

Where, When, and How

- Most organized sports-related injuries (62%) occur during practice rather than games.

- Collision and contact sports are associated with higher rates of injury. However, injuries from individual sports tend to be more severe.

- Each year, approximately 715,000 sports and recreation injuries occur in school settings alone.

- A national survey revealed that approximately 33% of parents often do not take the same safety precautions during their child's practice as they would for a game.

Who

- Older children are more likely to suffer from bicycle- and sports-related injuries and overexertion than younger children.

- Black children are one and a half times more likely than white children to suffer sports-related injuries.

- Children ages 5 to 14 years account for nearly 40% of all sports-related injuries treated in hospital emergency departments. The rate and severity of sports-related injury increases with a child's age.

- Children who do not wear or use protective equipment are at greater risk of sustaining sports-related injuries. Inappropriate or unavailable equipment are reasons for children's not wearing protective gear.

- The highest rates of injury for boys, in regards to sports, are ice hockey, rugby, and soccer. Soccer, basketball, and gymnastics seem to incur the highest rates of injury in girls.

Proven Interventions

- Children should have access to and consistently use the appropriate gear necessary for each respective sport.

- Children enrolled in organized sports through schools, community clubs, and recreation areas that are properly maintained assist in injury prevention.

- Coaches should be trained in first aid and CPR, and should have a plan for responding to emergencies. Coaches should be well versed in the proper use of equipment, and should enforce rules on equipment use.

- Sports programs with adults on staff who are Certified Athletic Trainers are ideal because they are trained to prevent or provide immediate care for athletic injuries.

Section 51.2

Playground Injuries

"Playground Safety Fact Sheet," © 2011 Safe Kids Worldwide
(www.safekids.org). Reprinted with permission.

Key Facts

- Non-fatal playground injuries are most often due to falls. The leading cause of death related to the playground and playground equipment is strangulation, and the majority of these deaths occur on home playgrounds.

- From 1990 to 2000, at least 147 children have died from playground equipment–related injuries. Nearly 70% of these deaths occurred on home playgrounds.

- About 45% of playground-related injuries are severe, which include fractures, internal injuries, concussions, dislocations, and amputations.

- In 2004, nearly 206,900 children ages 14 and under were treated in hospital emergency rooms for playground equipment–related injuries; children ages 5 to 14 accounted for nearly 75% of these injuries.

- The public playground injury rate among children ages 5 and under has doubled since 1980.

- In 2001, an estimated 8,250 children under the age of 2 years were treated in hospital emergency rooms for injuries associated with playground equipment; 95% of the injured were between 1 and 2 years old. Ninety-five percent of the injured children were 12 to 23 months of age.

Who

- Children ages 5 to 9 account for more than half of all playground-related injuries. The majority of these injuries occur at school.

- Children less than 4 are more likely to suffer head and face injuries, while children ages 5 to 14 are more likely to suffer injuries to the arm and hand.

- Female children hold a slightly higher risk of experiencing playground-related injuries than males.

How

- Falls are the most common mode of playground injury accounting for approximately 80% of all playground-related injuries.

- Strangulation is the primary cause of playground fatalities, accounting for over 50% of the deaths.

- Falls to the ground are responsible for an additional 20% of the deaths.

- Head injuries are involved in 75% of all fall-related deaths associated with playground equipment.

- In a study conducted by CPSC [U.S. Consumer Product Safety Commission], it was found that only 9% of home playgrounds had proper protective surfacing. About 80% of public playgrounds in the study had proper protective surfacing.

- Lack of supervision is associated with approximately 40% of playground injuries.

- A recent study found that children play without adult supervision more often on school playgrounds (32%), following park playgrounds (22%) and, lastly, childcare centers (5%).

Where and When

- It is estimated that one-third of playground deaths and 75% of playground injuries occur on public playgrounds.

- Nearly 40% of playground injuries occur during the months of May, June, and September.

- On public playgrounds, over half of the injuries occur as a result of the child climbing on equipment and falling, and 67% of injuries that occur on home playgrounds involve swings.

Prevention Strategies

- Increasing adult active supervision of children on playgrounds.

- Decreasing the height of playground equipment and using protective surfaces on the playground (energy-absorbing materials)—such as shredded rubber, wood chips, wood fiber, and sand—that reduce injuries related to falls. Both have shown to markedly reduce injury risk to children.

- Educating the public about the need for playgrounds to have separate age-appropriate playground areas for children. Only 42% of U.S. playgrounds have separate play areas for children ages 2 to 5 and children ages 5 to 12, and only 9% have signs indicating the age-appropriateness of equipment.

- A recent study found that the rate of playground-related injuries at North Carolina childcare centers dropped 22% after a law was passed requiring new playground equipment and surfacing in childcare facilities to conform to U.S. Consumer Product Safety Commission guidelines.

Laws and Regulations

- Playground equipment guidelines and standards have been developed by the U.S. Consumer Product Safety Commission and the American Society for Testing and Materials. Fifteen states have enacted some form of playground safety legislation.

- The CPSC has issued voluntary guidelines for drawstrings on children's clothing to prevent children from strangling or getting entangled in the neck and waist drawstrings of outerwear garments, such as jackets and sweatshirts. Children are at risk from strangulation when drawstrings on clothing become entangled in playground equipment.

Chapter 52

Sports Physicals

You already know that playing sports helps keep you fit. You also know that sports are a fun way to socialize and meet people. But you might not know why the physical you may have to take at the beginning of your sports season is so important.

What Is a Sports Physical?

In the sports medicine field, the sports physical exam is known as a preparticipation physical examination (PPE). The exam helps determine whether it's safe for you to participate in a particular sport. Most states actually require that kids and teens have a sports physical before they can start a new sport or begin a new competitive season. But even if a PPE isn't required, doctors still highly recommend getting one.

The two main parts to a sports physical are the medical history and the physical exam.

Medical History

This part of the exam includes questions about:

- serious illnesses among other family members;
- illnesses that you had when you were younger or may have now, such as asthma, diabetes, or epilepsy;
- previous hospitalizations or surgeries;
- allergies (to insect bites, for example);
- past injuries (including concussions, sprains, or bone fractures);
- whether you've ever passed out, felt dizzy, had chest pain, or had trouble breathing during exercise;
- any medications that you are on (including over-the-counter medications, herbal supplements, and prescription medications).

The medical history questions are usually on a form that you can bring home, so ask your parents to help you fill in the answers. If possible, ask both parents about family medical history.

Looking at patterns of illness in your family is a very good indicator of any potential conditions you may have. Most sports medicine doctors believe the medical history is the most important part of the sports physical exam, so take time to answer the questions carefully. It's unlikely that any health conditions you have will prevent you from playing sports completely.

Answer the questions as well as you can. Try not to guess the answers or give answers you think your doctor wants.

Physical Examination

During the physical part of the exam, the doctor will usually:

- record your height and weight;
- take a blood pressure and pulse (heart rate and rhythm) reading;
- test your vision;
- check your heart, lungs, abdomen, ears, nose, and throat;
- evaluate your posture, joints, strength, and flexibility.

Although most aspects of the exam will be the same for males and females, if a person has started or already gone through puberty, the doctor may ask girls and guys different questions. For example, if a girl is heavily involved in a lot of active sports, the doctor may ask her about her period and diet to make sure she doesn't have something like female athlete triad.

A doctor will also ask questions about use of drugs, alcohol, or dietary supplements, including steroids or other "performance enhancers" and weight-loss supplements, because these can affect a person's health.

At the end of your exam, the doctor will either fill out and sign a form if everything checks out okay or, in some cases, recommend a follow-up exam, additional tests, or specific treatment for medical problems.

Why Is a Sports Physical Important?

A sports physical can help you find out about and deal with health problems that might interfere with your participation in a sport. For example, if you have frequent asthma attacks but are a starting forward in soccer, a doctor might be able to prescribe a different type of inhaler or adjust the dosage so that you can breathe more easily when you run.

Your doctor may even have some good training tips and be able to give you some ideas for avoiding injuries. For example, he or she may recommend specific exercises, like certain stretching or strengthening activities, that help prevent injuries. A doctor also can identify risk factors that are linked to specific sports. Advice like this will make you a better, stronger athlete.

When and Where Should I Go for a Sports Physical?

Some people go to their own doctor for a sports physical; others have one at school. During school physicals, you may go to half a dozen or so "stations" set up in the gym; each one is staffed by a medical professional who gives you a specific part of the physical exam.

If your school offers the exam, it's convenient to get it done there. But even if you have a PPE at school, it's a good idea to see your regular doctor for an exam as well. Your doctor knows you—and your health history—better than anyone you talk to briefly in a gym.

If your state requires sports physicals, you'll probably have to start getting them when you're in ninth grade. Even if PPEs aren't required by your school or state, it's still smart to get them if you participate in school sports. And if you compete regularly in a sport before ninth grade, you should begin getting these exams even earlier.

Getting a sports physical once a year is usually adequate. If you're healing from a major injury, like a broken wrist or ankle, however, get checked out after it's healed before you start practicing or playing again.

You should have your physical about six weeks before your sports season begins so there's enough time to follow up on something, if necessary. Neither you nor your doctor will be very happy if your PPE is the day before baseball practice starts and it turns out there's something that needs to be taken of care before you can suit up.

What If There's a Problem?

What happens if you don't get the okay from your own doctor and have to see a specialist? Does that mean you won't ever be able to letter in softball or hockey? Don't worry if your doctor asks you to have other tests or go for a follow-up exam—it could be something as simple as rechecking your blood pressure a week or two after the physical.

Your doctor's referral to a specialist may help your athletic performance. For example, if you want to try out for your school's track team but get a slight pain in your knee every time you run, an orthopedist or sports medicine specialist can help you figure out what's going on. Perhaps the pain comes from previous overtraining or poor running technique. Maybe you injured the knee a long time ago and it never totally healed. Or perhaps the problem is as simple as running shoes that don't offer enough support. Chances are, a doctor will be able to help you run without the risk of further injury to the knee by giving you suggestions or treatment before the sports season begins.

It's very unlikely that you'll be disqualified from playing sports. The ultimate goal of the sports physical is to ensure safe participation in sports, not to disqualify the participants. Most of the time, a specialist won't find anything serious enough to prevent you from playing your sport. In fact, fewer than 1% of students have conditions that might limit sports participation, and most of these conditions are known before the PPE takes place.

Do I Still Have to Get a Regular Physical?

In a word, yes. It may seem like overkill, but a sports physical is different from a standard physical.

The sports physical focuses on your well-being as it relates to playing a sport. It's more limited than a regular physical, but it's a lot more specific about athletic issues. During a regular physical, however, your doctor will address your overall well-being, which may include things that are unrelated to sports. You can ask your doctor to give you both types of exams during one visit; just be aware that you'll need to set aside more time.

Even if your sports physical exam doesn't reveal any problems, it's always wise to monitor yourself when you play sports. If you notice changes in your physical condition—even if you think they're small, such as muscle pain or shortness of breath—be sure to mention them to a parent or coach. You should also inform your phys-ed teacher or coach if your health needs have changed in any way or if you're taking a new medication.

Just as professional sports stars need medical care to keep them playing their best, so do teenage athletes. You can give yourself the same edge as the pros by making sure you have your sports physical.

Chapter 53

Preventing Children's Sports Injuries

Causes of Sports Injuries

Participation in any sport, whether it's recreational bike riding or Pee-Wee football, can teach kids to stretch their limits and learn sportsmanship and discipline. But any sport also carries the potential for injury.

By knowing the causes of sports injuries and how to prevent them, you can help make athletics a positive experience for your child.

Kids can be particularly susceptible to sports injuries for a variety of reasons. Kids, particularly those younger than eight years old, are less coordinated and have slower reaction times than adults because they are still growing and developing.

In addition, kids mature at different rates. Often there's a substantial difference in height and weight between kids of the same age. And when kids of varying sizes play sports together, there may be an increased risk of injury.

As kids grow bigger and stronger, the potential for injury increases, largely because of the amount of force involved. For example, a collision between two 8-year-old Pee-Wee football players who weigh 65 or 70 pounds each does not produce as much force as that produced by two 16-year-old high school football players who may each weigh up to 200 pounds.

"Preventing Children's Sports Injuries," November 2008, reprinted with permission from www.kidshealth.org. Copyright © 2008 The Nemours Foundation. This information was provided by KidsHealth, one of the largest resources online for medically reviewed health information written for parents, kids, and teens. For more articles like this one, visit www.KidsHealth.org, or www.TeensHealth.org.

Also, kids may not assess the risks of certain activities as fully as adults might. So they might unknowingly take risks that can result in injuries.

Preventing Sports Injuries

You can help prevent your child from being injured by following some simple guidelines:

Use of Proper Equipment

It's important for kids to use proper equipment and safety gear that is the correct size and fits well. For example, kids should wear helmets for baseball, softball, bicycle riding, and hockey. They also should wear helmets while they're inline skating or riding scooters and skateboards.

For racquet sports and basketball, ask about any protective eyewear, like shatterproof goggles. Ask your child's coach about the appropriate helmets, shoes, mouth guards, athletic cups and supporters, and padding.

Protective equipment should be approved by the organizations that govern each of the sports. Hockey facemasks, for example, should be approved by the Hockey Equipment Certification Council (HECC) or the Canadian Standards Association (CSA). Bicycle helmets should have a safety certification sticker from the Consumer Product Safety Commission (CPSC).

Also, all equipment should be properly maintained to ensure its effectiveness. In the United States, the National Operating Committee on Standards for Athletic Equipment (NOCSAE) sets many of the standards for helmets, facemasks, and shin guards. In addition to meeting the NOSCAE standards, all equipment should be properly maintained to ensure its effectiveness over time.

Maintenance and Appropriateness of Playing Surfaces

Check that playing fields are not full of holes and ruts that might cause kids to fall or trip. Kids doing high-impact sports, like basketball and running, should do them on surfaces like tracks and wooden basketball courts, which can be more forgiving than surfaces like concrete.

Adequate Adult Supervision and Commitment to Safety

Any team sport or activity that kids participate in should be supervised by qualified adults. Select leagues and teams that have the same commitment to safety and injury prevention that you do.

The team coach should have training in first aid and CPR [cardio-pulmonary resuscitation], and the coach's philosophy should promote players' well-being. A coach with a win-at-all-costs attitude may encourage kids to play through injury and may not foster good sportsmanship. Be sure that the coach enforces playing rules and requires that safety equipment be used at all times.

Additionally, make sure your kids are matched for sports according to their skill level, size, and physical and emotional maturity.

Proper Preparation

Just as you wouldn't send a child who can't swim to a swimming pool, it's important not to send kids to play a sport that they're unprepared to play. Make sure that your child knows how to play the sport before going out on the field.

Your child should be adequately prepared with warm-ups and training sessions before practices as well as before games. This will help ensure that your child has fun and reduce the chances of an injury.

In addition, your child should drink plenty of fluids and be allowed to rest during practices and games.

Common Types of Sports Injuries

Three common types of sports injuries in children are acute injuries, overuse injuries, and reinjuries.

Acute Injuries

Acute injuries occur suddenly and are usually associated with some form of trauma. In younger children, acute injuries typically include minor bruises, sprains, and strains. Teen athletes are more likely to sustain more severe injuries, including broken bones and torn ligaments.

More severe acute injuries that can occur, regardless of age, include: eye injuries, including scratched corneas, detached retinas, and blood in the eye; broken bones or ligament injuries; brain injuries, including concussions, skull fractures, brain hemorrhages; and spinal cord injuries.

Acute injuries often occur because of a lack of proper equipment or the use of improper equipment. For example, without protective eyewear, eye injuries are extremely common in basketball and racquet sports. In addition, many kids playing baseball and softball have suffered broken legs or ankles from sliding into immobile bases.

551

Overuse Injuries

Overuse injuries occur from repetitive actions that put too much stress on the bones and muscles. Although these injuries can occur in adults as well as kids, they're more problematic in a child athlete because of the effect they may have on bone growth.

All kids who play sports can develop an overuse injury, but the likelihood increases with the amount of time a child spends on the sport.

Some of the most common types of overuse injuries are:

- **Anterior knee pain:** Anterior knee pain is pain in the front of the knee under the kneecap. The knee will be sore and swollen due to tendon or cartilage inflammation. The cause is usually muscle tightness in the hamstrings or quadriceps, the major muscle groups around the thigh.

- **Little League elbow:** Repetitive throwing sometimes results in pain and tenderness in the elbow. The ability to flex and extend the arm may be affected, but the pain typically occurs after the follow-through of the throw. In addition to pain, pitchers sometimes complain of loss of velocity or decreased endurance.

- **Swimmer's shoulder:** Swimmer's shoulder is an inflammation (swelling) of the shoulder caused by the repeated stress of the overhead motion associated with swimming or throwing a ball. The pain typically begins intermittently but may progress to continuous pain in the back of the shoulder.

- **Shin splints:** Shin splints are characterized by pain and discomfort on the front of the lower parts of the legs. They are often caused by repeated running on a hard surface or overtraining at the beginning of a season.

- **Spondylolysis:** Spondylolysis often results from trauma or from repetitive flexing, then overextension, twisting, or compression of the back muscles. This can cause persistent lower back pain. Spondylolysis is commonly seen in kids who participate in soccer, football, weight lifting, gymnastics, wrestling, and diving.

Overuse injuries can be caused or aggravated by:

- growth spurts or an imbalance between strength and flexibility;

- inadequate warm-up;

- excessive activity (for example, increased intensity, duration, or frequency of playing and/or training);

- playing the same sport year-round or multiple sports during the same season;

- improper technique (for example, overextending on a pitch);

- unsuitable equipment (for example, nonsupportive athletic shoes).

Reinjuries

Reinjury occurs when an athlete returns to the sport before a previous injury has sufficiently healed. Athletes are at a much greater risk for reinjury when they return to the game before recovering fully. Doing so places stress upon the injury and forces the body to compensate for the weakness, which can put the athlete at greater risk for injuring another body part.

Reinjury can be avoided by allowing an injury to completely heal. Once the doctor has approved a return to the sport, make sure that your child properly warms up and cools down before and after exercise.

Sudden exertion can also cause reinjury, so your child should re-enter the sport gradually. Explain that easing back into the game at a sensible pace is better than returning to the hospital!

Treating Sports Injuries

Treatment of sports injuries varies by the type of injury.

For acute injuries, many pediatric sports medicine specialists usually take a "better safe than sorry" approach. If an injury appears to affect basic functioning in any way—for example, if your child can't bend a finger, is limping, or has had a change in consciousness—first aid should be administered immediately. A doctor should then see the child. If the injury seems to be more serious, it's important to take your child to the nearest hospital emergency department.

For overuse injuries, the philosophy is similar. If a child begins complaining of pain, it's the body's way of saying there's a problem. Have the child examined by a doctor who can then determine whether it's necessary to see a sports medicine specialist. A doctor can usually diagnose many of these conditions by taking a medical history, examining the child, and ordering some routine tests.

It's important to get overuse injuries diagnosed and treated to prevent them from developing into larger chronic problems. The doctor may advise the child to temporarily modify or eliminate an activity to limit stress on the body.

In some cases, the child may not be able to resume the sport without risking further injury. Because overuse injuries are characterized by swelling, the doctor may prescribe rest, medications to help reduce inflammation, and physical therapy. When recovery is complete, your child's technique or training schedule may need to be adjusted to prevent the injury from flaring up again.

Chapter 54

Overtraining Burnout in Young Athletes

Burnout, or overtraining syndrome, is a condition in which an athlete experiences fatigue and declining performance in his/her sport despite continuing or increased training. Overtraining can result in mood changes, decreased motivation, frequent injuries, and infections.

How It Occurs

Burnout is thought to be a result of the physical and emotional stress of training. Many athletes have some initial decrease in performance when they increase their level of training. Generally, however, after a short recovery period the athlete will see an improvement in performance. Overtraining syndrome happens when an athlete fails to recover adequately from training and competition. The symptoms are due to a combination of changes in hormones, suppression of the immune system (which decreases the athlete's ability to fight infection), physical fatigue, and psychological changes.

Risk Factors

There are many factors that are thought to increase the risk of developing overtraining syndrome including:

- specializing in one sport;
- sudden and large increases in training;
- participation in endurance sports;
- high anxiety level;
- low self-esteem;
- pressure from parents/coaches.

Signs and Symptoms

In the young athlete, signs and symptoms of burnout can be highly variable and can include:

- chronic muscle and joint pain;
- weight loss and loss of appetite;
- increased heart rate at rest;
- decreased sports performance;
- fatigue;
- prolonged recovery time;
- lack of enthusiasm;
- frequent illnesses;
- difficulty completing usual routines;
- decreased school performance;
- personality or mood changes;
- increased anger or irritability;
- sleep disturbances (difficulty sleeping, or sleeping without feeling refreshed).

These are warning signs of unhealthy sports participation, which may increase the risk of burnout:

- The athlete is no longer having fun playing sports.
- The athlete's sport is dominating his/her and his/her family's life.
- The only topic of conversation at home or at the dinner table is the child's sports.
- The athlete is rewarded on how they perform in sports.

- The athlete has missed 10% of his/her season and has not yet seen a doctor.
- The only important thing to the athlete or parent is winning.
- A female athlete is now 16 and has not yet started her period.
- The athlete is dieting just to become a faster runner.
- A young athlete only plays one sport and is unwilling to try any others.

Diagnosis

There is no test for overtraining syndrome. The diagnosis is based on an athlete's story, the symptoms that he/she reports, and the absence of an alternative explanation for these symptoms.

Treatment

The only treatment for burnout is rest. The athlete should stop participation in training/competition for a set period of time. The time required varies (generally 4–12 weeks) depending on several factors, including the type of sport, level of skill and competition, and severity of symptoms. During the rest period, the athlete can participate in short intervals of low-intensity aerobic exercise to help keep active and fit; this type of activity should be unrelated to his/her sport.

Returning to Activity and Sports

When the signs and symptoms of burnout have resolved completely (including physical symptoms, mood changes, sleep disturbances, etc.), the athlete may begin slowly to reintroduce training. Athletes should increase the duration of activity before increasing the intensity of activity. If symptoms begin to recur when training is restarted, the athlete should again initiate a rest period and reevaluate the training approach.

Preventing Burnout

Specific guidelines for trainers/coaches/parents include:

1. Make training fun and interesting with age-appropriate games and workouts.

2. Keep the training regimen flexible with planned breaks one to two days per week and longer breaks every few months to allow for complete recovery.

3.   Maintain a supportive environment for the athlete.

4.   Teach the athlete to be aware of the cues from their body that indicate a need to slow down or change their training routine. Discuss the importance of overall health and wellness and be open to conversations about these issues.

Specific guidelines for the athlete include:

1.   Spend one to two days per week resting from organized sport participation or participating in alternate activities.

2.   Allow slightly longer breaks (a couple of weeks) from training and competition every three months. This time could be spent focusing on other activities and cross-training without intensive training or competition.

3.   Maintain a healthy, balanced diet. Drink plenty of water.

4.   Listen to your body. Take a short break or alter your training if your body needs a change.

5.   Try to be a well-rounded athlete who participates in many different activities.

Chapter 55

Preventing Child Abuse in Youth Sports

Abuse Defined

Your child is being abused when someone uses his or her power or position to harm them emotionally, physically, or sexually or as a result of neglect.

Emotional Abuse

- Is a verbal attack on a child's self-esteem by a person in a position of power, authority, or trust such as a parent or coach

- Occurs even if the attack is intended as a form of discipline or is not intended by the adult to cause harm

- Takes many forms, including any of the following:

  - Name calling ("Hey, Fatty!" or "Hey, Shorty" or "Hey, Mr. Klutz")

  - Threatening ("If you don't win, you can forget about me buying that new CD you want")

  - Insulting ("You're stupid" or "You're clumsy" or "You're an embarrassment to our family" or "You don't deserve to wear that uniform")

"Abuse in Youth Sports Takes Many Different Forms" by Brooke de Lench, Founder and Editor-in-Chief of MomsTeam.com: the Trusted Source for Youth Sports Parents. © 2011 MomsTeam.com. All rights reserved. Reprinted with permission.

- Criticizing or ridiculing ("You are a loser" or "I thought you were better than that. I guess I was wrong.")

- Intimidating ("Watch out kid, my son is going to break your nose")

- Yelling at a child for losing or not playing up to the adult's expectations

- Hazing

- Negative questioning ("Why didn't you win?" or "How could you let that guy beat you?")

- Shunning or withholding love or affection (not speaking to, hugging, or comforting your child after she plays poorly in a game or practice, or her team loses; showing obvious signs of disappointment)

- Punishing a child for not playing up to your expectations or when her team loses

Physical Abuse

- Occurs when a person in a position of power, authority, or trust such as a parent or coach purposefully injures or threatens to injure a child

- Takes many forms, including any of the following:
  - Slapping
  - Hitting
  - Shaking
  - Throwing equipment
  - Kicking
  - Pulling hair
  - Pulling ears
  - Striking
  - Shoving
  - Grabbing
  - Hazing
  - Punishing "poor" play or rules violations through the use of excessive exercise (extra laps etc.)[1] or by denying fluids

Sexual Abuse

- Occurs when a person in a position of power, authority, or trust engages in "sexualized" touching or sex with a child

- "Sexualized touching" is where touching, instead of being respectful and nurturing, is done in a sexual manner. Examples include:

  - Fondling instead of a hug

  - Long kiss on the lips instead of a peck on the cheek

  - Seductive stroking of any area of the child's body instead of a simple pat on the rear-end for a good play

What Is Harassment?

Your child is being harassed when she or he is threatened, intimidated, taunted, or subjected to racial, homophobic, or sexist slurs. Sexual harassment includes comments, contact, or behavior of a sexual nature that is offensive, uninvited, or unwelcome.

Neglect

Neglect is a chronic inattention to the basic necessities of life such as supervision, medical and dental care, adequate rest, safe environment, exercise, and fresh air.

Neglect in a sports setting may take the following forms:

- Injuries are not properly treated.

- Athletes are forced to play hurt.

- Equipment is inadequate, poorly maintained, or unsafe.

- Road trips are not properly supervised.

Surprisingly Common

According to a widely reported 1993 survey conducted by the Minnesota Amateur Sports Commission:

- almost half (45.3%) of those surveyed (both males and females) said they had been emotionally abused while participating in sports (i.e. called names, yelled at, or insulted);

- slightly more than 1 out of 6 (17.5%) said they had suffered physical abuse while playing sports (i.e. hit, kicked, or slapped);

- more than 1 in 5 (21%) said they had suffered neglect while playing sports (pressured to play with an injury);

- 1 in 12 (8%) said they had been sexually harassed while playing sports (called names with sexual connotations);

- 1 in 30 (3.4%) said they had been pressured into sex or sexual touching.

Twelve years later, a 2005 study by researchers at the University of Missouri, the University of Minnesota, and Notre Dame University reported in the *Journal of Research in Character Education* found that emotional abuse in youth sports was still widespread:

- More than 4 in 10 coaches have loudly argued with a ref or sport official following a bad call (youth athletes said 48% of coaches engaged in this behavior, although only 20% of parents said they did so).

- 7 out 10 youth athletes have heard a fan (most likely a parent) angrily yell at an official.

- 4 in 10 youth athletes have heard a fan angrily yell at a coach.

- 1 in 8 parents has angrily criticized their child's sports performance (another study, this one conducted in fall 2005 by Blue Cross and Blue Shield of Minnesota, reported that more than 4 in 10 parents had seen a verbal altercation between a parent and their child that they thought was inappropriate).

- One third of coaches have angrily yelled at a player for making a mistake, a high rate "of significant concern" to the study's authors, who wondered, "What would we think if a third of our teachers yelled at students for making mistakes, and 1 in 10 made fun of a student?"

- 1 in 7 athletes made fun of a less-skilled opponent. About 1 in 10 coaches admitted to making fun a team member. These numbers suggest that on most teams there is a high probability that one or more of the lesser skilled players has been at least mildly victimized.

- More than 4 in 10 youth athletes reported having been teased or yelled at by a fan or seeing a fan angrily yell at or tease another player.

Emotional Abuse: The Damage Is No Less Real

Perhaps because the damage caused by emotional abuse is not obvious, like sexual abuse, or immediately apparent, like a physical injury, its effect is often overlooked and minimized. But, says San Francisco child psychologist Maria Pease, the damage is no less real, and, in fact, may be much more damaging and long-lasting:

- Children are deeply affected by negative comments from parents, coaches, and other adults to whom they look up and respect. One comment can turn a child off to sports forever.

- Children are much more sensitive than adults to criticism: being yelled at, put down, or embarrassed is much more likely to have negative psychological consequences and to cause the child to feel humiliated, shamed, and degraded and to damage her feelings of self-worth and self-esteem.

- If the abuse becomes chronic, a pattern of negative comments can destroy a child's spirit, motivation, and self-esteem. Over time, the young athlete will begin to believe what adults say about him. Abusive comments intended to improve athletic performance are likely to have precisely the opposite effect.

- Children who experience screaming on a regular basis will react in certain ways to protect or defend themselves. This may be adaptive in the moment to survive the screaming, but ultimately be maladaptive and constrict their ability to be psychologically healthy over time.

- A more anxious, sensitive child may be intolerant of screaming very early on and remove himself from the sport (he may be the lucky one). However, he is also more likely to endure the screaming without telling a parent or responding to the coach directly out of fear of reprisal from the coach. A more sensitive child who stays in this situation may be more affected physiologically with overall heightened arousal levels as previously discussed.

- A more secure child will likely have the same physiological responses but be less vulnerable to them. He may find a way to tune out the coach, but this may come at a cost of emotional sensitivity. As the child becomes less sensitive to his own fearful feelings, he can become less sensitive to the feelings of others, leading to loss of empathy. He will also become less sensitive to emotions in general and have a loss of sensitivity to positive emotions as well. He is also likely to resent the coach for putting him in such a psychologically vulnerable position.

Children involved in sports often make strong connections and develop a special trusting relationship with their coaches and instructors, and if the coaches' power is abused, children can suffer severe psychological injuries that may last a lifetime. In a 2004 study of emotional abuse of elite child athletes in the United Kingdom, for instance, athletes reported that the abuse by their coaches created a climate of fear and made them feel stupid, worthless or upset, lacking in self-confidence, angry, depressed, humiliated, fearful, and hurt and left long-lasting emotional scars.

1. Gershoff, E.T. (2008). *Report on Physical Punishment in the United States: What Research Tells Us About Its Effects on Children.* Columbus, OH: Center for Effective Discipline ("compelling a child to engage in excessive exercise or physical exertion" is physical punishment).

Adapted from *Home Team Advantage: The Critical Role of Mothers in Youth Sports* (HarperCollins 2006) by Brooke de Lench, founder and editor-in-chief of MomsTeam.com.

Chapter 56

Growth Plate Injuries

What is the growth plate?

The growth plate, also known as the epiphyseal plate or physis, is the area of growing tissue near the ends of the long bones in children and adolescents. Each long bone has at least two growth plates: one at each end. The growth plate determines the future length and shape of the mature bone. When growth is complete—sometime during adolescence—the growth plates close and are replaced by solid bone.

Because the growth plates are the weakest areas of the growing skeleton—even weaker than the nearby ligaments and tendons that connect bones to other bones and muscles—they are vulnerable to injury. Injuries to the growth plate are called fractures.

Who gets growth plate injuries?

Growth plate injuries can occur in growing children and adolescents. In a child, a serious injury to a joint is more likely to damage a growth plate than the ligaments that stabilize the joint. Trauma that would cause a sprain in an adult might cause a growth plate fracture in a child.

This chapter excerpted from "Questions and Answers about Growth Plate Injuries," National Institute of Arthritis and Musculoskeletal and Skin Diseases (www.niams.nih.gov), August 2007.

Growth plate fractures occur twice as often in boys as in girls, because girls' bodies mature at an earlier age than boys. As a result, their bones finish growing sooner, and their growth plates are replaced by stronger, solid bone.

One-third of all growth plate injuries occur in competitive sports such as football, basketball, or gymnastics, while about 20% of growth plate fractures occur as a result of recreational activities such as biking, sledding, skiing, or skateboarding.

Fractures can result from a single traumatic event or from chronic stress and overuse. Most growth plate fractures occur in the long bones of the fingers (phalanges) and the outer bone of the forearm (radius). They are also common in the lower bones of the leg (the tibia and fibula).

What causes growth plate injuries?

Growth plate injuries can be caused by an event such as a fall or blow to the limb, or they can result from overuse. For example, a gymnast who practices for hours on the uneven bars, a long-distance runner, and a baseball pitcher perfecting his curve ball can all have growth plate injuries.

Although many growth plate injuries are caused by accidents that occur during play or athletic activity, growth plates are also susceptible to other disorders, such as bone infection, that can alter their normal growth and development. Other possible causes of growth plate injuries include child abuse, injury from extreme cold (for example, frostbite), radiation and medications, certain neurological disorders, genetics, and metabolic disease.

How are growth plate fractures diagnosed?

A child who has persistent pain, or pain that affects athletic performance or the ability to move and put pressure on a limb, should never be allowed or expected to "work through the pain." Whether an injury is acute or due to overuse, it should be evaluated by a doctor, because some injuries, if left untreated, can cause permanent damage and interfere with proper growth of the involved limb.

The doctor will begin the diagnostic process by asking about the injury and how it occurred and by examining the child. The doctor will then use X-rays to determine if there is a fracture, and if so, the type of fracture. Often the doctor will X-ray not only the injured limb but the opposite limb as well. Because growth plates have not yet hardened into solid bone, neither the structures themselves nor injuries to them show up on X-rays. Instead, growth plates appear as gaps between the shaft of a long bone, called the metaphysis, and the end of the bone, called the epiphysis. By comparing X-rays of the injured limb to those of the noninjured limb, doctors can look for differences that indicate an injury.

Very often the X-ray is negative, because the growth plate line is already there, and the fracture is undisplaced (the two ends of the broken bone are not separated). The doctor can still diagnose a growth plate fracture on clinical grounds because of tenderness of the plate. Children do get ligament strains if their growth plates are open, and they often have undisplaced growth plate fractures.

Other tests doctors may use to diagnose a growth plate injury include magnetic resonance imaging (MRI), computed tomography (CT), and ultrasound.

Because these tests enable doctors to see the growth plate and areas of other soft tissue, they can be useful not only in detecting the presence of an injury, but also in determining the type and extent of the injury.

How are growth plate injuries treated?

Treatment for growth plate injuries depends on the type of injury. In all cases, treatment should be started as soon as possible after injury and will generally involve a mix of the following:

Immobilization: The affected limb is often put in a cast or splint, and the child is told to limit any activity that puts pressure on the injured area.

Manipulation or surgery: If the fracture is displaced (meaning the ends of the injured bones no longer meet as they should), the doctor will have to put the bones or joints back in their correct positions, either by using his or her hands (called manipulation) or by performing surgery. Sometimes the doctor needs to fix the break and hold the growth plate in place with screws or wire. After the procedure, the bone will be set in place (immobilized) so it can heal without moving. This is usually done with a cast that encloses the injured growth plate and the joints on both sides of it. The cast is left in place until the injury heals, which can take anywhere from a few weeks to two or more months for serious injuries. The need for manipulation or surgery depends on the location and extent of the injury, its effect on nearby nerves and blood vessels, and the child's age.

Strengthening and range-of-motion exercises: These are exercises designed to strengthen the muscles that support the injured area of the bone and to improve or maintain the joint's ability to move in the way that it should. Your child's doctor may recommend these after the fracture has healed. A physical therapist can work with your child and his or her doctor to design an appropriate exercise plan.

Long-term follow-up: Long-term follow-up is usually necessary to monitor the child's recuperation and growth. Evaluation includes X-rays of matching limbs at three- to six-month intervals for at least two years. Some fractures require periodic evaluations until the child's bones have finished growing. Sometimes a growth arrest line (a line on the X-ray where the bone stopped growing temporarily) may appear as a marker of the injury. Continued bone growth away from that line may mean there will not be a long-term problem, and the doctor may decide to stop following the patient.

Will the affected limb of a child with a growth plate injury still grow?

About 85% of growth plate fractures heal without any lasting effect. Whether an arrest of growth occurs depends on the treatment provided, and the following factors, in descending order of importance:

- **Severity of the injury:** If the injury causes the blood supply to the epiphysis to be cut off, growth can be stunted. If the growth plate is shifted, shattered, or crushed, the growth plate may close prematurely, forming a bony bridge or "bar." The risk of growth arrest is higher in this setting. An open injury in which the skin is broken carries the risk of infection, which could destroy the growth plate.

- **Age of the child:** In a younger child, the bones have a great deal of growing to do; therefore, growth arrest can be more serious, and closer surveillance is needed. It is also true, however, that younger bones have a greater ability to heal.

- **Which growth plate is injured:** Some growth plates, such as those in the region of the knee, are more involved in extensive bone growth than others.

- **Type of fracture:** There are six fracture types, and types IV, V, and VI are the most serious.

The most frequent complication of a growth plate fracture is premature arrest of bone growth. The affected bone grows less than it would have without the injury, and the resulting limb could be shorter than the opposite, uninjured limb. If only part of the growth plate is injured, growth may be lopsided and the limb may become crooked.

Growth plate injuries at the knee have the greatest risk of complications. Nerve and blood vessel damage occurs most frequently there. Injuries to the knee have a much higher incidence of premature growth arrest and crooked growth.

Chapter 57

Developmental Diseases and Sports Injuries

Chapter Contents

Section 57.1

Osgood-Schlatter Disease

Chris is about to take part in his first soccer championship. Lately, though, he's had swelling, tenderness, and aching pain beneath his right knee joint. He seems to feel better when he takes a break from sports and other physical activities for a few days.

After visiting his doctor, Chris discovered that he has a condition called Osgood-Schlatter disease (OSD), a common cause of knee pain in teens. The condition most often affects guys between 13 and 14 years old and girls between 10 and 11 years old.

What Is Osgood-Schlatter Disease?

In 1903, doctors Robert Osgood and Carl Schlatter first described OSD after recognizing a pattern of symptoms in their patients. The doctors found that OSD was a growth-related problem seen mostly in young, athletic guys. It's more likely to happen during a growth spurt.

Osgood-Schlatter disease is an overuse injury of the knee. Frequent use and physical stress cause inflammation (pain and swelling) at the point where the tendon from the kneecap (called the patella) attaches to the shinbone (tibia).

Because the area is stressed by frequent use, it often leads to inflammation (pain and swelling) or even a tiny fracture of the shin bone. The pain usually worsens with exercise, jumping, and sports such as basketball, volleyball, soccer, figure skating, and gymnastics. In some people, both knees are affected.

The condition affects guys more than girls, especially guys who are active in sports involving deep knee bends, jumping, and running. But OSD affects girls, too, and the number of girls with OSD is increasing since more and more girls are participating in competitive sports.

What is a growth spurt? For about two years during adolescence, guys and girls grow more rapidly. This rapid growth period is often called a growth spurt. Although all people go through this spurt in height, the age at which it begins and the length of time it continues vary.

Signs and Symptoms of OSD

The symptoms of OSD include:

- pain, swelling, or tenderness below the knee;
- pain that becomes worse during activities such as running and jumping;
- limping after physical activity.

With OSD, these symptoms usually go away or feel better when a person rests.

OSD can cause very different symptoms in different people; it all depends on the severity of the condition. Some people may feel mild knee pain only when they play sports. Others may feel constant pain that makes playing any sport difficult.

What Do Doctors Do?

If a doctor thinks someone has OSD, he or she will examine the knee carefully and might take an X-ray to help find the cause of pain. In addition to doing a physical examination, the doctor probably will ask about any concerns and symptoms you have, your past health, your family's health, any medications you're taking, any allergies you may have, and other issues. This is called the medical history.

Most people with OSD are able to continue playing sports. If someone's pain is severe, the doctor might recommend taking a short break or trying activities with less jumping and running for a while. Ask your doctor about stretching exercises that can help relieve some of the pain while keeping the area strong and toned. These exercises often include quadriceps and hamstring stretches.

Icing the affected area after sports can help to relieve pain and swelling. A doctor might also prescribe anti-inflammatory medications, like ibuprofen, to treat the pain.

The good news is that OSD usually goes away on its own after the growth spurt has ended.

Section 57.2

Sever's Disease

Although the name might sound pretty frightening, Sever's disease is really a common heel injury that occurs in kids. It can be painful, but is only temporary and has no long-term effects.

About Sever's Disease

Sever's disease, also called calcaneal apophysitis, is a painful bone disorder that results from inflammation (swelling) of the growth plate in the heel. A growth plate, also called an epiphyseal plate, is an area at the end of a developing bone where cartilage cells change over time into bone cells. As this occurs, the growth plates expand and unite, which is how bones grow.

Sever's disease is a common cause of heel pain in growing kids, especially those who are physically active. It usually occurs during the growth spurt of adolescence, the approximately two-year period in early puberty when kids grow most rapidly. This growth spurt can begin any time between the ages of 8 and 13 for girls and 10 and 15 for boys. Sever's disease rarely occurs in older teens because the back of the heel usually finishes growing by the age of 15, when the growth plate hardens and the growing bones fuse together into mature bone.

Sever's disease is similar to Osgood-Schlatter disease, a condition that affects the bones in the knees.

Causes

During the growth spurt of early puberty, the heel bone (also called the calcaneus) sometimes grows faster than the leg muscles and tendons. This can cause the muscles and tendons to become very tight and overstretched, making the heel less flexible and putting pressure on the growth plate. The Achilles tendon (also called the heel cord) is the strongest tendon that attaches to the growth plate in the heel. Over time, repeated stress (force or pressure) on the already tight Achilles tendon damages the growth plate, causing the swelling, tenderness, and pain of Sever's disease.

Such stress commonly results from physical activities and sports that involve running and jumping, especially those that take place on hard surfaces, such as track, basketball, soccer, and gymnastics. It can even result from standing too long, which puts constant pressure on the heel. Poor-fitting shoes can contribute to the condition by not providing enough support or padding for the feet or by rubbing against the back of the heel.

Although Sever's disease can occur in any child, these conditions increase the chances of it happening:

- Pronated foot (a foot that rolls in at the ankle when walking), which causes tightness and twisting of the Achilles tendon, thus increasing its pull on the heel's growth plate

- Flat or high arch, which affects the angle of the heel within the foot, causing tightness and shortening of the Achilles tendon

- Short leg syndrome (one leg is shorter than the other), which causes the foot on the short leg to bend downward to reach the ground, pulling on the Achilles tendon

- Overweight or obesity, which puts weight-related pressure on the growth plate

Signs and Symptoms

The most obvious sign of Sever's disease is pain or tenderness in one or both heels, usually at the back. The pain also might extend to the sides and bottom of the heel, ending near the arch of the foot.

A child also may have these related problems:

- Swelling and redness in the heel

- Difficulty walking

- Discomfort or stiffness in the feet upon awaking

- Discomfort when the heel is squeezed on both sides

- An unusual walk, such as walking with a limp or on tiptoes to avoid putting pressure on the heel

Symptoms are usually worse during or after activity and get better with rest.

Diagnosis

A doctor can usually tell that a child has Sever's disease based on the symptoms reported. To confirm the diagnosis, the doctor will probably examine the heels and ask about the child's activity level and participation in sports. The doctor might also use the squeeze test, squeezing the back part of the heel from both sides at the same time to see if doing so causes pain. The doctor might also ask the child to stand on tiptoes to see if that position causes pain.

Although imaging tests such as X-rays generally are not that helpful in diagnosing Sever's disease, some doctors order them to rule out other problems, such as fractures. Sever's disease cannot be seen on an X-ray.

Treatment

The immediate goal of treatment is pain relief. Because symptoms generally worsen with activity, the main treatment for Sever's disease is rest, which helps to relieve pressure on the heel bone, decreasing swelling and reducing pain.

As directed by the doctor, a child should cut down on or avoid all activities that cause pain until all symptoms are gone, especially running barefoot or on hard surfaces because hard impact on the feet can worsen pain and inflammation. The child might be able to do things that do not put pressure on the heel, such as swimming and biking, but check with a doctor first.

The doctor might also recommend that a child with Sever's disease:

- perform foot and leg exercises to stretch and strengthen the leg muscles and tendons;

- elevate and apply ice (wrapped in a towel, not applied directly to the skin) to the injured heel for 20 minutes two or three times per day, even on days when the pain is not that bad, to help reduce swelling;

- use an elastic wrap or compression stocking that is designed to help decrease pain and swelling;

- take an over-the-counter medicine to reduce pain and swelling, such as acetaminophen (Tylenol) or ibuprofen (Advil, Motrin, Nuprin).

Note: Children should not be given aspirin for pain due to the risk of a very serious illness called Reye syndrome.

In very severe cases, the doctor might recommend that the child wear a cast for anywhere from 2 to 12 weeks to immobilize the foot so that it can heal.

Recovery and Recurrence

One of the most important things to know about Sever's disease is that, with proper care, the condition usually goes away within two weeks to two months and does not cause any problems later in life. The sooner Sever's disease is addressed, the quicker recovery is. Most kids can return to physical activity without any trouble once the pain and other symptoms go away.

Although Sever's disease generally heals quickly, it can recur if long-term measures are not taken to protect the heel during a child's growing years. One of the most important is to make sure that kids wear proper shoes. Good quality, well-fitting shoes with shock-absorbent (padded) soles help to reduce pressure on the heel. The doctor may also recommend shoes with open backs, such as sandals or clogs, that do not rub on the back of the heel. Shoes that are heavy or have high heels should be avoided. Other preventive measures include continued stretching exercises and icing of the affected heel after activity.

If the child has a pronated foot, a flat or high arch, or another condition that increases the risk of Sever's disease, the doctor might recommend special shoe inserts, called orthotic devices, such as:

- heel pads that cushion the heel as it strikes the ground;

- heel lifts that reduce strain on the Achilles tendon by raising the heel;

- arch supports that hold the heel in an ideal position.

If a child is overweight or obese, the doctor will probably also recommend weight loss to decrease pressure on the heel.

The risk of recurrence goes away on its own when foot growth is complete and the growth plate has fused to the rest of the heel bone, usually around age 15.

Chapter 58

Return to Play

Chapter Contents

Section 58.1

Return to Play Issues

"Return to Play: A Common Sense Guide for Coaches," reprinted with permission of the American College of Sports Medicine. Copyright © 2005 American College of Sports Medicine (www.acsm.org). Reviewed by David A. Cooke, MD, FACP, August 2011.

Return to Play

Injuries are a common occurrence for those who exercise. Whether it be an overuse problem (tendinitis) or an acute traumatic injury (fracture or sprain), many injuries require restriction of and/or change in your exercise program.

The amount of time away from exercise varies according to the type of injury, severity of injury, body part involved, and other situational factors. Although there are steps to promote healing, it still takes time.

Injuries involve dysfunction or disruption of some component of the musculoskeletal system. Depending on the type and severity of the injury, these may cause pain, swelling, stiffness, weakness, or decreased range of motion. Improvement in these symptoms occurs with the healing process, but this does not necessarily mean the injury is completely healed.

Actions You Can Take to Decrease or Control the Initial Symptoms

Protect: Protect the affected area from further injury.

Rest: Initially resting and protecting the injured part will result in less swelling and a more rapid recovery.

Ice: Ice packs on the affected area decrease swelling and help control pain. This is especially helpful in the first 48 to 72 hours after injury, but can continue to be used to minimize discomfort.

Compression: Wrapping or bracing of the injured part allows for control of initial swelling and decreases motion.

Elevation: Elevation of the injured part, especially if it is kept above the heart, helps decrease swelling and pain.

Healing Time

As stated before, healing time depends on site, severity, and type of injury. For example, a mild ankle sprain may heal in 2 to 4 weeks, while a fracture of the leg may take 8 to 12 weeks. However, healing usually proceeds in certain stages.

- Swelling and pain decreases or disappears in the first 24 to 72 hours.

- Discoloration (bruising) usually subsides within 10 to 14 days.

- Range of motion increases over 7 to 14 days, although stiffness and weakness may persist.

When an injury occurs, it may result in weakness due to tissue damage and disuse, in addition to decreased control over the damaged body part. Regaining strength and coordination of the injured body part should be considered part of the rehabilitation and healing process, and an injury should not be considered healed until this process is accomplished. Attempting to return to an activity before proper healing of the injury puts you at risk for reinjury or an additional injury. Consultation with a sports medicine professional may aid in the initial treatment and rehabilitation, and the determination of when to return to play.

Guidelines for Return to Play

- **Pain-free full range of motion:** The injured body part should have full movement and flexibility with little or no discomfort.

- **Return of strength:** The injured body part should be approximately equal (90%–95%) to the opposite side before returning to full activity.

- **Minimal pain or swelling:** Some mild discomfort, stiffness, and/or swelling during or after exercise is to be expected during the initial return to activity. This responds well to ice therapy.

- **Functional retraining:** You should be able to perform the specific motions and actions required for your sport effectively before returning to activity. For example, retraining a lower-extremity injury in basketball should involve the ability to run, stop, change directions, and jump.

581

- **Progressive return to activity:** Consider starting at 50% of normal activity and progress up as tolerated. An informal guideline you can use is to progress activity 10%–15% increase per week if the previous level of activity does not result in increased symptoms during exercise or the day after exercise.

- **Continue general conditioning with cross-training:** Using an alternative exercise allows maintenance of general cardiovascular fitness while not interfering with the healing of an injury. For example, ankle and knee injuries may do well with bicycling or swimming.

- **Mental confidence in ability to do exercise:** You must feel that you and your injury are ready to perform at the level required for your particular activity.

If you have any questions about how these guidelines apply to your particular injury, consultation with a sports medicine professional would be advisable.

Section 58.2

Mentally Preparing Athletes to Return to Play

"Mentally Preparing Athletes to Return to Play Following Injury,"
by Windee M. Weiss, Ph.D., ATC. © 2007 Association for Applied Sport
Psychology (http://appliedsportpsych.org). Reprinted with permission.

Mentally Ready to Return to Play?

The vast majority of athletes are ready to return to full practice and
competition as soon as they are medically cleared by the team physician or sports medicine staff. That is, once they are cleared physically,
most athletes have no problem re-entering the sport arena. However,
some athletes may be ready physically, but are not prepared mentally
to return, which could result in the following:

- Decreased confidence which leads to a decline in performance

- Reinjury or further injury

- Feelings of stress and anxiety due to lack of confidence in their
  physical condition

- Fear of injury and fear of returning to play

How Can You Help Mentally Prepare Your Athletes to Return to Play?

Athletic trainers play an important role in the rehabilitation of any
athlete's injury, not only in the physical rehabilitation of the injury,
but also helping athletes mentally get prepared to play. Due to the
day-to-day interaction that we have with our athletes, athletic trainers become important sources of social support for any injured athlete,
play a key role in helping athletes maintain their confidence, and can
encourage the use of mental strategies to "keep their head in the game"
even though their body is not.

Here are some easy ways to incorporate mental training skills into
a rehabilitation program:

1. **Incorporating imagery:** One way to keep athletes "in the game" is to implement an imagery training program during their rehab sessions. Athletes could mentally rehearse sport specific skills, plays, strategies, or a series of plays during a rehab session. The most likely time may be when they are icing at the end of the session. For example, this would be a great time for a basketball player to externally image (e.g., seeing themselves as if they were on TV) themselves successfully completing five times in a row each of the team's offensive plays. The same could be done with specific sport skills (e.g., the athlete visualizes him- or herself successfully shooting 10 free throws).

2. **Sport specific skill:** Whenever possible we need to be creative and keep our injured athletes active in their sport, despite the fact they may be immobilized in some form or fashion. "Think outside the box" and modify sport skills to keep the injured athlete participating in their sport. This will dramatically help with their motivation to return, mental preparation for playing the game, and interest and enjoyment of rehabilitation. For example, a basketball player recovering from ACL reconstruction can easily work on all passing drills, shooting drills (e.g., free throws, three-point shots), and ball-handling drills while seated in a chair. Additionally, during practice the injured athlete can follow their teammate who plays a similar position providing feedback and mentally engaging in practice drills and skills.

3. **Incorporating goal setting:** The injured athlete should be setting goals on a weekly, if not daily, basis for both rehabilitation skills and the modified sport specific skills. A goal is some standard they would like to achieve by a given deadline. For example, a rehabilitation goal may be: "Achieving zero degrees of extension by Friday of this week." Keep track of these goals, as well as when the athlete achieves each goal. This will give the athletic trainer a record of all the injured athlete has achieved, thus providing "evidence" of how far they have come during rehabilitation. By setting goals for their sport specific skills, this will help injured athletes focus and perceive these skills and drills as important. Lastly, by providing some rewards or positive feedback for accomplishing these goals we can help injured athletes maintain their motivation during the many months of rehabilitation.

Part Eleven

Additional Help and Information

Chapter 59

Glossary of Terms Related to Sports Injuries

Acromioclavicular (AC) joint: The joint of the shoulder located between the acromion (part of the scapula that forms the highest point of the shoulder) and the clavicle (collarbone).

Analgesics: Medications designed to relieve pain. Analgesics include both prescription and over-the-counter products. Some are made to be taken orally, and others are rubbed onto the skin.

Anterior cruciate ligament: A ligament in the knee that crosses from the underside of the femur to the top of the tibia. The ligament limits rotation and the forward movement of the tibia.

Arthrogram: A diagnostic test in which a contrast fluid is injected into the shoulder joint and an X-ray is taken to view the fluid's distribution in the joint. Leaking of fluid into an area where it does not belong may indicate a tear or opening.

Arthroscopic surgery: Repairing the interior of a joint by inserting a microscope-like device and surgical tools through small cuts rather than one large surgical cut.

This chapter is compiled from glossaries from the following documents produced by the National Institute of Arthritis and Musculoskeletal and Skin Diseases (www.niams.nih.gov): "Questions and Answers about Bursitis and Tendinitis," March 2011; "Knee Problems," May 2010; and "Questions and Answers about Shoulder Problems," May 2010.

Biopsy: A procedure in which tissue is removed from the body and studied under a microscope. A biopsy of joint tissue may be used to diagnose some forms of arthritis.

Bone scan (radionuclide scanning): A technique for creating images of bones on a computer screen or on film. Before the procedure, a very small amount of radioactive dye is injected into the bloodstream. The dye collects in the bones, particularly in abnormal areas of the bones, and is detected by a scanner. This test detects blood flow to the bone and cell activity within the bone, and it can show abnormalities in these processes that may aid diagnosis.

Bursa: A small sac of tissue located between a bone and other moving structures such as muscles, skin, or tendons. The bursa contains a lubricating fluid that allows these structures to glide smoothly.

Bursitis: Inflammation or irritation of a bursa.

Cartilage: A tough, elastic material that covers the ends of the bones where they meet to form a joint. In the knee, cartilage helps absorb shock and allows the joint to move smoothly.

Cervical spine: The upper portion of the spine closest to the skull. The cervical spine comprises seven vertebrae.

Computerized tomography (CT) scan: A painless procedure in which X-rays are passed through the body at different angles, detected by a scanner, and analyzed by a computer. This produces a series of clear cross-sectional images (slices) of the tissues on a computer screen. CT scan images show soft tissues such as ligaments or muscles more clearly than conventional X-rays. The computer can combine individual images to give a three-dimensional view.

Corticosteroids: Synthetic preparations of cortisol, which is a hormone produced by the body. Corticosteroids block the immune system's production of substances that trigger allergic and inflammatory responses. These drugs may be injected directly into the inflammation site. Generally, symptoms improve or disappear within several days. Frequent injections into the same site are not recommended.

Epicondylitis: A painful and sometimes disabling swelling of the tissues of the elbow.

Glenohumeral joint: The joint where the rounded upper portion of the humerus (upper arm bone) joins the glenoid (socket in the shoulder blade). This is commonly referred to as the shoulder joint.

Hamstring: Prominent tendons at the back of the knee. Each knee has a pair of hamstrings that connect to the muscles that flex the knee. The hamstring muscles, which bend at the knee, run along the back of the thigh from the hip to just below the knee.

Herniated disk: A potentially painful problem in which the hard outer coating of the disk is damaged, allowing the disk's jelly-like center to leak and cause irritation to adjacent nerves.

Iliotibial band syndrome: An inflammatory condition in the knee caused by the rubbing of a band of tissue over the outer bone (lateral condyle) of the knee. Although iliotibial band syndrome may be caused by direct injury to the knee, it is most often caused by the stress of long-term overuse, which sometimes results from sports training.

Impingement syndrome: When the rotator cuff becomes inflamed and thickened, it may get trapped under the acromion, resulting in shoulder pain or loss of motion.

Inflammation: The characteristic reaction of tissue to injury or disease. It is marked by four signs: swelling, redness, heat, and pain.

Joint: A junction where two bones meet. Most joints are composed of cartilage, joint space, the fibrous capsule, the synovium, and ligaments.

Lateral collateral ligament: The ligament that runs along the outside of the knee joint. It provides stability to the outer (lateral) part of the knee.

Ligament: A tough band of connective tissue that connects bones to bones.

Lumbar spine: The lower portion of the spine. The lumbar spine comprises five vertebrae.

Magnetic resonance imaging (MRI): A procedure that uses a powerful magnet linked to a computer to create pictures of areas inside the body. Magnetic energy stimulates the tissue to produce signals that are detected by a scanner and analyzed by a computer. This creates a series of cross-sectional images of a specific part of the body. An MRI is particularly useful for detecting soft tissue damage or disease.

Medial collateral ligament: The ligament that runs along the inside of the knee joint, providing stability to the outer (medial) part of the knee.

Meniscus: A pad of connective tissue that separates the bones of the knee. The menisci are divided into two crescent-shaped discs (lateral and medial) positioned between the tibia and femur on the outer and inner sides of each knee. The two menisci in each knee act as shock absorbers, cushioning the lower part of the leg from the weight of the rest of the body as well as enhancing stability.

Muscle: A tissue that has the ability to contract, producing movement or force. There are three types of muscle: striated muscle, which is attached to the skeleton; smooth muscle, which is found in such tissues as the stomach and blood vessels; and cardiac muscle, which forms the walls of the heart. For striated muscle to function at its ideal level, the joint and surrounding structures must all be in good condition.

Nonsteroidal anti-inflammatory drugs (NSAIDs): A class of medications that ease pain and inflammation and are available over the counter or with a prescription. Commonly used NSAIDs include ibuprofen (Advil, Motrin), naproxen sodium (Aleve), and ketoprofen (Actron, Orudis KT).

Orthopedic surgeon: A doctor who has been trained in the nonsurgical and surgical treatment of bones, joints, and soft tissues such as ligaments, tendons, and muscles.

Osteochondritis dissecans: A condition that results from a loss of the blood supply to an area of bone underneath a joint surface. The condition usually involves the knee. In osteochondritis dissecans, the affected bone and its covering of cartilage gradually loosen and cause pain. This problem usually arises spontaneously in an active adolescent or young adult. It may be due to a slight blockage of a small artery or to an unrecognized injury or tiny fracture that damages the overlying cartilage. A person with this condition may eventually develop osteoarthritis.

Patella: The bone that sits over the other bones at the front of the knee joint and slides when the leg moves. Commonly referred to as the kneecap, the patella protects the knee and gives leverage to muscles.

Plica syndrome: A syndrome that occurs when plicae (bands of synovial tissue) are irritated by overuse or injury. Synovial plicae are the remains of tissue pouches found in the early stages of fetal development. As the fetus develops, these pouches normally combine to form one large synovial cavity. If this process is incomplete, plicae remain as four folds or bands of synovial tissue within the knee. Injury, chronic overuse, or inflammatory conditions are associated with this syndrome.

Quadriceps muscle: The large muscle at the front of the thigh.

Range of motion: The extent to which a joint can move freely and easily.

RICE: An acronym for rest, ice, compression, and elevation. These are the four steps often recommended for treating musculoskeletal injuries.

Rotator cuff: A set of muscles and tendons that secures the arm to the shoulder blade and permits rotation of the arm.

Sciatica: Pain felt down the back and outer side of the thigh. The usual cause is a herniated disc that is pressing on a nerve root.

Tendonitis: Inflammation or irritation of a tendon.

Tendons: Fibrous cords that connect muscle to bone.

Transcutaneous electrical nerve stimulation (TENS): A technique that uses a small battery-operated unit to send electrical impulses to the nerves to block pain signals to the brain.

X-ray (radiography): A procedure in which an X-ray (high-energy radiation with waves shorter than those of visible light) beam is passed through the body to produce a two-dimensional picture of the bones. X-rays are often used in diagnosing musculoskeletal problems.

Chapter 60

Directory of Resources Related to Sports Injuries

General Organizations and Resources

American Academy of Family Physicians
PO Box 11210
Shawnee Mission, KS 66207-1210
Phone: 913-906-6000
Toll Free: 800-274-2237
Website: http://www.aafp.org

American Academy of Pediatrics
141 Northwest Point Boulevard
Elk Grove Village, IL 60007
Phone: 847-434-4000
Fax: 847-434-8000
Website: http://www.aap.org

American Academy of Orthopaedic Surgeons (AAOS)
6300 North River Road
Rosemont, IL 60018-4262
Phone: 847-823-7186
Fax: 847-823-8125
Website: http://www.aaos.org
E-mail: custserv@aaos.org

American Academy of Physical Medicine and Rehabilitation
9700 W. Bryn Mawr Ave.
Suite 200
Rosemont, Illinois 60018
Phone: 847-737-6000
Fax: 847-737-6001
Website: http://www.aapmr.org

The information in this chapter was compiled from sources deemed accurate. Inclusion does not imply endorsement, and the list is not intended to be comprehensive. All contact information was verified and updated in August 2011.

American Association of Neurological Surgeons
5550 Meadowbrook Drive
Rolling Meadows, IL 60008-3852
Phone: 847-378-0500
Toll Free: 888-566-AANS (2267)
Fax: 847-378-0600
E-mail: info@aans.org
Website: http://www.aans.org

American Chiropractic Association (ACA)
1701 Clarendon Boulevard
Arlington, VA 22209
Phone: 703-276-8800
Fax: 703-243-2593
E-mail: memberinfo@acatoday.org
Website: http://www.acatoday.org

American College of Sports Medicine (ACSM)
P.O. Box 1440
Indianapolis, IN 46206-1440
Phone: 317-637-9200
Fax: 317-634-7817
Website: http://www.acsm.org

American Council on Exercise (ACE)
4851 Paramount Drive
San Diego, CA 92123
Toll-Free: 888-825-3636
Phone: 858-279-8227
Fax: 858-576-6564
Website: http://www.acefitness.org
E-mail: support@acefitness.org

American Medical Athletic Association
4405 East-West Highway
Suite 405
Bethesda, MD 20814
Phone: 301-913-9517
Toll Free: 800-776-2732
Fax: 301-913-9520
Website: http://www.amaasportsmed.org

American Medical Society for Sports Medicine
4000 W. 114th Street
Suite 100
Leawood, KS 66211
Phone: 913-327-1415
Fax: 913-327-1491
E-mail: office@amssm.org
Website: http://www.amssm.org

American Orthopaedic Society for Sports Medicine (AOSSM)
6300 North River Road
Suite 500
Rosemont, IL 60018
Phone: 847-292-4900
Website: http://www.sportsmed.org
E-mail: aossm@aossm.org

American Osteopathic Academy of Sports Medicine
2424 American Lane
Madison, WI 53704
Phone: 608-443-2477
Fax: 608-443-2474
Website: http://www.aoasm.org

American Physical Therapy Association (APTA)
1111 North Fairfax Street
Alexandria, VA 22314-1488
Toll-Free: 800-999-2782
Phone: 703-684-APTA
(684-2782)
TDD: 703-683-6748
Fax: 703-684-7343
E-mail: Research-dept@apta.org
Website: http://www.apta.org

American Running Association
4405 East-West Highway
Suite 405
Bethesda, MD 20814
Phone: 800-776-2732
(ext. 13 or 12)
Fax: 301-913-9520
Website:
http://www.americanrunning.org

American Sports Medicine Institute
2660 10th Avenue South
Suite 505
Birmingham, AL 35205
Phone: 205-918-0000
Fax: 205-918-0800
Website: http://www.asmi.org

AthleticAdvisor
Website:
http://athleticadvisor.com

Centers for Disease Control and Prevention (CDC)
Division of Nutrition, Physical
Activity, and Obesity (DNPAO)
1600 Clifton Road
Atlanta, GA 30333
Toll-Free: 800-CDC-INFO
(232-4636)
Toll-Free TTY: 888-232-6348
Website: http://www.cdc.gov/
nccdphp/dnpao/index.html
E-mail: cdcinfo@cdc.gov

Cleveland Clinic
9500 Euclid Avenue
Cleveland, OH 44195
Toll-Free: 800-223-2273
Phone: 216-444-2200
TTY: 216-444-0261
Website:
http://www.clevelandclinic.org

Consumer Product Safety Commission
4330 East West Highway
Bethesda, MD 20814
Toll-Free: 800-638-2772
(Hotline: 8:00 a.m.–5:30 p.m. EST)
Toll-Free TTY: 800-638-8270
(Hotline: 8:00 a.m.–5:30 p.m. EST)
Phone: 301-504-7923 (General
Information: Monday–Friday
8:00 a.m.–4:30 p.m. EST)
Fax: 301-504-0124
and 301-504-0025
Website: http://www.cpsc.gov

Gatorade Sports Science Institute
617 West Main Street
Barrington, IL 60010
Toll Free: 800-616-GSSI
(616-4774)
Website:
http://www.gssiweb.com

Hughston Health Alert
Hughston Foundation
6262 Veterans Pkwy
Columbus, GA 31908-9517
Phone: 706-324-6661
Toll Free: 800-331-2910
Website:
http://www.hughston.com/haa

National Athletic Trainers' Association
2952 Stemmons Freeway #200
Dallas, TX 75247
Phone: 214-637-6282
Fax: 214-637-2206
Website: http://www.nata.org

National Center for Sports Safety
2316 1st Avenue South
Birmingham, Alabama 35233
Phone: 205-329-7535
Toll Free: 866-508-NCSS (6277)
Fax: 205-329-7526
E-mail: info@SportsSafety.org
Website:
http://www.sportssafety.org

National Institute of Arthritis and Musculoskeletal and Skin Diseases (NIAMS)
Information Clearinghouse
National Institutes of Health
1 AMS Circle
Bethesda, MD 20892-3675
Toll Free: 877-22-NIAMS
(226-4267)
Phone: 301-495-4484
TTY: 301-565-2966
Fax: 301-718-6366
Website:
http://www.niams.nih.gov
E-mail:
NIAMSinfo@mail.nih.gov

National Strength and Conditioning Association (NSCA)
1885 Bob Johnson Drive
Colorado Springs, CO 80906
Toll-Free: 800-815-6826
Phone: 719-632-6722
Fax: 719-632-6367
Website: http://www.nsca-lift.org
E-mail: nsca@nsca-lift.org

Orthosports
Website:
http://www.orthosports.com.au

President's Council on Physical Fitness and Sports (PCPFS)
Department W
Tower Building
Suite 560
1101 Wootton Parkway
Rockville, MD 20852
Phone: 240-276-9567
Fax: 240-276-9860
Website: http://www.fitness.gov
E-mail: fitness@hhs.gov

St. John's Hospital
800 E. Carpenter St.
Springfield, Illinois 62769
Phone: 217-544-6464
Website: http://www.st-johns.org

University of Pittsburgh Medical Center Sports Medicine
200 Lothrop St.
Pittsburgh, PA 15213-2582
Phone: 412-647-UPMC (8762)
Toll Free: 800-533-UPMC (8762)
Website: http://www
.sportsmedicine.upmc.com

Children and Sports Injuries

Children's Memorial Hospital
2300 Children's Plaza
Chicago, IL 60614-3363
Phone: 773-880-4000
Website:
http://www.childrensmemorial.org

Kidshealth.org
Nemours Foundation
Website: http://www.kidshealth.org

Safe Kids Worldwide
1301 Pennsylvania Avenue NW
Suite 1000
Washington, DC 20004-1707
Phone: 202-662-0600
Website: http://www.safekids.org

Dental Injuries

Academy for Sports Dentistry
118 Faye Street
PO Box 364
Farmersville, IL 62533
Toll Free: 800-273-1788
Fax: 217-227-3438
E-mail: info@
academyforsportsdentistry.org
Website: http://www
.academyforsportsdentistry.org

American Dental Association
211 East Chicago Ave.
Chicago, IL 60611-2678
Phone: 312-440-2500
Website: http://www.ada.org

Exercise-Induced Asthma

American Academy of Allergy, Asthma, and Immunology
555 East Wells Street
Suite 1100
Milwaukee, WI 53202-3823
Phone: 414-272-6071
E-mail: info@aaaai.org
Website: http://www.aaaai.org

American College of Allergy, Asthma, and Immunology
85 West Algonquin Road
Suite 550
Arlington Heights, IL 60005
Phone: 847-427-1200
Fax: 847-427-1294
E-mail: mail@acaai.org
Website: http://www.acaai.org

American Lung Association
1301 Pennsylvania Ave. NW
Suite 800
Washington, DC 20004
Phone: 202-785-3355
Fax: 202-452-1805
E-mail: info@lungusa.org
Website: http://www.lungusa.org

Asthma and Allergy Foundation of America (AAFA)
8201 Corporate Drive
Suite 1000
Landover, MD 20785
Toll-Free: 800-7-ASTHMA (727-8462)
Website: http://www.aafa.org
E-mail: info@aafa.org

Eye Injuries

Coalition to Prevent Sports Eye Injuries
5 Summit Avenue
Hackensack, NJ 07601
Toll Free: 866-265-3582
Fax: 201-621-4352
Website:
http://www.sportseyeinjuries.com

Prevent Blindness America
211 West Wacker Drive, Suite 1700
Chicago, Illinois 60606
Toll Free: 800-331-2020 (8:30 a.m. to 5:00 p.m. CST, Monday through Friday)
Website:
http://www.preventblindness.org

Facial Injuries

American Academy of Otolaryngology—Head and Neck Surgery
1650 Diagonal Road
Alexandria, VA 22314-2857
Phone: 703-836-4444
Website: http://www.entnet.org

Foot Injuries

American Academy of Podiatric Sports Medicine
Phone: 301-845-9887
E-mail: info@aapsm.org
Website: http://www.aapsm.org

American Podiatric Medical Association
9312 Old Georgetown Road
Bethesda, MD 20814-1621
Phone: 301-581-9200
Website: http://www.apma.org

Hand Injuries

American Society for Surgery of the Hand
6300 North River Road
Suite 600
Rosemont, IL 60018
Phone: 847-384-8300 (between 7:30 a.m. and 5:30 p.m. CST, Monday through Friday)
Fax: 847-384-1435
E-mail: info@assh.org
Website: http://www.assh.org

Skin Conditions

American Academy of Dermatology
PO Box 4014
Schaumburg, IL 60168
Phone: 847-240-1280
Toll Free: 866-503-SKIN (7546)
Fax: 847-240-1859
Website: http://www.aad.org

Spinal Cord Injuries

Christopher & Dana Reeve Foundation
636 Morris Turnpike
Suite 3A
Short Hills, NJ 07078
Toll Free: 800-225-0292
Phone: 973-379-2690
Website:
http://www.christopherreeve.org

North American Spine Society
7075 Veterans Blvd.
Burr Ridge, IL 60527
Phone: 630-230-3600
Fax: 630-230-3700
Website: http://www.spine.org

Index

Index

Page numbers followed by 'n' indicate a footnote. Page numbers in *italics* indicate a table or illustration.

603